Functional Electrical Stimulation Cycling in Clinical Practice

Murillo Frazão
Editor

Functional Electrical Stimulation Cycling in Clinical Practice

Springer

Editor
Murillo Frazão
Lauro Wanderley University Hospital – EBSERH/UFPB
João Pessoa, PB, Brazil

ISBN 978-3-032-23936-5 ISBN 978-3-032-23937-2 (eBook)
https://doi.org/10.1007/978-3-032-23937-2

This Springer imprint is published by the registered company Springer Nature Switzerland AG
The registered company address is: Gewerbestrasse 11, 6330 Cham, Switzerland

To all engineers, healthcare professionals, patients, and scientists who have contributed to the evolution of FES cycling over more than four decades. Your curiosity, persistence, and commitment to innovation have transformed a promising concept into a life-changing clinical reality.

*To my dear friend, **Luís Augusto Werlang**, for always believing in me and for joining me on this journey of FES-cycling development. Your partnership and trust have been invaluable.*

*To my family—**Wanessa**, my beloved wife, and **Lucca** and **Pedro**, my wonderful sons—thank you for your unwavering support, patience, and love. All my efforts are for you!*

Foreword

Functional Electrical Stimulation cycling (FES cycling) has evolved from a promising concept into a clinically relevant modality with a growing body of evidence across rehabilitation and critical care contexts. Despite this progress, its adoption in routine practice remains limited. A major reason is practical. The technique sits at the intersection of stimulation engineering, muscle physiology, and cycle ergometry. Many professionals have access to equipment, but do not have access to consolidated guidance on how to select parameters, define dose, monitor responses, and ensure safety across different patient profiles. This book was written to address that gap.

A dedicated technical reference on FES cycling has been needed for years. The literature is extensive, but it is distributed across disciplines and publication formats. Clinicians often find isolated protocols without the underlying rationale. Researchers often find methodological variability that complicates reproducibility and comparison. Industry professionals often find that device specifications do not translate directly into clinical decision-making. By integrating foundational principles with applied protocols, this volume provides a structured framework that supports both implementation and scientific rigor.

One of the strengths of this book is its systematic coverage of the determinants of therapeutic and training response. The reader is guided through the biophysical basis of stimulation, including waveform characteristics, current delivery, electrode placement considerations, and the implications of pulse width, frequency, and intensity for recruitment, fatigue, and tolerability. The text also emphasizes variables that are sometimes treated superficially in clinical discussions, such as torque, power output, cadence, resistance profiles, and the mechanical constraints of cycle ergometry. These are not secondary details. They are central to dose quantification, progression planning, and interpretation of outcomes.

The clinical sections are equally important. FES cycling is used in heterogeneous scenarios, with different goals and constraints. In neurological rehabilitation, priorities may include motor relearning, cardiovascular conditioning, and mitigation of secondary complications. In musculoskeletal or metabolic contexts, the focus may shift toward training load management and functional performance. In the intensive care unit, the constraints are unique. Patients may have profound weakness, altered consciousness, hemodynamic instability, and high risk of complications from immobility. In such settings, safe delivery requires explicit operational criteria, careful monitoring, and a clear understanding of what constitutes an appropriate dose. This book recognizes these differences and provides guidance that is both evidence informed and operationally oriented.

A consistent theme throughout the volume is that FES cycling outcomes depend on precision. Dose is not defined by session duration alone. It is defined by the interaction of stimulation parameters with mechanical work, patient state, and timing within the clinical course. Insufficient intensity can produce minimal recruitment and limited benefit. Excessive intensity can accelerate fatigue, compromise adherence, or increase risk. Improper synchronization between stimulation and crank position can reduce efficiency and increase discomfort. Without standardized measurement of torque and power, it is difficult to quantify training load, evaluate progression, or compare protocols between studies and centers. The book's emphasis on quantification and monitoring therefore supports both better clinical results and better science.

The author of this work, Prof. Dr. Murilo Frazão, is exceptionally well positioned to write it. Over the last decade, he has built a focused research and development trajectory in neuromuscular electrical stimulation and FES cycling, contributing to the scientific literature and translating findings into practical applications. His academic background includes master's and doctoral training at the Federal University of Paraíba and postdoctoral work at the University of Brasília, with a consistent focus on clinical exercise physiology and electrical stimulation. This combination of physiological expertise and methodological discipline is reflected in the clarity of the book's conceptual structure and the practicality of its recommendations.

My professional relationship with Prof. Frazão began more than 15 years ago and has developed into a long-term collaboration characterized by shared scientific priorities and mutual trust. Approximately 10 years ago, he invited me to collaborate on the development of a new FES cycling device, the Mobitronics/Mobi Light systems by INBRAMED. At that time, the market was dominated by high-cost solutions that did not fully meet the requirements of many clinical services, particularly those that needed accurate dose delivery, integrated measurement, and operational robustness for settings such as intensive care. The goal was to support precise stimulation and cycling control, enable meaningful performance metrics, and improve accessibility without compromising safety or effectiveness. That development experience reinforced the central message of this book. FES cycling is most effective when it is engineered and applied as a dosed intervention, not as a generic technology.

I also had the opportunity to contribute to the development of this volume at the conceptual level, through discussions on structure and the prioritization of themes that clinicians and researchers repeatedly face in implementation. This perspective, informed by two decades of work in peripheral electrical stimulation and clinical exercise physiology, strengthened my conviction that the field benefits from a single, coherent technical reference. This book fulfills that role.

For the clinician, this text supports implementation. It provides the rationale behind parameter selection and practical guidance for safe application across patient populations. For the researcher, it supports methodological consistency. It clarifies variables that should be reported, monitored, and standardized to improve reproducibility and facilitate comparison across studies. For educators and industry professionals, it offers a shared language that can align training, device development, and clinical protocols.

FES cycling is no longer an experimental curiosity. It is a modality with meaningful clinical potential when applied with appropriate technique, dose, and timing. The value of this book is that it makes that application more achievable. It translates a complex intersection of physiology and engineering into an organized approach that can be taught, implemented, and studied. I expect it to become a key reference for professionals who want to use FES cycling safely, precisely, and effectively.

It has been an honor and a privilege to contribute this foreword.

Paulo Eugênio Silva
PhD in Health Sciences and Technologies
University of Brasília
Brasília, Brazil
Postdoctoral Training, Department of Physical Medicine and Rehabilitation
University of São Paulo
São Paulo, SP, Brazil

Preface

Over the past decades, Functional Electrical Stimulation cycling (FES cycling) has evolved from a pioneering concept for individuals with spinal cord injury into a versatile and increasingly sophisticated technology for clinical rehabilitation, functional evaluation, and performance enhancement. What was once limited to specialized research centers is now progressively entering hospitals, rehabilitation clinics, intensive care units, and even sports environments.

Yet, despite thousands of scientific publications since the 1980s, there has been no comprehensive book dedicated exclusively to guiding clinicians in the practical and evidence-based use of FES cycling. This book was conceived to fill that gap.

FES cycling represents more than the application of electrical pulses to induce pedaling. It integrates neurophysiology, exercise science, biomedical engineering, and clinical reasoning into a single therapeutic and assessment platform. By depolarizing motoneurons through computer-controlled transcutaneous stimulation, it enables muscle contractions independent of voluntary neural pathways. This capacity makes FES cycling uniquely positioned to address situations in which movement is severely impaired (ranging from neurological disorders to critical illness and chronic systemic diseases).

Beyond therapy, FES cycling offers an objective and nonvolitional method for evaluating muscle performance. Through real-time measurement of torque, power output, and stimulation cost, clinicians can quantify neuromuscular function with a level of precision that was previously difficult to achieve in patients unable to perform voluntary effort. In this sense, FES cycling bridges treatment and assessment, rehabilitation and technology.

The motivation for this book arises from three central observations:

First, the scientific evidence supporting FES cycling continues to grow, demonstrating benefits in metabolic regulation, cardiovascular conditioning, ventilatory responses, muscle preservation, and functional recovery across multiple clinical populations.

Second, technological innovation has accelerated. Modern systems incorporate advanced control strategies, adaptive stimulation patterns, data analytics, and integration with digital platforms. However, many professionals lack structured guidance to translate these technological advances into safe and effective clinical protocols.

Third, there is a clear interdisciplinary need. Healthcare professionals require a solid theoretical and physiological foundation to implement FES cycling responsibly in practice.

The chapters are organized to provide a logical progression. We begin with historical development, fundamental concepts, and terminology. We then explore the principles of electrical stimulation and cycle ergometry, followed by detailed discussion of equipment characteristics and technological innovations. The physiological bases (metabolic, cardiovascular, and ventilatory responses) are examined to ground clinical decisions in scientific rationale.

Functional assessment methods are presented alongside clinical applicability in neurological and non-neurological conditions, as well as perspectives in sports and performance contexts. The book concludes with a dedicated discussion on technological innovations and future perspectives in FES cycling, highlighting emerging developments, evolving control strategies, and the directions that may shape the next generation of rehabilitation and performance technologies.

Throughout the book, emphasis is placed on clinical applicability, practical guidance, and integration of evidence with experience. Didactic elements are incorporated to enhance understanding and facilitate implementation.

This work is the result of collaboration among clinicians and researchers from different institutions and countries. Each author brings expertise in electrical stimulation, rehabilitation sciences, exercise physiology, and clinical practice. The diversity of perspectives reflects the interdisciplinary nature of FES cycling itself.

We hope this book serves not only as a reference but as a catalyst. A catalyst for safer and more effective rehabilitation programs. A catalyst for technological refinement driven by clinical insight. And ultimately, a catalyst for improving the lives of patients whose mobility and functional capacity can be meaningfully enhanced through innovation.

Functional Electrical Stimulation cycling stands at the intersection of physiology and technology. Its future will depend on informed professionals capable of understanding both. It is our sincere expectation that this book contributes to that mission.

João Pessoa, Brazil Murillo Frazão

Contents

1 **Introduction to FES-Cycling Technology: Concepts and Historical Context of the Development of the First Equipment** 1
Murillo Frazão

2 **Principles of Electrical Stimulation** 11
Victor Hugo de Souza Ribeiro, Leandro Andrade Moreira, Vitória dos Santos Nogueira, and João Luiz Quagliotti Durigan

3 **Technical Characteristics of FES-Cycling Systems** 31
Murillo Frazão

4 **Physiological Bases of FES-Cycling Therapy: Metabolic, Cardiovascular, and Ventilatory Responses** 47
Murillo Frazão and Gerson Cipriano Jr

5 **Functional Assessment Based on FES-Cycling Technology** 63
Murillo Frazão, Thainá de Gomes Figueiredo, Rafael Michel de Macedo, and Juliana Goulart Prata Oliveira Milani

6 **FES-Cycling Clinical Applicability in Neurological Diseases** 101
Lara A. Pilutti, Ashwini Sansare, Laurie Magerfleisch, Colleen Connaughton, and Murillo Frazão

7 **Clinical Applicability of FES-Cycling in Non-neurological Diseases** 151
Murillo Frazão

8 **FES-Cycling for Competition and Leisure** 183
Efe Anil Aksöz and Kenneth J. Hunt

9 **Practical FES-Cycling Guideline Based on Functional Outcomes** 201
Murillo Frazão

10 **Technological Innovations and Future Perspectives in FES-Cycling** . . . 215
Murillo Frazão

Index 233

Contributors

Efe Anil Aksöz rehaLab—The Laboratory for Rehabilitation Engineering, Division of Mechatronics and Systems Engineering, School of Engineering and Computer Science, HuCE—Institute for Human Centred Engineering, Bern University of Applied Sciences, Biel, Switzerland

Gerson Cipriano Jr Physical Therapy Department, University of Brasilia – UNB, Brasilia, DF, Brazil

Colleen Connaughton Restorative Therapies, Nottingham, MD, USA

João Luiz Quagliotti Durigan Faculty of Health Sciences and Technologies, Rehabilitation Sciences Program, Laboratory of Muscle and Tendon Plasticity, University of Brasilia, Brasília, DF, Brazil

Murillo Frazão Lauro Wanderley University Hospital – EBSERH/UFPB, João Pessoa, PB, Brazil

Thainá de Gomes Figueiredo Oswaldo Crus University Hospital, UPE, Recife, PE, Brazil
Agamenon Magalhães Hospital, Recife, PE, Brazil
Tiradentes University, Recife, PE, Brazil

Kenneth J. Hunt rehaLab—The Laboratory for Rehabilitation Engineering, Division of Mechatronics and Systems Engineering, School of Engineering and Computer Science, HuCE—Institute for Human Centred Engineering, Bern University of Applied Sciences, Biel, Switzerland

Rafael Michel de Macedo Agamenon Magalhães Hospital, Recife, PE, Brazil
Costantini Cardiologic Hospital, Curitiba, PR, Brazil

Laurie Magerfleisch Restorative Therapies, Nottingham, MD, USA

Juliana Goulart Prata Oliveira Milani Faculty of Rehabilitation Sciences, Rehabilitation Research Center (REVAL), Hasselt University, Hasselt, Belgium
Graduate Programme in Health Sciences and Technologies, University of Brasilia (UnB), Brasilia, DF, Brazil

Leandro Andrade Moreira Laboratory of Muscle and Tendon Plasticity, Rehabilitation Sciences Program, University of Brasilia, Brasília, DF, Brazil

Lara A. Pilutti Interdisciplinary School of Health Sciences, Brain and Mind Research Institute, University of Ottawa, Ottawa, ON, Canada
Thomas Edwards, Northern Ontario School of Medicine, Thunder Bay, ON, Canada

Ashwini Sansare Texas A&M University, College Station, TX, USA

Vitória dos Santos Nogueira Laboratory of Muscle and Tendon Plasticity, Rehabilitation Sciences Program, University of Brasilia, Brasília, DF, Brazil

Victor Hugo de Souza Ribeiro Laboratory of Muscle and Tendon Plasticity, Physical Education College, University of Brasilia, Brasília, DF, Brazil

Introduction to FES-Cycling Technology: Concepts and Historical Context of the Development of the First Equipment

1

Murillo Frazão

Introduction

Functional Electrical Stimulation (FES) has emerged as a transformative technology in the field of rehabilitation, offering promising solutions for individuals with neuromuscular disorders, spinal cord injuries, or other motor impairments. Among the various applications of FES, Functional Electrical Stimulation cycling (FES-cycling) stands out as an innovative approach that combines electrical stimulation with exercise to improve muscle strength, cardiovascular health, and overall functional capacity. By stimulating muscles to produce contractions while cycling, FES-cycling enables individuals who are unable to engage in traditional physical activities due to paralysis or weakness to achieve therapeutic benefits. This chapter provides an overview of the underlying principles of FES-cycling, exploring how it works, and traces the historical development of FES-cycling since its experimental roots.

The concept of FES-cycling dates back to the 1970–1980s when pioneering researchers like Dr. Jerrold S. Petrofsky recognized the potential of electrical stimulation not only to maintain muscle tone but also to induce functional movement. Petrofsky and his colleagues hypothesized that electrical stimulation could simulate the effects of exercise in patients with severe motor deficits, such as those suffering from spinal cord injuries. They explored the use of FES devices in combination with stationary cycling, leading to the creation of FES-cycling, a technique designed to stimulate the muscles of the lower limbs while cycling, even when voluntary movement was not possible. Over time, FES-cycling evolved from a novel concept to a promising rehabilitative technology, attracting attention from researchers, clinicians, and patients alike.

M. Frazão (✉)
Lauro Wanderley University Hospital – EBSERH/UFPB, João Pessoa, PB, Brazil
e-mail: murillo.frazao@gmail.com

M. Frazão (ed.), *Functional Electrical Stimulation Cycling in Clinical Practice*,
https://doi.org/10.1007/978-3-032-23937-2_1

Concept of Functional Electrical Stimulation (FES)

Definition of FES

Functional electrical stimulation (FES) refers to the use of electrical currents to stimulate muscles, generating contractions that enable functionally beneficial movements, particularly in individuals with impaired motor control. Before we can go on, two key points must be clarified:

1. FES is not a specific type of electrical current; it is the intended application of electrical currents that generate muscle contractions to promote functional movement [1].
2. Electrically induced muscle contractions without resulting movement do not constitute FES.

FES aims to help individuals regain functional movement, such as walking, cycling, grasping objects, or breathing, by activating muscles that might otherwise be paralyzed or weakened.

Overview of How FES Works in Stimulating Muscles

FES works by applying low-frequency electrical impulses to the motor nerves that control specific muscles. These electrical impulses mimic the natural signals sent by the brain to the muscles during voluntary movements. When the electrical current reaches the nerves, it stimulates the muscles to contract, producing movement or assisting in muscle re-education. This can help retrain the muscles and nerves to function properly or enhance the movement capability of the patient.

In the case of paralyzed or weakened muscles, FES can be used to stimulate the muscles repeatedly, facilitating improvements in muscle strength, endurance, and coordination. The stimulation can be tailored in terms of intensity, frequency, and timing to match the patient's specific needs, promoting functional movement patterns.

Differences Between FES and Other Forms of Electrical Stimulation

While FES is a type of electrical stimulation, there are several key differences between FES and other forms of electrical stimulation techniques. Some of these include:

Purpose

- FES is primarily aimed at restoring or improving functional movement, targeting specific muscles that help in daily tasks or mobility (e.g., walking, grasping, cycling).
- TENS (Transcutaneous Electrical Nerve Stimulation) is used mainly for pain relief by stimulating sensory nerves and reducing pain signals.
- NMES (Neuromuscular Electrical Stimulation) focuses on maintaining or increasing muscle strength through the stimulation of motor nerves without targeting functional movement. It is commonly used for muscle rehabilitation and prevention of atrophy.

Application Context

- FES is used in rehabilitation settings for patients with conditions like spinal cord injury, stroke, or brain injury to help them perform daily tasks and improve mobility.
- TENS is mainly used for pain management in patients with chronic or acute pain conditions.
- NMES is often applied for muscle strengthening and rehabilitation, such as in cases of muscle wasting or to prevent muscle degeneration in immobilized patients.

In summary, FES is a specialized technique that is used to help individuals regain specific functional movements, while other forms of electrical stimulation like TENS and NMES may have different therapeutic goals, such as pain relief or muscle strengthening.

The Concept of FES-Cycling

What Is FES-Cycling?

FES-cycling is a support technology for physical training and rehabilitation in situations of muscle weakness and/or inability to move voluntarily. FES-cycling has gained popularity in several situations of immobility. The technology was originally developed in the 1980s for patients with spinal cord injury [2], and has been greatly improved since then.

In FES-cycling, electrical impulses are delivered through electrodes placed on the skin over specific muscles, causing them to contract in a way that mimics natural movement. The concept is to promote the cycling exercise induced by the depolarization of the motor neuron and, consequently, all the physiological stages of muscle contraction. There is direct activation of muscle contractions, regardless of the functionality of the physiological pathway [3]. This muscle contraction must be synchronized, harmonious and adequate to promote the cycling movement. As the muscles contract, the individual is able to pedal the bike, engaging in cycling exercises that improve muscle strength, endurance, and cardiorespiratory fitness.

Overview of the Technology: How It Combines FES with Cycling

The FES-cycling system is a device composed of hardware and software designed to perform multichannel functional electrical stimulation for coordinated activation of the main muscles involved in pedaling. The therapy provides electrical pulses through transcutaneous self-adhesive electrodes. The equipment consists of a dedicated computer system, a pedaling dynamics assessment system (a sensor precisely detects the positioning of the pedals) and a multichannel neuromuscular stimulator module for coordinated activation of the main muscles involved in pedaling.

The electrostimulation is synchronized to trigger according to the pedal position. It is coordinated by a computational algorithm embedded in the equipment's microprocessor that follows the biomechanical activation sequence observed in the target task—pedaling. It is important to emphasize that the entire task is coordinated by the angular position of the crank. Figure 1.1 shows one of the possible channel activation sequences that the system can perform. In this configuration, eight muscle groups are activated.

In stationary commercial equipment's, the entire system is controlled and monitored through a graphical interface in computer software. With the graphical interface, the most appropriate therapy, and the intensity, frequency and pulse width of the electrostimulation can be chosen. The interface also allows adjustments to the rotation cadence and workload of the cycle ergometer.

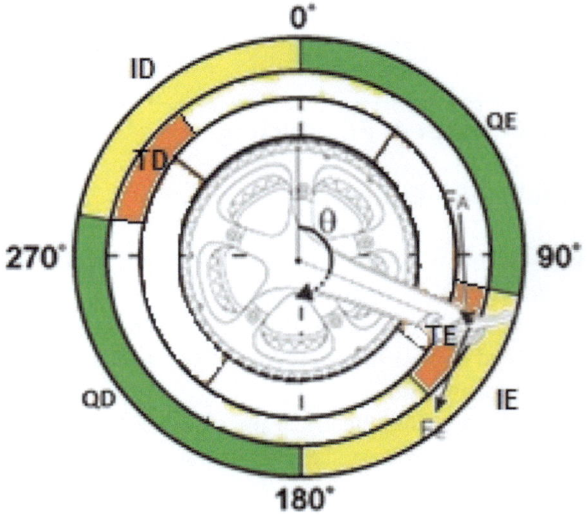

Fig. 1.1 A possible channel activation sequences that the FES-cycling system can perform. Right Quadriceps—QD (vastus medialis and lateralis); Left Quadriceps—QE (vastus medialis and lateralis); Right Hamstring—ID; Left Hamstring—IE; Right Tibial—TD and Left Tibial—TE, coordinated by the angular position of the cycle ergometer pedal

Historical Development of the First FES-Cycling Equipment

Early Beginnings of Electrical Stimulation and Pathway for FES-Cycling Development

Since 1940s decade, in many forms of disability due to paralysis, researchers studied possibilities to regain some function through direct electrical stimulation of paralyzed muscles. At that moment, some animal model studies were developed. Initially, finding the most suitable type of current and method of application seemed like a big challenge. In 1946, Fischer and Ramsey [4] studied the effects of daily (twice a day) electrical stimulation on muscles protein content. In 1947, Kosman et al. [5] analyzed the influence of duration and frequency of treatment in electrical stimulation of paralyzed muscle. Additionally, in 1948 the same researchers group analyzed the importance of current form [6].

In the 1960s decade, an explosion of electrical stimulation studies happened. Beyond paralyzed muscles studies, researches with healthy subjects were directed to determine the nature of electrical signals which produce the maximum stimulation effects with minimum discomfort and pain. In this sense, Vodovnik et al. [7] analyzed the pain response to different direct and alternate currents waveforms (sine, rectangular and exponential waves) for tetanic muscle contractions. Until then, the researches had been concerned with isometric muscle contraction. However, some devices began to be developed to allow the analysis of the dynamic behavior of isotonic contraction against external loads [8].

The 1970s were a pivotal decade for the development of Functional Electrical Stimulation, as this was when the technology transitioned from basic muscle stimulation to a more therapeutic and functional approach for individuals with neurological impairments, particularly for those with paralysis. In this context, Dr. Jerrold S. Petrofsky along with his colleagues were great pioneers in this field. They led groundbreaking research on the use of electrical stimulation for muscle paralysis. They initially focused on muscle re-education by applying electrical currents to stimulate muscle contraction, hoping to restore motor function in individuals with spinal cord injuries or other forms of paralysis.

Why FES-Cycling Was Created?

Dr. Jerrold S. Petrofsky and his colleagues focused their research on the use of electrical stimulation to treat muscle paralysis. Over time, they realized that merely inducing muscle contraction was not sufficient to achieve meaningful functional outcomes for individuals with paralysis.

In few years, the team advanced their work by exploring the concept of electrically induced exercise. Their hypothesis was that combining electrical stimulation with exercise might provide additional benefits. They believed that this approach could stimulate not just muscle contraction, but also enhance neuromuscular and cardiovascular function—critical components for individuals with long-term disabilities, especially those who had been confined to a wheelchair for years.

FES-cycling emerged as a potential therapeutic intervention. The idea was that by using electrical stimulation to activate the leg muscles while cycling, individuals could achieve not only improved muscle strength but also enhanced cardiovascular fitness and circulation, which are typically compromised in individuals with paralysis. This method held promise for improving the overall health, mobility, and quality of life for those with limited motor control, and it paved the way for advancements in rehabilitative treatments that integrate electrical stimulation.

Who Created the FES-Cycling?

The scientific article that provides the detailed description of the first equipment [2] outlines the contributions of four key scientists who played a pivotal role in developing FES-cycling in the early 1980s:

Jerrold S. Petrofsky, Ph.D.

Jerrold S. Petrofsky earned a Bachelor's degree in Biology from Washington University, St. Louis, in 1970. He earned his doctorate in Physiology from the St. Louis University Medical School in 1974. He completed post-doctoral research at that institution in 1976 and then joined its faculty as an Assistant Professor of Physiology. In 1979, Petrofsky came to Wright State, where he is a Professor of Biomedical Engineering and also the Director of the WSU National Center for Rehabilitation Engineering. He has received numerous awards, including the Dayton Section, Institute for Electrical and Electronics Engineers 1981 Noble Award for Engineering and IEEE's 1983 "Special Award" for continuing outstanding work; the ADD (Abilities Demonstrated by the Disabled) 1982 Research Project of the Year award, ADD's highest annual award for service to the disabled; the Spinal Cord Society's 1982 "Scientist of the Year" award; and the 1966 University of Missouri curator's award. Petrofsky has had nearly 200 scholarly papers published and holds 12 patents. He is a member of numerous professional societies, including the American Physiological Society, the Ohio Academy of Science, the Institute of Electrical and Electronics Engineers, the Biomedical Engineering Society (fellow), Sigma Xi, the Aerospace Medical Association, and others. In addition to his research into programmed electrical stimulation of paralyzed muscles, his current research interests include the mechanism of fatigue from both static and dynamic exercise as well as the mechanisms for cardiorespiratory responses to the two forms of exertion.

Chandler A. Phillips, M.D.

C.A. Phillips received the A.B. degree (1965) from Stanford University and the M.D. degree (1969) from the University of Southern California. He is a registered Professional Engineer (1974) in Electrical Engineering with the State of California. Phillips is currently Professor of Engineering and Physiology at Wright State University (Dayton, OH) and has been the Director of its Biomedical Engineering Program since 1975. He has been a co-investigator on the muscle paralysis project since 1977, and recently has been appointed Deputy Director of the newly established National Center for Rehabilitation Engineering at Wright State University. The author of over 100 scientific communications, his research interests include the biomechanics and energetics of skeletal and cardiac muscle with special emphasis on mathematical modeling.

Harry H. Heaton, III, B.S.

Harry H. Heaton, III is a Research Associate with the National Center for Rehabilitation Engineering at Wright State University. He received his B.S. in Biological Sciences from Wright State University and is currently continuing his studies in the field of biomedical engineering. While an undergraduate, he earned the national scholarship Of the National Micrographics Association, Wright State University's Frederick A. White scholarship and the Institute for Electrical and Electronics Engineers (IEEE) College Technology Award. As a researcher, he has been cited by the Wright State faculty and the IEEE for his work in rehabilitation engineering.

Roger M. Glaser, Ph.D.

Roger M. Glaser, Professor of Physiology and Director of the Laboratory for Applied Physiology, came to Wright State in 1972 as an Assistant Professor of Biological Sciences. After moving to the Physiology Department in 1974, Glaser was promoted to Associate Professor in 1976 and to full Professor in 1981. Roger Glaser earned a Bachelor's degree in Health and Physical Education in 1968 and a Master of Science in Exercise Physiology in 1969 from Queens College of the City University of New York. He earned his doctorate in Exercise Environmental Physiology from Ohio State University in 1971, where he was a post-doctoral fellow the following year. Author of Laboratory Procedures for Medical Physiology, with K.H. Mechlin, Glaser has received several awards, including the Military Order of the Purple Heart for Outstanding Research in Service to the Handicapped.

Where FES-Cycling Was Created?

The FES-cycling was created in the National Center for Rehabilitation Engineering & Departments of Engineering, Physiology, and Computer Science at Wright State University, Dayton, Ohio, USA.

How Was the First FES-Cycling Device?

In early 1980s, a FES-cycling equipment was detailed described for the first time [2]. The system purposed was a bicycle ergometer for exercising paralyzed muscle. The device was based upon a standard Monark™ bicycle ergometer. The ergometer has been modified with sensors for feedback of crank position that an Apple II™ computer then uses to coordinate stimulation of muscles [2].

This system was used for isotonic training for both the cardiovascular system and skeletal muscle for individuals who are paralyzed. The muscles used in the study were the iliacus and quadriceps. Exercise training to test the device was conducted on four paraplegic and quadriplegic subjects over a period of 30 days. Exercise was induced three times per week for a period of 15 min. Results of these experiments showed an increase in endurance and muscle size [2].

Bicycle Modifications

As mentioned above, a modification of the Monark™ cycle ergometer involved placing a sensor on the pedals of the bicycle to allow measurement of pedal rotation. Another change was replacing the pedals with breakaway shoes (Fig. 1.2). This involved making wooden shoe bottoms and bolting these to the bike. With Velcro™ on both the wooden shoe bottoms and the shoe of the subjects, any adverse movement would result in the feet coming off the pedals and thus prevent ankle injury [2].

Additionally, knee stabilizer bars were used to keep the knees in alignment, and a special high seatback with a shoulder harness and seatbelt are used to maintain the posture of the subject.

Computer Program [2]

The computer program to control movement on bicycle ergometer was developed in various stages. Because of weakness of bones and joints following years of no exercise due to paralysis, it was felt best to keep the exercise workload to a minimum. Consequently, the duty cycle was such that the quadriceps muscle was only

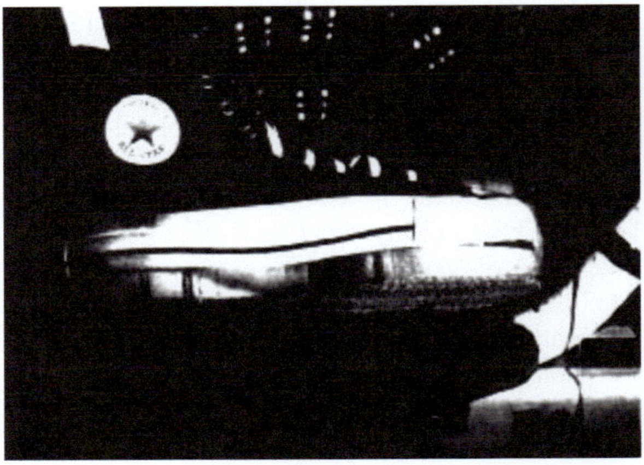

Fig. 1.2 Breakaway shoes [2]

functioning during 35% of any given cycle rotation. The iliacus muscles (used to lift the legs) functioned during 50% of the crank rotation.

The bicycle was timed such that the potentiometer read 0 V when the right leg was at the top of its rotations. For the next 90° of rotation of the right leg, the right quadriceps muscle was stimulated; this was the only time the right quadriceps muscle was stimulated. For both legs, the iliacus muscles were stimulated at the bottom of the crank rotation (180°), and this continued until the top of the crank rotation (0°). The result was that the rotation of a bicycle crank was divided into four phases of 90° each (during which time different muscles were activated).

Operationally, the subjects were passively pedaled at 40 RPM to begin rotation, and the voltage to the quadriceps muscles was increased until they could maintain the rotation at that speed. The iliacus muscles were the activated to bring them up to appropriate voltage to increase the speed to 50 RPM. Voltage on the two muscle groups was adjusted by varying the two Apple™ game paddle inputs. Therefore, by alternately adjusting the quadriceps and the iliacus stimulation, the bicycle speed could be adjusted. Too much stimulation of the iliacus muscle resulted in inward rotation of the knees. Therefore, the voltage was adjusted to increase the speed of cycling but not to the point where knees started moving inward during pedaling.

References

1. Wood D, Swain I. Functional electrical stimulation. In: Taktak A, Ganney P, Long D, White P, editors. Clinical Engineering: A Handbook for Clinical and Biomedical Engineers. London: Academic Press; 2014.
2. Petrofsky JS, Phillips C, Heaton HH, Glaser RM. Bicycle ergometer for paralyzed muscle. J Clin Eng. 1984;9(1):13–20.
3. Gojda J, Waldauf P, Hrušková N, Blahutová B, Krajčová A, Urban T, Tůma P, Řasová K, Duška F. Lactate production without hypoxia in skeletal muscle during electrical cycling: crossover study of femoral venous-arterial differences in healthy volunteers. PLoS One. 2019;14(3):1–15.
4. Fischer E, Ramsey VW. The effect of daily electrical stimulation of normal and denervated muscles upon their protein content and upon some of the physicochemical properties of the protein. Am J Phys. 1946;1945:583–6.
5. Kosman AJ, Osborne SL, Ivy AC. The influence of duration and frequency of treatment in electrical stimulation of paralyzed muscle. Arch Phys Med Rehabil. 1947;28(1):12–7.
6. Kosman AJ, Osborne SL, Ivy AC. Importance of current form and frequency in electrical stimulation of muscles; studies in retardation of muscle atrophy in the dog. Archives of physical medicine. 1948;29(9):559–62.
7. Vodovnik L, Long C 2nd, Lippay A. Pain response to different tetanizing currents. Arch Phys Med Rehabil. 1965;46:187.
8. Crochetiere WJ, Vodovnik L, Reswick JB. Electrical stimulation of skeletal muscle--a study of muscle as an actuator. Med Biol Eng. 1967;5(2):111–25.

Principles of Electrical Stimulation 2

Victor Hugo de Souza Ribeiro, Leandro Andrade Moreira,
Vitória dos Santos Nogueira,
and João Luiz Quagliotti Durigan

Introduction

Electrotherapy is well known as an effective tool for rehabilitation in various conditions, including increasing muscle strength in cases of atrophy, as well as for training and recovery [1, 2]. Electrotherapy involves the application of an electrical current to the skin via electrodes positioned on the targeted region [3] to depolarize motor neurons, causing involuntary muscle contractions [4]. Especially in physical therapy, neuromuscular electrical stimulation (NMES) is widely used primarily to preserve or maintain neuromuscular function during periods of reduced muscle use caused by orthopedic injuries, disease, or the aging process. It is also used to restore neuromuscular function after its decline and to improve neuromuscular performance in both individuals with certain diseases and those who are apparently healthy [5].

Basic Principles of Electrical Stimulation

An electric current is a basic physical form of energy and can interact with biological tissues, promoting physiological and therapeutic effects. Electric charge is the fundamental unit that gives rise to current, a continuous and orderly flow of charges

V. H. de Souza Ribeiro
Laboratory of Muscle and Tendon Plasticity, Physical Education College,
University of Brasilia, Brasília, DF, Brazil

L. A. Moreira · V. dos Santos Nogueira
Laboratory of Muscle and Tendon Plasticity, Rehabilitation Sciences Program,
University of Brasilia, Brasília, DF, Brazil

J. L. Q. Durigan (✉)
Faculty of Health Sciences and Technologies, Rehabilitation Sciences Program,
Laboratory of Muscle and Tendon Plasticity, University of Brasilia, Brasília, DF, Brazil

M. Frazão (ed.), *Functional Electrical Stimulation Cycling in Clinical Practice*,
https://doi.org/10.1007/978-3-032-23937-2_2

through conductive material. In electrotherapy, this concept refers to the flow of charges transferred through an electrode, which may be made of silicone or aluminum, into the body [2, 8, 11, 12]. The purpose of this current flow is to depolarize motor (peripheral activation) and sensory (central activation) axons. However, this recruitment pattern is preserved only when the patient's innervation remains intact. If the muscle is denervated, NMES can be used to recruit fibers directly within the muscle. However, conducting an electrodiagnostic test is essential for the physiotherapist to determine the intensity (rheobase) and pulse duration (chronaxie) needed for sarcolemma depolarization [13, 14].

Types of Electrical Stimulation

There are several objectives for which NMES is used, and the main ones are discussed below.

- *TENS (Transcutaneous Electrical Nerve Stimulation)*

TENS is a safe, non-invasive, and low-cost non-pharmacological intervention with minimal adverse effects and well-established contraindications. It delivers a low-voltage current to the skin to relieve pain and can be applied either by the patient or by a physical therapist. There are two types of TENS: high frequency (≥50 Hz), also known as conventional TENS, and low frequency (1–10 Hz), also called acupuncture TENS. It promotes analgesia by activating ascending and descending inhibitory neuronal pathways, stimulating large-diameter (Aβ) primary afferent fibers from the skin and deep (articular) structures. These fibers send signals that activate areas involved in the descending inhibitory pain pathway. Both types act on the opioidergic system and are commonly used in cases of postoperative pain, as well as in the clinical management of acute and chronic pain [15–20].

- *NMES (Neuromuscular Electrical Stimulation)*

It is used to recruit muscles for strength development and to prevent atrophy in bedridden patients or individuals with significant muscle weakness. It works by directly stimulating motor neurons, eliciting muscle contractions. Typically, the current frequency is adapted to a value close to 20 Hz, aiming to reduce neuromuscular fatigue, combined with higher intensities are applied to generate effective muscle force. This method is widely utilized in rehabilitation following injuries, muscle weakness, and post-surgical recovery.

- *FES (Functional Electrical Stimulation)*

It is used in patients with neuromuscular deficits to elicit functional movements, thereby enhancing autonomy and improving motor function. Electrical stimulation is precisely applied to activate specific muscles, enabling purposeful movements such as walking or grasping objects. In the context of FES, different current delivery strategies are used to optimize muscle activation and reduce fatigue. Among the most common are synchronous stimulation, in which all channels are activated simultaneously, providing global contraction, and asynchronous stimulation, in which channels are triggered at different times, mimicking the natural recruitment of fibers and reducing muscle fatigue. More advanced techniques, such as SDSS (Spatially Distributed Sequential Stimulation), use multiple small electrodes over the same muscle, activated sequentially, distributing the load and increasing patient comfort [45].

Physiological Basis of Electrical Stimulation

There are notable differences between voluntary contractions and those induced by electrical stimulation. Voluntary contractions follow the Henneman recruitment principle [21–23], which states that smaller-caliber axons are activated first due to their lower activation threshold, whereas larger-caliber axons require a higher depolarization threshold and more neurotransmitters to recruit the motor unit. When examining muscle fibers, they can be classified by contraction speed into slow-twitch fibers, which are resistant to fatigue, and fast-twitch fibers, which fatigue more quickly. This difference in fatigue resistance aligns with the Henneman recruitment principle [21–23], whereby smaller-caliber nerve fibers, innervating the less fatigable type I muscle fibers, are recruited first, followed by larger-caliber fibers that activate the more fatigable type II muscle fibers. Unlike voluntary contractions, NMES-evoked contractions do not follow the recruitment principle, as the fibers activated depend on the depolarization of motor axons located beneath (or closest to) the electrode on the skin surface. This characteristic makes the evoked contraction more fatiguing because it recruits all fiber types simultaneously [24, 25], been this is a handicap.

Electrical Parameter

It is crucial to understand the physical parameters that guide the application and effectiveness of electrical stimulation. The main parameters are related to:

- *Amplitude or intensity of current*

It is measured in amperes (A) and its most used range for electrotherapy is from 20 μA to 150 mA. Pulse amplitude and duration determine which nerve fibers are recruited: low amplitude activates sensory fibers, moderate amplitude recruits motor fibers, and high amplitude can cause pain. There is a direct relationship between the intensity of the electrical current, the pulse width (sum of the positive and the negative phase), and the resulting electric field within the tissues. As the intensity of the current increases, the electric field expands in size and penetrates deeper into the underlying tissues, affecting a larger volume and reaching nerve fibers located further from the electrode. When the pulse width is low, meaning each pulse lasts a very short time, a higher current intensity is required to stimulate sensory, motor, and pain fibers effectively. This is because shorter pulses deliver less energy per pulse, so the intensity must be increased to reach the activation thresholds of these nerves. Conversely, when the pulse width is longer, more energy is delivered in each pulse, allowing sensory, motor, and peripheral fibers to be recruited at lower current intensities. The interplay between pulse width and intensity is crucial in determining which nerve fibers are activated and how effectively. By adjusting these parameters, clinicians can target specific fibers for different therapeutic goals, such as pain relief, muscle activation, or functional movement. Understanding this relationship helps optimize electrical stimulation treatments to achieve the best clinical results while minimizing discomfort.

- *Pulse width*

Pulse width is measured in microseconds (μs) or milliseconds (ms) and it is the sum of the positive phase and the negative phase. Pulse width determines how long the current flows during each pulse and is closely related to current intensity. As mentioned previously, shorter pulses require greater current intensity/amplitude, whereas wider pulses require lower intensity (less energy) to achieve the same effect. When pulse durations exceed 500 μs, the sensory, motor, and pain thresholds are reached more quickly, even at low amplitudes, which may result in considerable discomfort for the patient. This parameter requires careful control because it has a direct impact on muscle strength production, pain modulation, and tissue repair. The balance between pulse duration and current amplitude is especially important for optimizing force generation while maintaining current efficiency. The pulse duration can vary from 1 to 1000 μs; however, the most used range is between 200 and 500 μs. In practice, pulse widths between 200 and 500 μs are the most used in scientific research. Nonetheless, some studies indicate that applying longer pulses (around 1000 μs) combined with high frequencies (approximately 100 Hz) to the nerve may help reduce muscle fatigue caused by NMES [2, 13, 26, 27],

- *Frequency*

Selecting the stimulation frequency is crucial for muscle contraction, analgesia, and tissue repair, as it directly affects the functioning of neural pathways. This influence occurs through changes in the bioelectric potentials of nerve cell membranes. The resulting frequency of this interference in the membrane potential determines the activation pattern and the way in which the targeted pathways will respond to electrical stimulation. The available literature includes well-conducted studies showing that higher frequencies (around 100 Hz) used to generate contractions result in greater muscle recruitment, producing more force but also leading to greater fatigue. Conversely, at lower frequencies (approximately 20–50 Hz), muscle fatigue is significantly reduced, although contraction force decreases accordingly

[13, 28]. For muscle contraction, the most used frequency range for muscle recruitment is between 20 and 100 Hz, which produces tetanic (sustained) contractions. Frequencies below 10 Hz produce non-tetanic (non-sustained) contractions, which are typically used for edema drainage and muscle relaxation.

- *WAVEFORMS*

There are five types of waveforms: continuous, quadratic or rectangular, sinusoidal, triangular, and peaked or exponential. The waveform defines the amount of energy transmitted to the patient and, consequently, the perception of the current. In NMES, the waveform also determines whether the current is direct or alternating. If the current is unidirectional, it will have a monophasic characteristic. In NMES, the current may flow in a single direction, known as monophasic or direct current (Fig. 2.1), in which the electrode polarities are fixed, one positive and one negative. In contrast, when the pulse alternates directions without a fixed polarity, the current is referred to as alternating or biphasic [29]. It is well established that direct current is recommended for tissue repair, particularly in the treatment of ulcers, to assist in inflammatory processes, reduce edema, and for use in iontophoresis [12, 29, 30], and on the other hand, biphasic currents are employed for purposes such as pain relief, muscle strengthening, tissue repair, and minimizing fatigue [13]. Biphasic currents can be either symmetrical, having the same waveform and equal charge in both phases, or asymmetrical, with different waveforms between phases. They may also be classified as balanced, when the charge is equal in both phases, and unbalanced, when the charge differs between phases [31] (Fig. 2.2). Symmetrical biphasic currents are generally perceived as more comfortable than monophasic currents, as monophasic stimulation lacks pole alternation, leading to an accumulation of electrical charge at the electrodes [32].

It's also important to understand the concepts of low, medium, and high frequencies. Low-frequency currents operate in the 1–1000 Hz range and are used for therapeutic purposes, such as TENS. Medium-frequency currents operate in the range of 1001–10,000 Hz and are used therapeutically when modulated within the 1–200 Hz

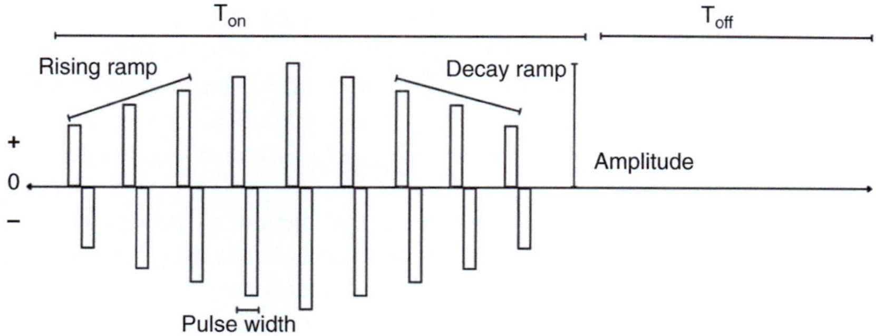

Fig. 2.1 Ilustration of Ton and Toff modulation, rise ramp and fall ramp in a biphasic rectangular current

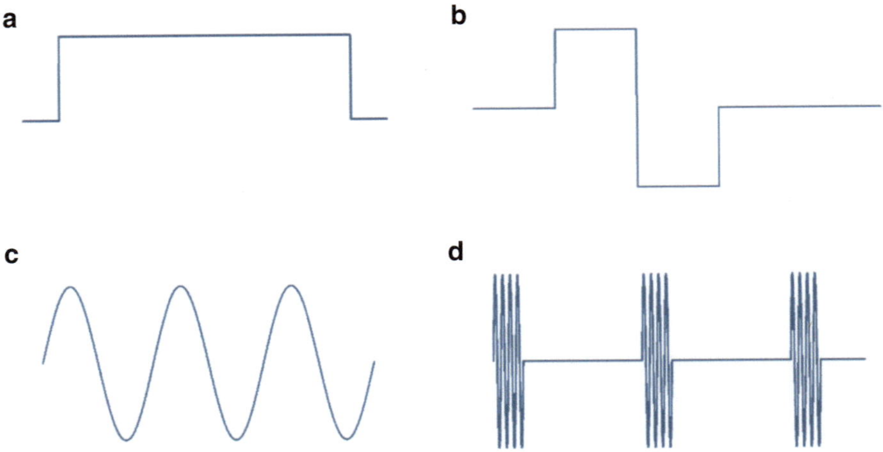

Fig. 2.2 (**a**) Representation of a quadratic monophasic current. (**b**) Rectangular biphasic current. (**c**) Sinusoidal biphasic current. (**d**) Sinusoidal biphasic pulsed current

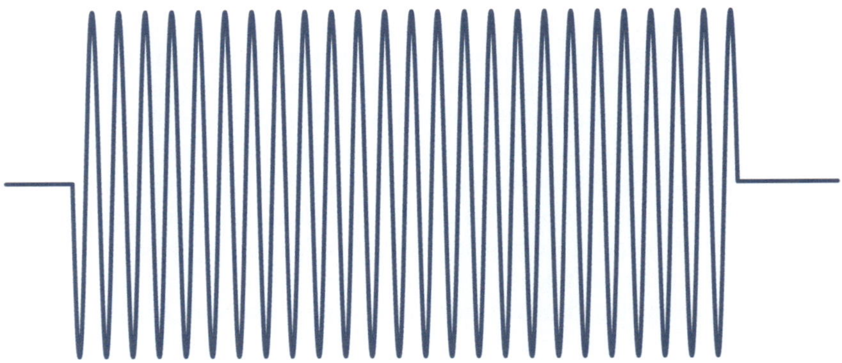

Fig. 2.3 The classical Russian Current is an alternating (biphasic) sinusoidal wave of 2.5 kHz frequency and 50 Hz pulse width

range [2]. The most well-known commercially available medium-frequency currents include Russian current (2500 Hz) (Fig. 2.3), Australian/Aussie current (1000 Hz) (Fig. 2.4), and heterodyne/vector interferential current (4000 Hz). High-frequency currents, operating at frequencies above 10,000 Hz and are applied in clinical settings for purposes such as producing deep tissue heating and generating electromagnetic radiation.

Both the current parameters and the precise placement of electrodes on the skin are critical for the effectiveness of NMES and for understanding the central and peripheral responses it elicits. To date, numerous studies have aimed to determine the optimal current type, waveform, and modulation parameters to maximize the effectiveness of electrical stimulation. Among the various options, two types of currents are most investigated due to their widespread use: alternating current (medium

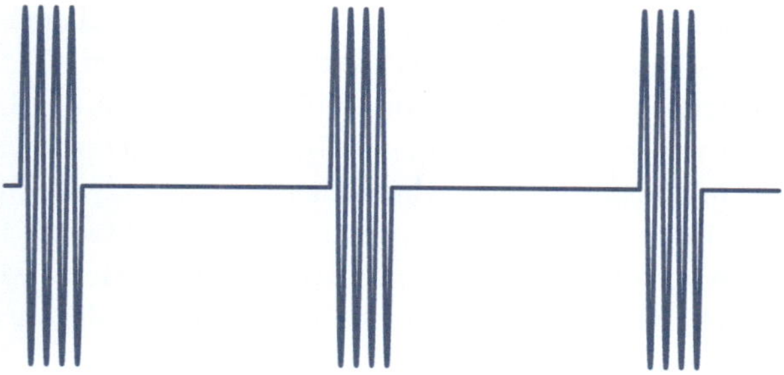

Fig. 2.4 The Australian current (Aussie) is a medium-frequency AC (typically 1 kHz) modulated in short bursts, classic: 4 ms ON/16 ms OFF, which results in a 50 Hz modulation

frequency) and pulsed current (low frequency). Alternating current is characterized by delivering stimulation in bursts, with each burst consisting of multiple pulses. It is modulated at a carrier frequency ranging from 1000 to 10,000 Hz and burst frequencies in the low-frequency range (1–200 Hz) [13, 28, 33]. Pulsed current delivers intermittent pulses separated by significant intervals between each pulse. Its frequency varies from 1 to 200 Hz, and the stimulation can be modulated as either monophasic or biphasic [13, 28, 33]. The choice of current type must be made according to the objective to be achieved; however, there is no consensus on which of the two currents and which modulation parameters are more effective in inducing greater force production with less sensory discomfort.

- *Ramp time*

For better applicability of the current, some modulations can be performed, the most used being pulse trains (Ton/Toff), rising and falling ramps, intensity, frequency, phase/pulse width and burst [11]. It is recommended that the practitioner includes an off-time (Toff) interval and an on-time (Ton) current delivery period, because contractions induced by electrical current are more metabolically fatiguing than voluntary contractions, so this modulation promotes greater muscle adaptation to training while reducing fatigue. When using Ton and Toff periods, it is essential to adjust the contraction (Ton) and rest (Toff) durations, commonly referred to as the Ton/Toff ratio. Although many protocols exist, it is well established that a minimum contraction time of 5 s is necessary to induce muscle strength adaptations through electrical stimulation. Consequently, a 1:3 ratio (5 s of Ton followed by 15 s of Toff) is often applied initially, with the goal of progressing toward a 1:1 ratio as treatment advances [13]. Ramp-up and ramp-down modulation controls the time (in seconds) that the current takes to reach its maximum intensity and/or return to zero intensity. This modulation allows for a more physiological muscle contraction, as the number of recruited motor units is proportional to the gradual increase in current amplitude. To achieve smoother and more sequential contractions in both time and space, ramp-up and ramp-down phases are increasingly incorporated into the electrical stimulation parameters. This approach aims to mimic a more natural pattern of muscle recruitment and may also help improve fatigue tolerance [11]. The difference in contraction speed between fibers is largely due to their mitochondrial content. Slow-twitch fibers contain more mitochondria, allowing greater aerobic ATP production, which is slower due to the required chemical reactions. They also possess a specific myosin ATPase that breaks down ATP to release energy for force generation and transmission to the thin filaments [13, 28, 33]. Fast-twitch fibers have fewer mitochondria and rely on anaerobic pathways, producing ATP quickly but in limited amounts, which leads to faster fatigue. They contain more myofibrils, enabling greater force production than slow-twitch fibers. Smaller motor units (slow-twitch) sustain lower force for long durations, while larger motor units (fast-twitch) generate high force briefly, explaining why we can walk for hours but cannot sprint for long [13, 28, 33].

Electrode Placement

It is necessary to understand the concept of electrodes, considering the role they play in the context of electrical stimulation. These are conductive devices applied to the skin with the purpose of delivering electrical current to the body, or from it, for therapeutic purposes. They are typically made from conductive materials such as copper or silver, coated with layers of rubber or plastic. When connected to electrotherapy equipment, electrodes allow the transmission of electrical current to the target body regions, enabling the desired therapeutic effects of stimulation. Their non-invasive nature—in the case of surface electrodes—allows for a safe and effective interface between the electrostimulator and the skin tissue. This interface can be established through different types of electrodes, such as aluminum electrodes, silicone-carbon electrodes (often mistakenly referred to as "rubber" electrodes), and self-adhesive electrodes, all composed of distinct materials that influence current conduction and body conformity (Fig. 2.5).

Aluminum electrodes are primarily recommended for the application of polarized currents, being especially indicated for procedures such as galvanization and iontophoresis. However, their use in clinical settings aimed at muscle strength gain is quite limited [34]. On the other hand, silicone-carbon electrodes are widely used in clinical practice, both for muscle strengthening and analgesia applications. This popularity is largely due to their low cost, good electrical conductivity, and impedance considered acceptable for therapeutic purposes. Self-adhesive electrodes, although they offer lower impedance compared to silicone-carbon electrodes, which promotes greater patient tolerance to electrical currents, have a higher cost and are

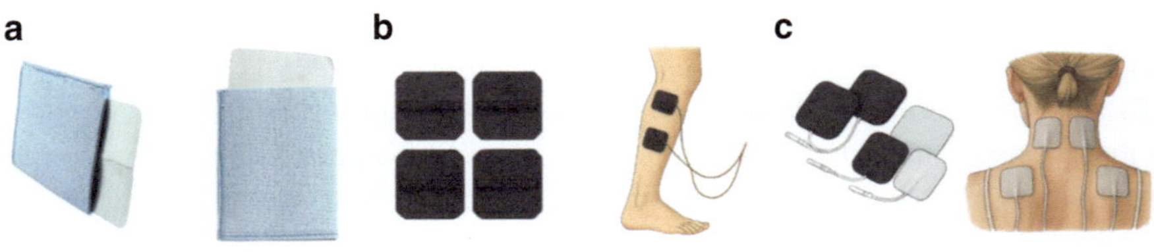

Fig. 2.5 Different types of electrodes. (**a**) Aluminum electrodes and sponges required for coupling; (**b**) Silicone–carbon electrodes; (**c**) Self-adhesive electrodes

designed for single use or limited reuse by the same patient. For this reason, they are more commonly used in laboratory settings and scientific research, being less frequently employed in routine clinical practice.

In addition to the choice of electrode type, other aspects must be carefully considered when planning a treatment involving electrical stimulation. Electrode size, for example, can directly influence factors such as skin impedance, current density, discrimination, and the perception of responses generated in biological tissue. Larger electrodes tend to reduce current density and skin impedance, providing a more comfortable and less painful motor response, and are especially recommended for larger muscle groups. However, their broader area of action results in less specific stimulation. On the other hand, smaller electrodes offer greater specificity in targeting particular regions or muscles, favoring more localized recruitment. Nevertheless, due to the concentration of current in a smaller area, they may lead to increased discomfort and pain, especially after the excitation of motor neurons [35].

Understanding the type of electrode application should also be explored. Scientific evidence indicates that identifying and placing electrodes directly over motor points can significantly improve patient comfort and enhance the therapeutic effects of electrical stimulation [36–38]. Despite this, some professionals adopt standardized placements, arguing that a greater distance between electrodes, especially with longitudinal orientation along the muscle fibers and placement at opposite ends of the muscle, favors the production of higher muscular torque [39, 40]. Another relevant placement strategy, although still utilized in clinical practice, involves applying stimulation over peripheral nerves (Fig. 2.6). This approach has proven to be highly effective in generating muscle force while simultaneously reducing the sensory discomfort associated with electrical current [2, 41]. Given these possibilities, it is recommended that electrode placement be personalized based on the individual anatomy of the target tissue, adjusting both the location and size of the electrodes according to the specific characteristics of each patient.

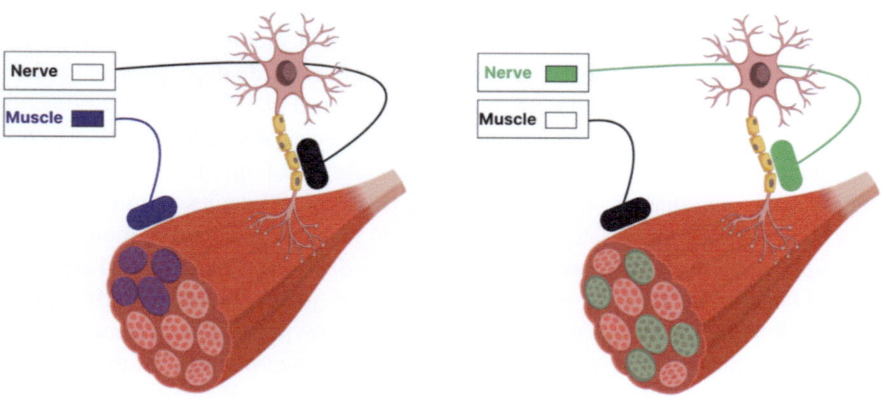

Fig. 2.6 Representation of the application of electrical stimulation directly on the muscle belly and on the nerve trunk

When developing a treatment plan, it is essential to consider several factors related to the electrodes, such as the manufacturing material, sizes and shapes, type of conductive medium (gel, water, adhesive), positioning relative to the target tissues, and the orientation between the electrodes. These elements directly influence the effectiveness and safety of the applied electrical stimulation.

Physiological Effects of Electrical Stimulation

When applied in a therapeutic context, electrical stimulation triggers a series of physiological effects that support its use in clinical practice. These effects are responsible for the benefits observed in various neuromuscular conditions and, therefore, form the basis for the clinical justification of this physical modality. However, physiological responses to electrical stimulation can vary significantly depending on the parameters used, the patient's clinical condition, and the specific goals of the treatment. Thus, understanding these mechanisms is essential for effective and safe application.

Muscle Strengthening

Muscle strengthening induced by electrical stimulation is based on the current's ability to generate muscle contractions, like physiological ones, through the direct activation of motor neurons. Physiological muscle contraction occurs through the depolarization of the motor neuron, with the propagation of the action potential to the neuromuscular junction, where the release of acetylcholine activates postsynaptic receptors and triggers the intracellular events responsible for muscle contraction, force production, and joint movement [42]. Although both share similar functional mechanisms, muscle contraction evoked by electrical stimulation presents some particularities, especially due to the supramaximal and simultaneous recruitment of motor units, without following the physiological principle of orderly recruitment. This non-selective recruitment pattern, independent of motor unit size, allows for high levels of muscle activation, promoting strength-related adaptations and reducing the occurrence of neuromuscular accommodation (Fig. 2.7).

Despite its effectiveness in generating force, electrically induced muscle contraction is inherently uncomfortable. This discomfort can limit the intensity of stimulation and, consequently, the strengthening potential. Strategies to minimize this sensation include appropriate electrode size and placement, targeting motor points (regions where motor units are more superficially distributed), and careful attention to joint positioning during application. For instance, joints placed in overly lengthened or shortened positions tend to increase sensitivity [43–45]. Additionally, individual anatomical factors, such as the depth of motor neurons and the thickness of the skinfold, also influence the effectiveness of stimulation. Patients with a greater

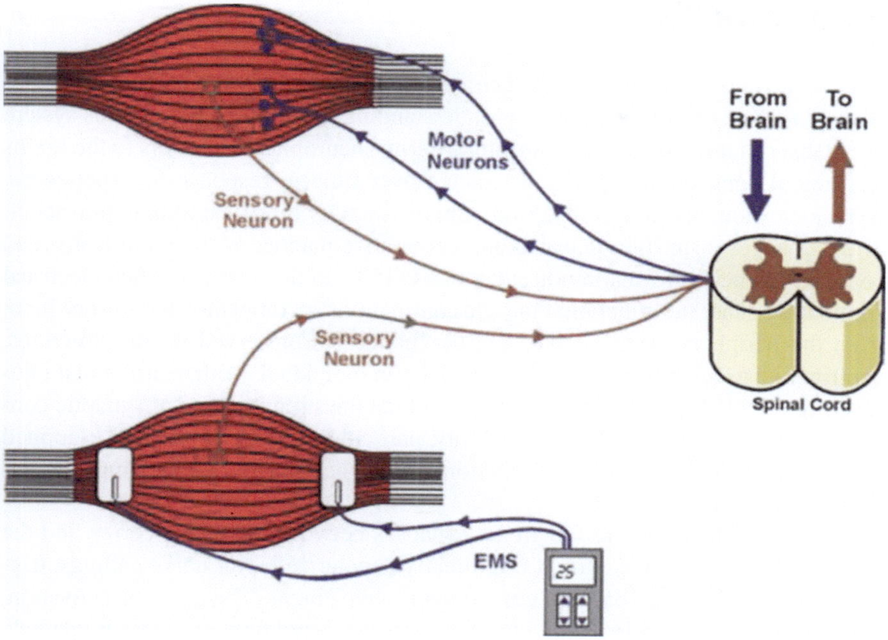

Fig. 2.7 Electrical stimulation of the afferent and efferent impulse of the motor neuron. Voluntary contraction vs. evoked contraction. (**Source:** Pavlovic and Stanislav [67])

amount of adipose tissue tend to experience lower evoked torque and higher discomfort, as fat acts as an electrical insulator, reducing current penetration.

When it comes to the stimulation parameters used to promote muscle hypertrophy, both low- and medium-frequency currents have proven to be effective. Current literature suggests that there are no significant differences between these modalities regarding the torque produced or the level of discomfort perceived during application, which provides the therapist with greater flexibility in choosing the most appropriate type of current for each context [46]. However, it is important to understand that electrical stimulation does not produce the same effects in all individuals. A significant portion of the population does not respond adequately to the stimuli, meaning it is not possible to evoke sufficient muscle torque to generate meaningful strength or hypertrophy adaptations. In such cases, the mechanical tension induced by electrical stimulation becomes insufficient to trigger the physiological processes responsible for the desired muscular adaptations. Additionally, electrical stimulation can enhance other therapeutic approaches aimed at muscle hypertrophy, especially in individuals with specific clinical conditions. When combined with physical exercise, it has been shown to increase muscle strength compared to active control groups [47–49].

Muscle Re-education

Muscle reeducation mediated by electrical stimulation is based on the principles of neuroplasticity, one of the pillars for understanding how the central nervous system is capable of reorganizing itself. In simple terms, neuroplasticity refers to the brains and neural connections' ability to change over time in response to experiences, behaviors, thoughts, and to external stimuli, such as electrical stimulation itself. These changes occur in a repeated and cumulative manner as the brain learns and consolidates new information throughout life [50]. In this context, when electrical stimulation generates functional muscle contractions accompanied by sensory input from the periphery, it can induce plastic changes in preserved neural structures, contributing to functional recovery, especially in individuals with neurological injuries (Fig. 2.7) [51–55]. Such adaptations include the strengthening of synaptic connections and increased cortical excitability, particularly when stimulation is applied repetitively, associated with real functions, and synchronized with attempts at voluntary movement.

Even when there are no functional synapses between the motor cortex and the motor neurons, electrical current can directly depolarize motor nerve endings, triggering muscle contraction and, consequently, movement. This type of activation, when repeated and applied with a functional purpose, not only produces immediate improvements during the intervention but can also lead to long-lasting effects, reflecting actual adaptations within neural circuits [56]. The continuous sensory input generated by each assisted contraction increases CNS excitability and strengthens the communication pathways between the brain and muscles, which helps explain why motor gains may persist even after the stimulation sessions have ended.

Finally, electrical stimulation has shown consistent evidence of its potential to enhance function in individuals with different neurological conditions. In stroke, for instance, this intervention has proven effective in improving activities of daily living, as well as promoting the recovery of motor skills even in cases of severe paresis [57]. In children with cerebral palsy undergoing botulinum toxin injections, electrical stimulation has also been shown to enhance the effects of the intervention, contributing to muscle re-education, functional gains, and, consequently, the promotion of neuroplasticity [58].

Pain Management

Pain control through electroanalgesia is based on neurophysiological mechanisms of pain modulation. Its effectiveness is anchored in classical neuroscience theories, such as the Gate Control Theory of Pain [59]. According to this theory, non-painful sensory stimuli activate larger, fast-conducting nerve fibers (A-β fibers), which compete with thinner, slower-conducting nociceptive fibers (C fibers and A-δ fibers) for the transmission of signals to the dorsal horn of the spinal cord. This competition

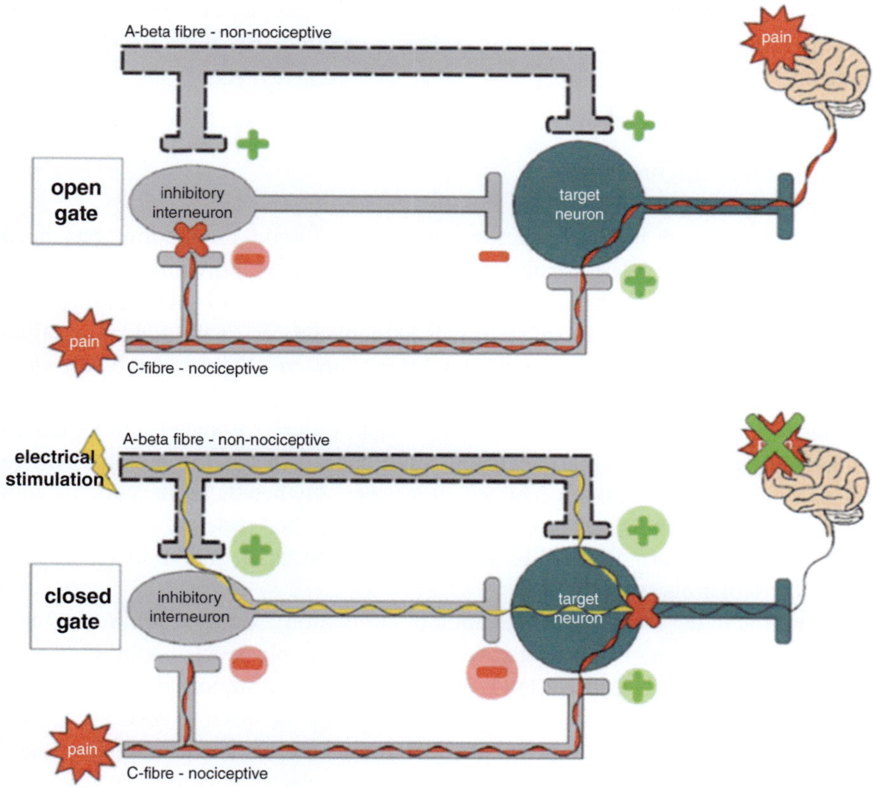

Fig. 2.8 Illustration of the Gate Control Theory of Pain. (**Source:** Vervaat et al. [68])

favors the inhibition of nociceptive signals, thereby reducing pain perception at the spinal level (Fig. 2.8).

Another proposed mechanism involves the endogenous release of opioids, such as endorphins, which are produced in the basal nuclei and act at both spinal and cortical levels. These natural opioids exert strong analgesic effects, and their release can be particularly stimulated by low-frequency currents. It is worth noting, however, that endorphin-mediated analgesic responses may vary according to individual predisposition, being more effective in patients with higher endogenous availability of these substances. Additionally, electrical stimulation may be as effective as oral analgesics in controlling pain in cases of acute trauma, with the advantage of not causing the side effects frequently associated with these medications [60]. Thus, individuals with contraindications to pharmacological treatment may benefit from this approach as an alternative for pain management.

Although this is a safe and widely used resource, there are some important clinical limitations. So-called analgesic tolerance may occur with repeated use, requiring frequent adjustments to stimulus intensity between applications [61]. In addition, patients using systemic opioids (such as morphine, codeine, or tramadol) tend to show a reduced response to electroanalgesia, particularly with low-frequency protocols.

Circulation Improvement

An improvement in fluid circulation, particularly blood circulation, has been observed with the use of electrical stimulation, especially in individuals with limitations for performing conventional exercise or those affected by immobility syndrome [62]. The primary mechanism involved in this process is the activation of the venous muscle pump, triggered by the rhythmic contractions generated by the electrical current. These contractions compress intramuscular and intermuscular vessels, facilitating venous return to the heart, which, in turn, contributes to increased cardiac output and peripheral perfusion—particularly in the lower limbs, where venous stasis is more common. This effect is especially beneficial for patients with reduced mobility, decreased autonomy, and prolonged bed rest, situations in which impaired venous return can lead to fluid accumulation, pain, and an increased risk of cardiovascular disease [63, 64].

In addition to the mechanical activation of circulation, electrical stimulation also promotes local biochemical effects. Among these, the release of vasodilatory substances—such as nitric oxide—stands out, as it acts on the smooth muscle of blood vessels, promoting vasodilation and reducing peripheral vascular resistance. This mechanism enhances regional blood flow and optimizes the delivery of oxygen and nutrients to the stimulated tissues. In the long term, electrical stimulation can also induce significant muscular and vascular adaptations, such as increased capillary density, improved endothelial function, and enhanced oxidative enzyme activity, thereby favoring the muscle's metabolic capacity [64]. Such adaptations contribute to sustained improvements in muscle oxygenation and metabolite removal, resulting in chronic benefits for circulation and vascular health.

Reduction of Muscle Spasticity

The physiological mechanisms by which electrical stimulation acts on muscle spasticity involve both spinal and supraspinal adaptations, promoting immediate and sustained effects on the modulation of involuntary motor activity [65]. At the spinal cord level, electrical stimulation primarily acts by reducing the excitability of alpha motor neurons, exerting an inhibitory effect on hyperactive spinal reflexes. This occurs through the activation of sensory afferents during electrically induced rhythmic contractions, which restore the sensory feedback pattern and reduce neural hyperexcitability. Furthermore, repeated stimulation may induce neurospinal plasticity processes, leading to the reorganization of intraspinal synapses, resulting in improved motor control and a reduction in spastic symptoms [66].

Complementarily, electrical stimulation exerts effects on the supraspinal nervous system, acting on cortical circuits through the facilitation of neuroplasticity. The modulation of functional connectivity between brain structures involved in motor control has been associated with a persistent reduction in spasticity, especially when electrical stimulation is combined with functional tasks [10, 66]. From a clinical perspective, there are two main strategies for applying electrical stimulation to manage spasticity, depending on the target muscle group. When stimulation is applied to the antagonist of the spastic muscle group, the goal is to exploit the mechanism of reciprocal inhibition, in which activation of the antagonist physiologically inhibits the spastic muscle via the spinal reflex arc. In this approach, a moderate frequency (around 20–30 Hz) is used to maintain function without inducing premature fatigue. Conversely, when stimulation is applied directly to the spastic muscle, the objective is to induce neuromuscular fatigue and autogenic inhibition, mediated by increased tension in the Golgi tendon organ. For this purpose, higher frequencies (approximately 100 Hz) and prolonged contraction times (10–15 s) are recommended, promoting relaxation of the hyperactive muscle and reducing tone.

Safety Considerations and Contraindications

Although electrical stimulation is widely used in the clinical management of various conditions, its application requires strict attention to safety, appropriate parameter settings, and assessment of contraindications. The effectiveness of the treatment is directly related to the correct selection of stimulation parameters, such as intensity, frequency, and duration of application. Inappropriate use of electrical stimulation may lead to adverse reactions, such as pain, hyperemia, skin irritation, and, in more severe cases, tissue injury. Among the absolute contraindications of electrical stimulation, the presence of implanted electronic devices, such as cardiac pacemakers and defibrillators, stands out. These devices may suffer electrical interference if stimulation is applied near the thoracic region, which can compromise their function and put the patient at risk [6, 7, 9, 10]. Additionally, there are specific anatomical areas, such as the carotid artery region and the glottis, where stimulation should be avoided. This is because stimulation in these locations can alter important autonomic reflexes, causing undesirable changes in heart rate and blood pressure [6].

Another point that deserves attention is the presence of metal implants at the application site. The use of polarized currents in these regions may generate local heating, increasing the risk of tissue injury. Patients with uncontrolled epilepsy also require careful evaluation, as electrical stimulation may, in some cases, trigger seizures. Furthermore, conditions such as active infections, open wounds, deep vein thrombosis, active neoplasms, and peripheral vascular disorders are considered relative contraindications; that is, the application of stimulation should be carefully assessed based on the clinical situation, lesion location, and treatment goals. In the case of pregnant women, it is recommended to avoid electrical stimulation over the abdominal and lumbosacral regions, except in specific cases with rigorous protocols and specialized supervision. This recommendation is due to the theoretical possibility of inducing uterine contractions, which may pose obstetric risks [6].

Moreover, electrical stimulation is not indicated for patients with severe cognitive impairments or communication difficulties, as they are unable to report discomfort or adverse effects, increasing the risk of injury. Young children, sedated patients, or those with sensory disorders should also be carefully evaluated to ensure the safety of the application. Finally, for patients with cardiovascular diseases, a more cautious approach is essential. Electrical stimulation should be performed carefully, especially in those with a history of arrhythmias, heart failure, or structural cardiopathies. Although safe protocols exist for stable patients, any treatment must always be preceded by a thorough medical evaluation and continuous monitoring, particularly when stimulation involves large muscle groups or high intensities.

In addition to clinical precautions, equipment care is an important component of safety in the application of electrical stimulation. Electrodes must be kept clean and in good condition, with carbon models washed using mild soap and air-dried naturally, avoiding friction to prevent damage to the conductive material. Equipment, cables, and accessories should be disinfected between sessions with appropriate solutions, avoiding abrasive substances or high-concentration alcohol that may compromise the integrity of the components. Preventive maintenance of the devices must be carried out by qualified professionals, including periodic inspections of calibration, cable insulation, leakage current, and electrical continuity of the electrodes. It is recommended that the devices undergo technical review annually or whenever they remain unused for extended periods, minimizing electrical risks and ensuring parameter stability.

Continuous monitoring is therefore critical to ensure the safe and effective application of the treatment. Direct observation of the patient's perceived discomfort, inspection of the skin before and after each session, assessment of the muscular response, and, when indicated, physiological monitoring—such as heart rate, blood pressure, and oxygen saturation—particularly in individuals with cardiovascular or neurological conditions, should be systematically conducted. Stimulation parameters must be adjusted in real time, taking into consideration both the patient's discomfort threshold and the quality of the evoked muscle contraction. Furthermore, in patients with a history of epilepsy, unstable cardiovascular conditions, or communication limitations, the procedure should be performed under the supervision of a qualified professional, adhering strictly to the absolute and relative contraindications previously described.

Potential adverse effects should also be addressed. Localized discomfort or pain, hyperemia, skin irritation, and paresthesia during stimulation represent the most commonly observed reactions. Less frequently, localized edema, superficial burns, or, in patients with metallic implants, excessive heating of the area may occur, potentially resulting in tissue damage. The incidence and severity of these effects are closely associated with current intensity, pulse width, stimulation frequency, total exposure duration, and the quality of electrode–skin contact.

Conclusion

Electrical stimulation is a versatile, evidence-based therapeutic resource with the potential to preserve and restore muscle function, improve venous return, optimize tissue perfusion, and assist in preventing complications associated with immobility. Its effectiveness, however, depends directly on the careful selection of stimulation parameters—including current type, frequency, pulse width, intensity, and application time—which must be adjusted according to the clinical objective and the patient's individual response. Inappropriate selection of these parameters can compromise both the effectiveness and the safety of the intervention, reinforcing the need for in-depth technical knowledge on the part of the clinician. Furthermore, its application must respect absolute and relative contraindications, as well as consider factors such as tolerance, neuromuscular integrity, and overall clinical status. When integrated in an individualized manner into the therapeutic plan, electrical stimulation can serve as an adjunct strategy capable of enhancing functional outcomes and accelerating the rehabilitation process. Ultimately, it is the combination of correct indication and precise parameter adjustment that determines the true effectiveness and safety of this therapeutic modality, making the physiotherapist's expertise a central element for treatment success.

References

1. Babault N, Cometti C, Maffiuletti NA, Deley G. Does electrical stimulation enhance post-exercise performance recovery? Eur J Appl Physiol. 2011;111(10):2501–7. https://doi.org/10.1007/s00421-011-2117-7. Epub 2011 Aug 17.
2. Bastos JAI, Martins WR, Júnior GC, Collins DF, Durigan JLQ. Contraction fatigue, strength adaptations, and discomfort during conventional versus wide-pulse, high-frequency, neuromuscular electrical stimulation: a systematic review. Appl Physiol Nutr Metab. 2021;46(11):1314–21. https://doi.org/10.1139/apnm-2021-0269. Epub 2021 July 14.
3. Ward AR, Robertson VJ. The variation in fatigue rate with frequency using kHz frequency alternating current. Med Eng Phys. 2000;22(9):637–46. https://doi.org/10.1016/s1350-4533(00)00085-0.
4. Veldman MP, Gondin J, Place N, Maffiuletti NA. Effects of neuromuscular electrical stimulation training on endurance performance. Front Physiol. 2016;7:544. https://doi.org/10.3389/fphys.2016.00544. PMID: 27899898; PMCID: PMC5110544.
5. Maffiuletti NA, Gondin J, Place N, Stevens-Lapsley J, Vivodtzev I, Minetto MA. Clinical use of neuromuscular electrical stimulation for neuromuscular rehabilitation: what are we overlooking? Arch Phys Med Rehabil. 2018;99(4):806–12. https://doi.org/10.1016/j.apmr.2017.10.028. Epub 2017 Dec 9.
6. Johnson MI, Paley CA, Howe TE, Sluka KA. Transcutaneous electrical nerve stimulation for acute pain. Cochrane Database Syst Rev. 2015;2015(6):CD006142. https://doi.org/10.1002/14651858.CD006142.pub3. Published 2015 June 15.
7. Suhail A, Cretnik A, Huemer M. Risk of occurrence of electromagnetic interference from the application of transcutaneous electrical nerve stimulation on the sensing function of implantable defibrillators. Europace. 2023;25(7). https://doi.org/10.1093/europace/euad206.
8. Basford JR. A historical perspective of the popular use of electric and magnetic therapy. Arch Phys Med Rehabil. 2001;82(9):1261–9. https://doi.org/10.1053/apmr.2001.25905.

9. Florian E. Influence of electrical stimulation therapy on permanent pacemaker function. Wien Klin Wochenschr. 2019;131(13–14):313–20. https://doi.org/10.1007/s00508-019-1494-5.
10. Ovadia-Caro S, Khalil AA, Sehm B, Villringer A, Nikulin VV, Nazarova M. Predicting the response to non-invasive brain stimulation in stroke. Front Neurol. 2019;10:302. https://doi.org/10.3389/fneur.2019.00302. Published 2019 Apr 2.
11. Robinson AJ, Snyder-Mackler L. Clinical electrophysiology: electrotherapy and electrophysiologic testing. 2nd ed. Philadelphia: Lippincott Williams & Wilkins; 1995.
12. Robertson V, Ward A, Low J, Reed A. Eletroterapia explicada: princípios e prática. 4th ed. Rio de Janeiro: Elsevier; 2009.
13. Silva VZM, Durigan JLQ, Arena R, Noronha M, Gurney B, Cipriano G Jr. Current evidence demonstrates similar effects of kilohertz-frequency and low-frequency current on quadriceps evoked torque and discomfort in healthy individuals: a systematic review with meta-analysis. Physiother Theory Pract. 2015;31(8):533–9.
14. Bergquist AJ, Clair JM, Lagerquist O, Mang CS, Okuma Y, Collins DF. Neuromuscular electrical stimulation: implications of the electrically evoked sensory volley. Eur J Appl Physiol. 2011;111(10):2409–26.
15. Woolf CJ, Barrett GD, Mitchell D, Myers RA. Naloxone-reversible peripheral electroanalgesia in intact and spinal rats. Eur J Pharmacol. 1977;45(3):311–4.
16. Garrison DW, Foreman RD. Decreased activity of spontaneous and noxiously evoked dorsal horn cells during transcutaneous electrical nerve stimulation (TENS). Pain. 1994;58(3):309–15.
17. Garrison DW, Foreman ED. Effects of prolonged transcutaneous electrical nerve stimulation (TENS) and variation of stimulus variables in dorsal horn cell activity. Eur J Phys Med Rehabil. 1997;216(2):87–94.
18. Lee KH, Chung JM, Willis WD Jr. Inhibition of primate spinothalamic tract cells by TENS. J Neurosurg. 1985;62(2):276–87.
19. Sjölund BH. Peripheral nerve stimulation suppression of C-fiber-evoked flexion reflex in rats: part 1: parameters of continuous stimulation. J Neurosurg. 1985;63(4):612–6.
20. Sjölund BH. Peripheral nerve stimulation suppression of C-fiber-evoked flexion reflex in rats: part 2: parameters of low-rate train stimulation of skin and muscle afferent nerves. J Neurosurg. 1988;68(2):279–83.
21. Henneman E. Relation between size of neurons and their susceptibility to discharge. Science. 1957;126(3287):1345–7.
22. Henneman E, Somjen G, Carpenter DO. Excitability and inhibitability of motoneurons of different sizes. J Neurophysiol. 1965;28(3):599–620.
23. Henneman E, Somjen G, Carpenter DO. Functional significance of cell size in spinal motoneurons. J Neurophysiol. 1965;28:560–80.
24. Maffiuletti NA. Physiological and methodological considerations for the use of neuromuscular electrical stimulation. Eur J Appl Physiol. 2010;110(2):223–34.
25. Barss TS, Ainsley EN, Claveria-Gonzalez FC, Luu MJ, Miller DJ, Wiest MJ, et al. Utilizing physiological principles of motor unit recruitment to reduce fatigability of electrically-evoked contractions: a narrative review. Arch Phys Med Rehabil. 2018;99(4):779–91.
26. Medeiros FV, Bottaro M, Vieira A, Lucas TP, Modesto KA, Bo APL, et al. Kilohertz and low-frequency electrical stimulation with the same pulse duration have similar efficiency for inducing isometric knee extension torque and discomfort. Am J Phys Med Rehabil. 2017;96(6):388–94.
27. Paternostro-Sluga T, Schuhfried O, Vacariu G, Lang T, Fialka-Moser V. Chronaxie and accommodation index in the diagnosis of muscle denervation. Am J Phys Med Rehabil. 2002;81(4):253–60.
28. Vaz MA, Frasson VB. Low-frequency pulsed current versus kilohertz-frequency alternating current: a scoping literature review. Arch Phys Med Rehabil. 2018;99(4):792–805.
29. Robinson AJ, Snyder-Mackler L. Clinical electrophysiology: electrotherapy and electrophysiologic testing. 3rd ed. Philadelphia: Lippincott Williams & Wilkins; 2008.
30. Kukulka CG. In: Gersh MR, editor. Electrotherapy in rehabilitation. Philadelphia: F.A. Davis; 1994.

31. Starkey C. Therapeutic modalities. 4th ed. Philadelphia: F. A. Davis Company; 2013.
32. Baker LL, Bowman BR, McNeal DR. Effects of waveform on comfort during neuromuscular electrical stimulation. Clin Orthop Relat Res. 1988;233:75–85.
33. Iijima H, Takahashi M, Tashiro Y, Aoyama T. Comparison of the effects of kilohertz- and low-frequency electric stimulations: a systematic review with meta-analysis. PLoS One. 2018;13(4):e0195236.
34. Robinson A. Clinical electrophysiology: electrotherapy and electrophysiologic testing. Philadelphia: Lippincott Williams & Wilkins; 2008.
35. Flodin J, Juthberg R, Ackermann PW. Effects of electrode size and placement on comfort and efficiency during low-intensity neuromuscular electrical stimulation of quadriceps, hamstrings and gluteal muscles. BMC Sports Sci Med Rehabil. 2022;14(1):11.
36. Botter A, Oprandi G, Lanfranco F, Allasia S, Maffiuletti NA, Minetto MA. Atlas of the muscle motor points for the lower limb: implications for electrical stimulation procedures and electrode positioning. Eur J Appl Physiol. 2011;111(10):2461–71. https://doi.org/10.1007/s00421-011-2093-y.
37. Glaviano NR, Saliba S. Can the use of neuromuscular electrical stimulation be improved to optimize quadriceps strengthening? Sports Health. 2016;8(1):79–85. https://doi.org/10.1177/1941738115618174.
38. Gobbo M. Muscle motor point identification is essential for optimizing neuromuscular electrical stimulation use. J Neuroeng Rehabil. 2014;11(17). https://doi.org/10.1186/1743-0003-11-17.
39. Lyons G. An investigation of the effect of electrode size and electrode location on comfort during stimulation of the gastrocnemius muscle. Med Eng Phys. 2004;26(10):873–8. https://doi.org/10.1016/j.medengphy.2004.08.003.
40. Vieira TM. Electrode position markedly affects knee torque in tetanic, stimulated contractions. Eur J Appl Physiol. 2016;116(2):335–42. https://doi.org/10.1007/s00421-015-3289-3.
41. Bergquist AJ. Neuromuscular electrical stimulation: implications of the electrically evoked sensory volley. Eur J Appl Physiol. 2011;111(10):2409–26. https://doi.org/10.1007/s00421-011-2087-9.
42. Wolpaw JR, Carp JS. Plasticity from muscle to brain. Prog Neurobiol. 2006;78(3–5):233–63. https://doi.org/10.1016/j.pneurobio.2006.03.001.
43. Bertolasi L. The influence of muscular lengthening on cramps. Ann Neurol. 1993;33(2):176–80. https://doi.org/10.1002/ana.410330207.
44. David H, Nicola AM, Prisca E. The application of neuromuscular electrical stimulation training in various non-neurologic patient populations: a narrative review. PM R. 2015;7(11):1167–78. https://doi.org/10.1016/j.pmrj.2015.03.022.
45. Cavalcante JGT, Ribeiro VHS, Marqueti RC, et al. Effect of muscle length on maximum evoked torque, discomfort, contraction fatigue, and strength adaptations during electrical stimulation in adult populations: a systematic review. PLoS One. 2024;19(6):e0304205. https://doi.org/10.1371/journal.pone.0304205. Published 2024 June 10.
46. Natália LP, Karenina AM, Ivo VS. Effects of different electrical stimulation currents and phase durations on submaximal and maximum torque, efficiency, and discomfort: a randomized crossover trial. Braz J Phys Ther. 2021;25(5):593–600. https://doi.org/10.1016/j.bjpt.2021.03.001.
47. Bispo VA, Bastos JAI, Almeida CCD, Modesto KAG. The effects of neuromuscular electrical stimulation on strength, pain, and function in individuals with knee osteoarthritis: a systematic review with meta-analysis. Fisioterapia Pesquisa. 2021;28(4):416–26. https://doi.org/10.1590/1809-2950/20028528042021.
48. de Paula Gomes CAF, Politti F, de Souza Bacelar Pereira C, et al. Exercise program combined with electrophysical modalities in subjects with knee osteoarthritis: a randomised, placebo-controlled clinical trial. BMC Musculoskelet Disord. 2020;21(1):258. https://doi.org/10.1186/s12891-020-03293-3. Published 2020 Apr 20.
49. Hammami N, Jdidi H, Khezami MA, et al. Isokinetic strengthening and neuromuscular electrical stimulation protocol impact on physical performances, functional status and quality

of life in knee osteoarthritis overweight/obese women. Knee. 2022;39:106–15. https://doi.org/10.1016/j.knee.2022.09.004.
50. Peter RH. Neural plasticity: the effects of environment on the development of the cerebral cortex. Cambridge: Harvard University Press; 2009.
51. Stein DG, Hoffman SW. Concepts of CNS plasticity in the context of brain damage and repair. J Head Trauma Rehabil. 2003;18(4):317–41. https://doi.org/10.1097/00001199-200307000-00004.
52. Bütefisch CM. Plasticity in the human cerebral cortex: lessons from the normal brain and from stroke. Neuroscientist. 2004;10(2):163–73. https://doi.org/10.1177/1073858403262152.
53. Kleim JA, Jones TA. Principles of experience-dependent neural plasticity: implications for rehabilitation after brain damage. J Speech Lang Hear Res. 2008;51(1):S225–39. https://doi.org/10.1044/1092-4388(2008/018).
54. Richards LG, Stewart KC, Woodbury ML, Senesac C, Cauraugh JH. Movement-dependent stroke recovery: a systematic review and meta-analysis of TMS and fMRI evidence. Neuropsychologia. 2008;46(1):3–11. https://doi.org/10.1016/j.neuropsychologia.2007.08.013.
55. Wittenberg GF. Experience, cortical remapping, and recovery in brain disease. Neurobiol Dis. 2010;37(2):252–8. https://doi.org/10.1016/j.nbd.2009.09.007.
56. Michael WO, Chi-Chang DL, Victoria H. Stroke rehabilitation: strategies to enhance motor recovery. Annu Rev Med. 2009;60(1):55–68. https://doi.org/10.1146/annurev.med.60.042707.104248.
57. Kristensen MGH, Busk H, Wienecke T. Neuromuscular electrical stimulation improves activities of daily living post stroke: a systematic review and meta-analysis. Arch Rehabil Res Clin Transl. 2021;4(1):100167. https://doi.org/10.1016/j.arrct.2021.100167. PMID: 35282150; PMCID: PMC8904887.
58. Yang FA, Mi Le JR, Lu CH, et al. Uma revisão sistemática e meta-análise da estimulação elétrica neuromuscular após injeção de toxina botulínica em crianças com paralisia cerebral. Sci Rep. 2025;15:4690.
59. Melzack R, Wall PD. Pain mechanisms: a new theory. Science. 1965;150(3699):971–9. https://doi.org/10.1126/science.150.3699.971.
60. Ordog GJ. Transcutaneous electrical nerve stimulation versus oral analgesic: a randomized double-blind controlled study in acute traumatic pain. Am J Emerg Med. 1987;5(1):6–10. https://doi.org/10.1016/0735-6757(87)90281-6.
61. Richard EL, Barbara R, Carol GTV. An investigation of the development of analgesic tolerance to TENS in humans. Pain. 2011;152(2):335–42. https://doi.org/10.1016/j.pain.2010.10.040.
62. Ishikawa M, Miura H, Tamura Y, Murakami A. Effect of electrical muscle stimulation on vascular endothelial function during prolonged sitting. Phys Ther Res. 2022;25(3):127–33. https://doi.org/10.1298/ptr.E10191.
63. Malek AM, Alper SL, Izumo S. Hemodynamic shear stress and its role in atherosclerosis. JAMA. 1999;282(21):2035–42. https://doi.org/10.1001/jama.282.21.2035.
64. Ploesteanu RL, Nechita AC, Turcu D, Manolescu BN, Stamate SC, Berteanu M. Effects of neuromuscular electrical stimulation in patients with heart failure – review. J Med Life. 2018;11(2):107–18.
65. Motta-Oishi AA, Magalhães FH, Mícolis de Azevedo F. Neuromuscular electrical stimulation for stroke rehabilitation: is spinal plasticity a possible mechanism associated with diminished spasticity? Med Hypotheses. 2013;81(5):784–8. https://doi.org/10.1016/j.mehy.2013.08.013. Epub 2013 Aug 22.
66. Senarath ID, Thalwathte RD, Pathirage M, Kularatne SAM. The effectiveness of radial extracorporeal shock wave therapy vs transcutaneous electrical nerve stimulation in the management of upper limb spasticity in chronic-post stroke hemiplegia-A randomized controlled trial. PLoS One. 2023;18(5):e0283321. https://doi.org/10.1371/journal.pone.0283321. PMID: 37235581; PMCID: PMC10218748.
67. Pavlovic R, Stanislav D. Electro-muscle stimulation - the application in practice. A Kin Int Sci J Kin. 2016;10:49–55.
68. Vervaat FE, van der Gaag A, Teeuwen K, van Suijlekom H, Wijnbergen I. Neuromodulation in patients with refractory angina pectoris: a review. Eur Heart J Open. 2022;3(1):oeac083. https://doi.org/10.1093/ehjopen/oeac083. PMID: 36632476; PMCID: PMC9825802.

Technical Characteristics of FES-Cycling Systems

3

Murillo Frazão

Introduction

Functional Electrical Stimulation (FES)-cycling is an innovative rehabilitation approach that combines neuromuscular electrical stimulation with cycling ergometry, enabling patients with neurological or musculoskeletal impairments to perform structured exercise and functional movements [1]. Unlike conventional electrical stimulation applied in static conditions, FES-cycling requires a precise integration between stimulation parameters and mechanical dynamics, ensuring that muscle activation is synchronized with the pedal cycle. This coordination is fundamental for generating effective torque, maintaining cadence, and providing a safe and physiologically meaningful workout.

Understanding the technical characteristics of FES-cycling systems is essential for both clinical application and technological development. These systems involve multiple components, including stimulation and control units, electrodes, sensors, and ergometer devices, all working in harmony through adaptive control algorithms and real-time feedback loops. Variations in design (such as motorized vs. non-motorized ergometers and static vs. non-static configurations) affect the therapeutic objectives, usability, and overall performance.

This chapter aims to provide a comprehensive overview of the technical aspects of FES-cycling, highlighting the interaction between electrical stimulation and ergometer systems, the importance of electrode design, synchronization strategies, and the role of advanced sensors in closed-loop control. Additionally, it explores different equipment configurations, resistance mechanisms, and control strategies that underpin safe, efficient, and adaptive neuromuscular rehabilitation.

M. Frazão (✉)
Lauro Wanderley University Hospital – EBSERH/UFPB, João Pessoa, PB, Brazil
e-mail: murillo.frazao@gmail.com

M. Frazão (ed.), *Functional Electrical Stimulation Cycling in Clinical Practice*,
https://doi.org/10.1007/978-3-032-23937-2_3

Electrical Stimulator Main Characteristics

The main components of electrical stimulation devices are a stimulation and control unit to generate and regulate the stimulation, and electrodes to deliver the electrical current [2].

Stimulation and Control Unit

A Functional Electrical Stimulation control unit is a sophisticated system designed to deliver precisely controlled electrical pulses to elicit muscle contractions. These systems typically consist of a control box, connecting wires, and may include sensors and advanced control algorithms to enhance performance and adaptability.

The control box serves as the central component, housing the power supply, board, signal generation circuitry, and a microprocessor responsible for regulating key stimulation parameters such as pulse width, frequency, and amplitude. Modern control boxes may also feature wireless communication, data logging, and programmable interfaces, offering greater flexibility for clinical and research applications. The connecting wires transmit electrical impulses from the control box to the electrodes, which are placed on or within the body to stimulate the targeted muscles or nerves.

Most FES-cycling systems incorporate sensors that provide essential feedback to optimize stimulation delivery and performance [3]. Basic setups typically include pedal or crank position sensors, which trigger or halt electrical stimulation at specific points in the pedaling cycle. More advanced systems integrate additional sensors such as inertial measurement units (IMUs), force-sensitive resistors (FSRs), or electromyography (EMG) sensors to monitor limb position, movement, torque, and muscle activity. These real-time data streams enable dynamic adjustment of stimulation timing and intensity, forming the basis of closed-loop control systems [4].

In closed-loop FES-cycling, embedded control algorithms continuously process sensor input to regulate key stimulation parameters (such as pulse width, frequency, and amplitude) in real time. This allows the system to automatically adapt stimulation patterns in response to the rider's physiological and biomechanical status. By maintaining target cycling parameters (e.g., cadence, torque, or range of motion), closed-loop systems enhance the effectiveness, safety, and comfort of neuromuscular stimulation, especially for users with fluctuating muscle responses or fatigue. This adaptive approach ensures that the stimulation remains aligned with therapeutic goals throughout the session.

Electrode

Electrodes are placed on the skin at locations where the underlying tissue is intended to be activated. Electrical current is injected through at least one pair of electrodes and generates a potential gradient in the underlying tissue. The potential gradient

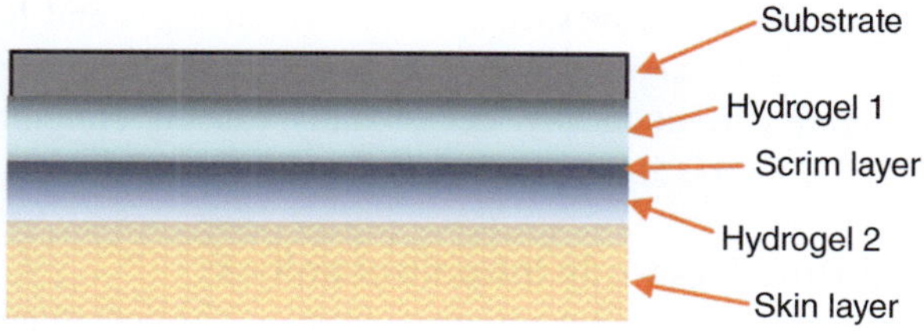

Fig. 3.1 Self-adhesive hydrogel stimulation electrodes are manufactured in a multi-layer configuration. Keller and Kuhn [5]

depolarizes excitable tissue under the electrodes that serve as cathode. Above a certain threshold potential excitable tissue is activated [5].

Electrode Characteristics

Material

Self-adhesive hydrogel electrodes are the most commonly used type of electrode for FES-cycling. It utilizes a conductive gel to establish contact between a conductive element and the subject's skin. These electrodes are constructed in a multilayer configuration, as illustrated in Fig. 3.1, comprising multiple hydrogel layers and a wiring cable that connects the electrical stimulator to the electrode substrate. The skin-contact layer features an electrically conductive gel with relatively low peel strength, allowing for secure yet easily removable contact with the skin. This gel has a moist texture and can be detached without causing discomfort or damage. It is typically composed of co-polymers synthesized from monomers such as acrylic acid and N-vinylpyrrolidone. Beneath the skin-contact layer, a second hydrogel layer serves as an interface between the skin-contacting gel and the electrode substrate [5].

Requirements

The essential requirements for conductive stimulation electrodes are clear: they must ensure effective stimulation with minimal discomfort, while avoiding permanent skin damage such as burns or irritation. For neuromuscular stimulation, optimal performance specifically refers to the reliable and localized activation of targeted muscle groups [6]. Effective skin contact is critical, as it maximizes the electrode–skin interface area and improves current transmission. On a microscopic level, the skin surface is highly irregular, featuring ridges, valleys, and loosely attached keratin layers. To overcome this unevenness and enhance contact, liquid or adhesive gel-based interfaces are commonly employed. A practical advantage of gel-based or sticky electrodes is their ability to temporarily adhere to the skin, ensuring consistent positioning during stimulation.

Ideally, current density should be evenly distributed across the entire electrode surface to avoid hotspots and discomfort. A tapered reduction in current density toward the edges further helps mitigate edge effects. Modern electrode designs often address this by incorporating a current redistribution layer (typically placed between two hydrogel layers) to promote uniform current spread. When the electrode or interface gel acts as the dominant source of electrical impedance, the influence of skin inhomogeneities (such as variations in stratum corneum thickness, minor abrasions, or structures like sweat ducts and hair follicles) is significantly diminished. However, sweat ducts filled with conductive saline fluid can still concentrate current locally, occasionally causing stinging or pain if not adequately dried prior to stimulation.

Skin and Electrode Inhomogeneities

Skin and electrode inhomogeneities play a critical role in shaping the distribution of current density, which directly influences both the effectiveness of neuromuscular stimulation and patient comfort. A key limitation in clinical and home use is the reduced patient compliance resulting from discomfort during stimulation sessions. Localized areas of elevated current density can lead to discomfort, skin irritation, or even burns if not properly managed [7]. It is well established that electrode size and placement significantly affect both the perceived comfort and the physiological outcomes [8].

Skin inhomogeneities are a major factor that contributes to the occurrence of current density peaks. The skin is inherently non-uniform, with localized resistance differences caused by its complex structure. Small-scale skin inhomogeneities are associated with structures such as pores and sweat glands [9] and larger-scale inhomogeneities are associated to variations in hydration levels and skin morphology [10].

Additionally, electrode edge effects play a significant role in the formation of current density peaks during electrical stimulation. This phenomenon refers to the uneven distribution of current, with higher current densities occurring at the edges of the electrode compared to its center. This edge concentration occurs because the electrical path at the edge offers less resistance, facilitating a greater flow of current [11]. As a result, localized electrochemical reactions may be intensified, potentially leading to tissue irritation, damage, or altered stimulation patterns. It is particularly prominent in disk-shaped electrodes, where the geometry causes the current to concentrate along the perimeter. As such, careful electrode design is essential to optimize stimulation efficiency while minimizing adverse effects [12].

Ergometer Devices Main Characteristics

FES-cycling ergometers used in rehabilitation can be broadly classified into motorized and non-motorized systems, each with distinct functional characteristics and clinical applications. Motorized FES-cycling ergometers are equipped with an integrated motor that drives the pedals, allowing passive or assisted [13], and even resisted cycling (Fig. 3.2). This feature makes them particularly suitable for individuals with severe motor impairments or complete paralysis, as the motor can maintain a constant pedaling motion even when voluntary muscle contribution is minimal or absent. These systems can also operate in isokinetic mode, enabling constant-speed pedaling when the user provides active input, which facilitates specific training protocols and controlled resistance levels. Additionally, motorized ergometers often incorporate advanced safety features, such as torque monitoring

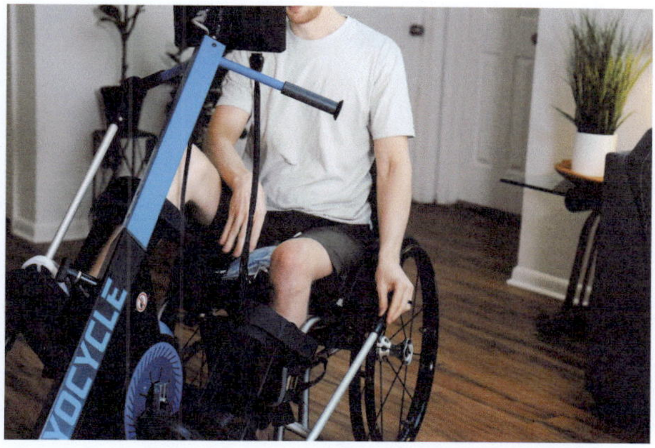

Fig. 3.2 Example of a motorized FES-cycling device. (Source: myolyn.com)

and automatic stop functions, to prevent joint overstrain or improper movement [14]. However, their complexity may involve higher cost, more sophisticated control algorithms, and longer setup time, especially when synchronizing FES stimulation with motor assistance.

In motorized FES-cycling systems, resistance is actively managed by an integrated electric motor that can both assist and oppose pedal motion. This dual capability enables a range of training modes: passive cycling (where the motor drives the pedals for severely impaired users), active-assisted cycling (where the motor supports voluntary or FES-driven movement), and resistive cycling (where the motor applies controlled braking force to increase training intensity). Resistance levels are typically adjusted via electronic control systems linked to the FES unit, allowing precise modulation based on cadence, torque, or predefined therapeutic protocols. Advanced systems can employ isokinetic modes, where resistance adapts to maintain a constant pedaling speed [15], and isotonic modes, where a fixed torque is applied regardless of cadence. Motorized resistance control ensures safety and adaptability, making these systems ideal for early rehabilitation and progressive training.

Non-motorized FES-cycling ergometers, in contrast, rely entirely on the user's own muscular effort induced by electrical stimulation to generate pedaling motion [16] (Fig. 3.3). These systems promote greater neuromuscular engagement and active participation, making them highly effective for improving muscle strength, cardiovascular fitness, and motor control in users with moderate to mild impairments. By requiring the muscles to overcome inertia without motor support, non-motorized systems can elicit more physiological muscle contractions, mimicking natural cycling patterns. However, this design also limits their use in patients with profound weakness or flaccid paralysis, as they may be unable to initiate or sustain effective pedaling without external assistance.

In non-motorized systems, resistance is generated through mechanical components, most commonly freewheel-based drivetrains combined with gear ratios or magnetic resistance units in stationary adaptations. On outdoor tricycles or bicycles, resistance comes naturally from terrain gradients, aerodynamic drag, and rolling

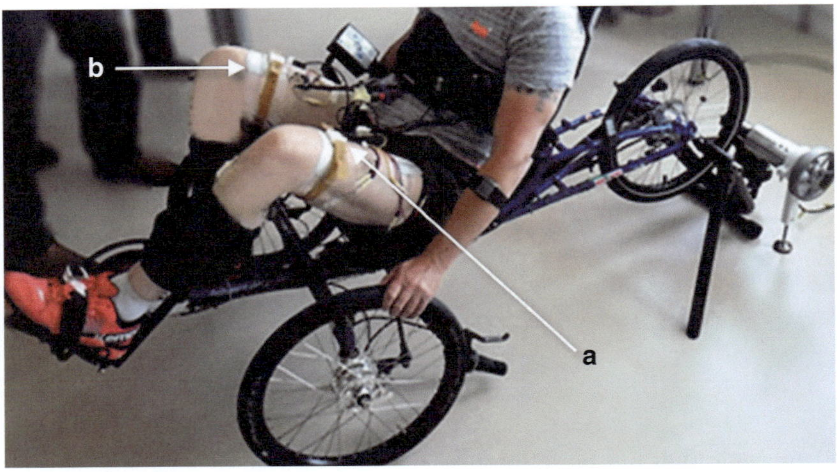

Fig. 3.3 Example of a non-motorized FES-cycling device. The participant was installed on a recumbent trike and was equipped with 2 IMUs (**a**) connected to the controller and 2 pairs of surface electrodes (**b**) connected to the electrical stimulator. (Sijobert et al. [16])

resistance, requiring the use of multi-speed gear systems to manage torque demands effectively. Lower gears are essential for starts or uphill segments, reducing load on electrically stimulated muscles, while higher gears increase challenge on flat surfaces. Some non-motorized setups incorporate friction or magnetic brakes to add resistance for conditioning purposes. Unlike motorized systems, non-motorized devices lack automated control, so resistance adjustment is manual, often requiring assistance or prior gear setup. This simplicity offers benefits in portability and cost, but it limits fine-tuned control and safety features available in motorized systems.

Electrical Stimulation and Ergometer Devices Interaction

Unlike conventional electrical stimulation, in FES-cycling, the triggering and stopping of electrical pulses cannot be controlled solely by time-based parameters. If stimulation were applied on a fixed temporal schedule, it would quickly lead to significant asynchrony between muscle activation and pedal motion, resulting in inefficient power generation, poor cycling biomechanics, and disrupted cadence.

To prevent this, the FES system must maintain precise synchronization between electrical stimulation and pedal position, which is achieved through real-time interaction between the stimulator and the ergometer, commonly referred to as a closed-loop control strategy. By integrating these sensing strategies with adaptive control algorithms, FES-cycling systems can ensure smooth, coordinated pedaling that mimics physiological movement patterns, maximizing both safety and therapeutic benefit.

Crank Position Sensors

The most common method uses a crank angle encoder or position sensor mounted on the ergometer's crank. Stimulation is triggered and stopped based on predefined angular windows for each muscle group (e.g., quadriceps, hamstrings, gluteals), ensuring activation only during the phases where the muscle contributes positively to pedaling torque [17, 18] (Fig. 3.4).

Inertial Measurements Units (IMUs)

IMUs mounted on the thighs or legs measure limb orientation, acceleration, and angular velocity. Using this kinematic data, the system determines when a limb is in the upward or downward phase of the pedal stroke, dynamically activating the appropriate stimulation channels [16, 19] (Fig. 3.5).

Electromyography (EMG) Sensors

In EMG-triggered systems, voluntary muscle activation is detected through surface EMG electrodes. When a contraction is identified, the system delivers electrical stimulation to amplify or assist the movement. This biofeedback-based approach is particularly useful in training for patients with total or partial motor function [20, 21] (Fig. 3.6).

Table 3.1 and Fig. 3.7 bring a resume of the synchronization methods.

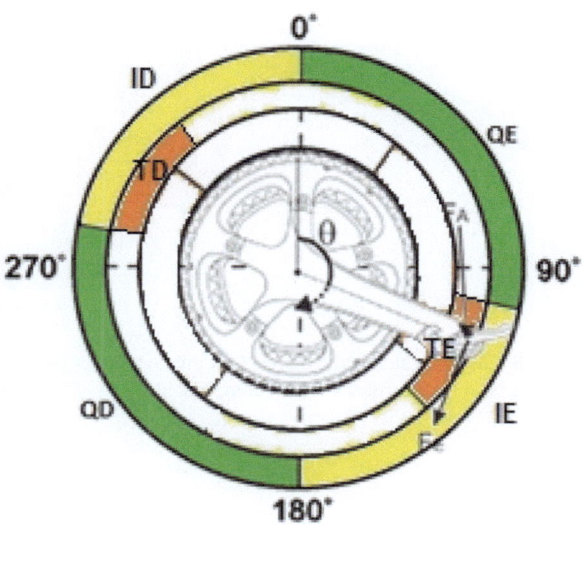

Fig. 3.4 A possible channel activation sequences that the FES-cycling system can perform. Right Quadriceps—QD (vastus medialis and lateralis); Left Quadriceps—QE (vastus medialis and lateralis); Right Hamstring—ID; Left Hamstring—IE; Right Tibial—TD and Left Tibial—TE, coordinated by the angular position of the cycle ergometer pedal

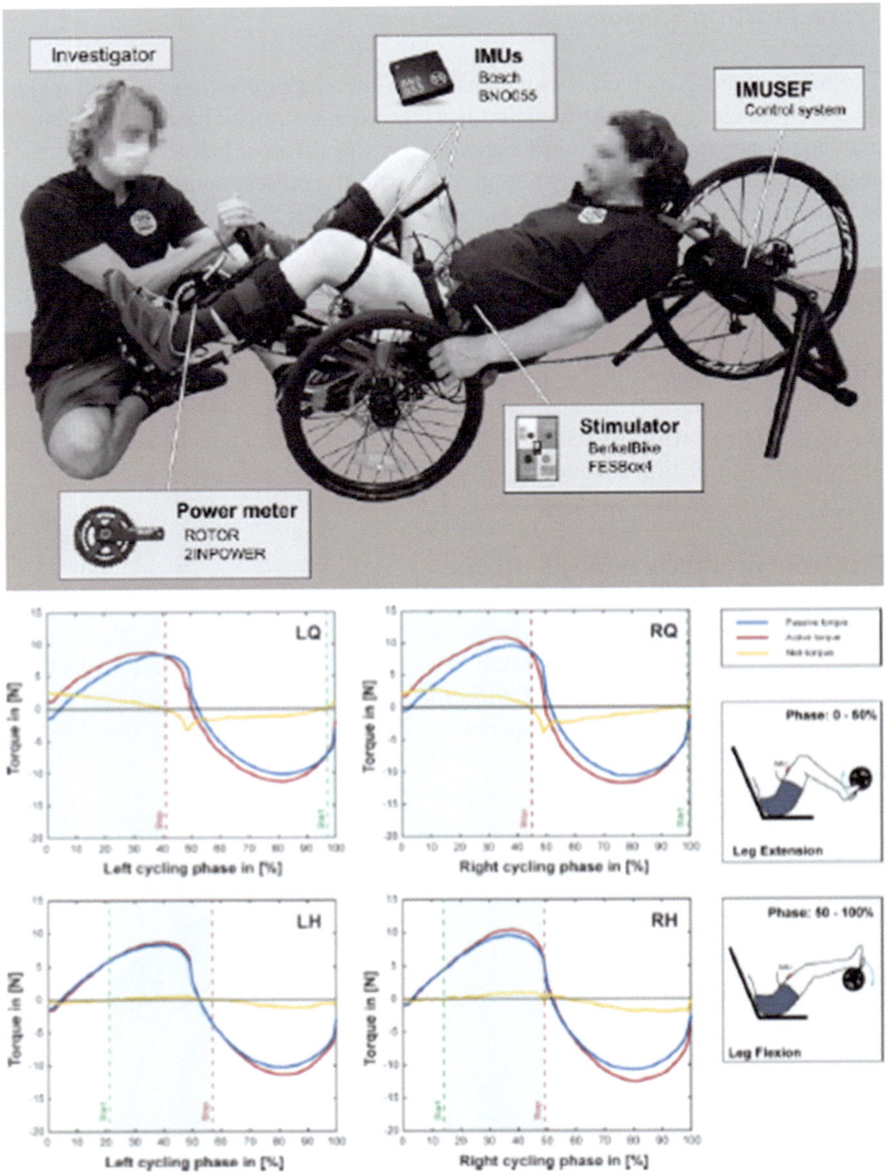

Fig. 3.5 IMUs located at the thighs. Left quadriceps (LQ), right quadriceps (RQ), left hamstrings (LH) and right hamstrings (RH). (Schmoll et al. [19])

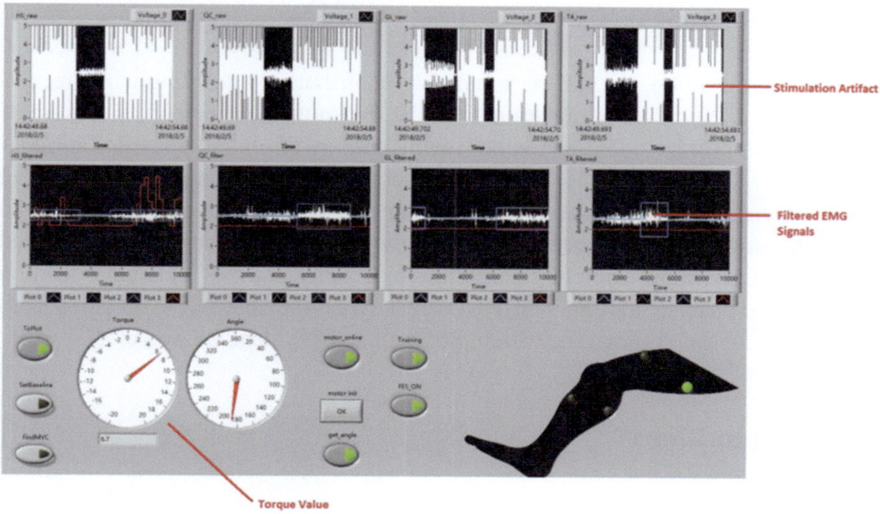

Fig. 3.6 Example of EMG signals and torque measurement during FES-cycling. (Wang et al. [21])

Fig. 3.7 FES-cycling synchronization methods. (Source: the author)

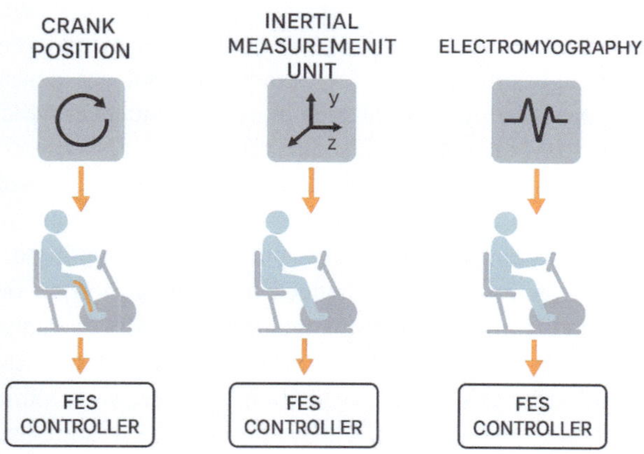

Table 3.1 FES-cycling synchronization methods

Method	Sensors used	Advantages	Limitations
Crank position	Rotary encoder / hall sensor	Simple, reliable, widely used in commercial devices	Requires mechanical integration; limited adaptability
IMUs	Inertial sensors (accelerometer + gyroscope)	Portable, works on mobile setups, no crank modification	Sensitive to drift, needs calibration
EMG	Surface EMG electrodes	Encourages active participation; adaptive to volitional input	Complex signal processing; less effective with flaccid paralysis

IMUs Inertial measurements units, *EMG* Electromyography

FES-Cycling Modes

In active FES-cycling, the patient voluntarily contributes to pedaling while receiving functional electrical stimulation to assist the movement or enhance exercise intensity. To optimize coordination between voluntary effort and electrical stimulation, active systems typically integrate sensors (crank position encoders, inertial measurement units, torque sensors, or electromyography). In passive mode, the ergometer motor drives the pedaling motion, while electrical stimulation is applied to the muscles without voluntary contribution. Usually, sensors like crank position encoders and cadence monitors ensure correct synchronization of stimulation with pedal position, even though the patient does not actively generate force.

Control Algorithms

Control algorithms in FES-cycling govern the timing, intensity, and duration of electrical stimulation to coordinate muscle contractions with the mechanical demands of cycling. The primary objective is to maintain smooth pedaling, achieve target cadence, and optimize energy efficiency while minimizing muscle fatigue. Early systems relied on open-loop algorithms, where stimulation was triggered based on pre-set time or rustic crank angle windows without real-time feedback. Although simple, open-loop control cannot compensate for variations in muscle response, fatigue, or changes in cycling cadence, which often results in asynchronous movement and reduced performance.

Modern FES-cycling devices increasingly use closed-loop control strategies that incorporate real-time feedback from sensors. These inputs enable adaptive algorithms to dynamically adjust pulse width, amplitude, frequency, and stimulation timing in response to changes in cadence, torque output, and voluntary effort. Advanced implementations include proportional-integral-derivative (PID) controllers [22], model predictive control (MPC) [23], and EMG-triggered control, which blend voluntary muscle activation with electrical stimulation for improved neuromuscular engagement [24]. By continuously adapting stimulation to patient-specific responses, closed-loop algorithms enhance safety, comfort, and therapeutic effectiveness during FES-cycling .

Equipment Types

Static

Static FES-cycling systems are primarily designed for rehabilitation purposes, providing controlled exercise sessions using stationary cycle ergometers. Conventional ergometers can be adapted for FES-cycling; however, numerous dedicated commercial FES-cycling devices are available on the market, offering enhanced integration and safety features. Table 3.2 brings the comparison between adapted conventional ergometers and commercial devices.

Based on patient positioning, these devices can be classified into three main categories:

1. Vertical with seat (Fig. 3.8)—The patient cycles in an upright or semi-recumbent position, using the equipment's seat.

Table 3.2 Comparison of adapted vs commercial FES-cycling systems

Feature	Adapted conventional ergometer	Commercial FES-cycling equipment
System integration	Basic: Standard ergometer retrofitted with stimulator	Fully integrated system combining ergometer and stimulator
Resistance type	Magnetic brake (manual or basic electronic adjustment)	Motor-assisted resistance with programmable settings
Motor assistance	Not available	Yes, for passive and assistive cycling
Sensor synchronization	Basic crank sensor (manual calibration)	Advanced: Crank sensor, IMUs, torque sensors
Safety features	Limited (no torque limit or spasm detection)	Built-in safety: Torque limits, spasm detection, auto-stop
Control modes	Open-loop (predefined timing windows)	Closed-loop: Adaptive control based on feedback
Software and feedback	Minimal or none	Advanced: Real-time feedback, progress tracking
Cost	Low to moderate (clinic adaptation)	High (specialized medical device)
Typical use case	Research, low-cost rehab, experimental setups	Clinical rehab (hospital, outpatient), home programs

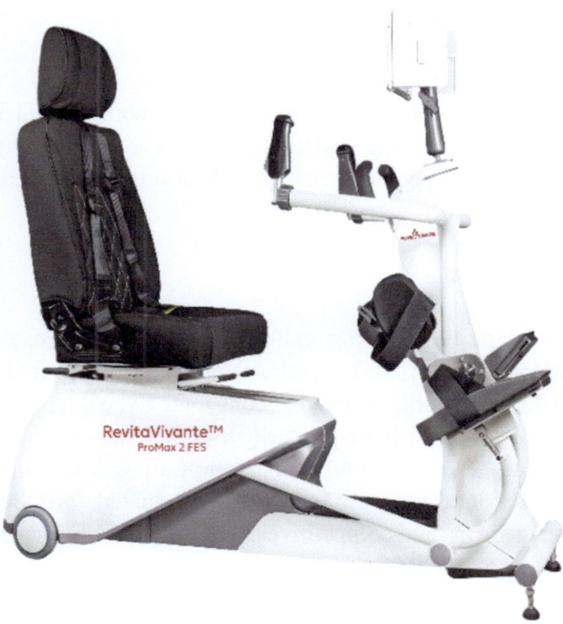

Fig. 3.8 Vertical with seat RevitaVivante™ equipment. (Source: https://www.robotimize.tech/product/revitavivante-fes-cycling-series/)

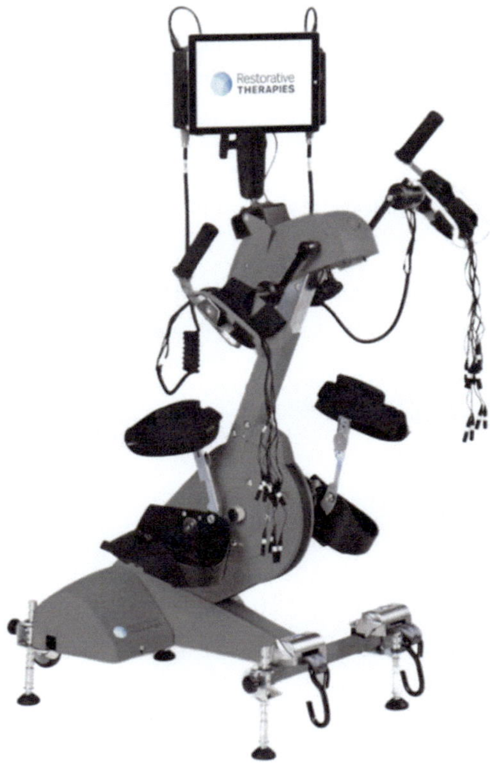

Fig. 3.9 Vertical without seat RT-300™ equipment. (Source: https://restorative-therapies.com/rt300/)

2. Vertical without seat (Fig. 3.9)—Designed for patients who use their own seating, typically wheelchairs, to engage with the device.
3. Horizontal (Fig. 3.10)—The patient cycles in a recumbent or lying position, often on a hospital bed.

The first two models are most commonly found in home-based or outpatient rehabilitation, while horizontal systems are primarily used in inpatient or intensive care settings, enabling early mobilization even for bedridden patients.

Non-static

Non-static FES-cycling equipment refers to systems designed to promote mobility, outdoor activity, and functional independence, often integrating recreational and competitive components that contribute to health and well-being [25]. Unlike static ergometers, which are primarily used in clinical or home-based rehabilitation, these systems extend beyond therapeutic purposes to enhance social participation and motivation. They are frequently associated with leisure activities, community engagement, and competitive events such as FES-assisted cycling races featured in the Cybathlon initiative [26].

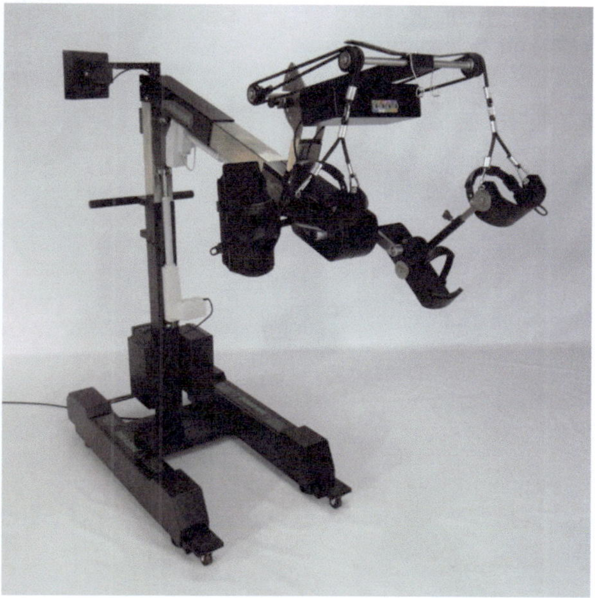

Fig. 3.10 Horizontal recumbent or lying position MOBITRONICS™ equipment. (Source: https://inbramed.med.br/produtos/fes-cycling/mobitronics/)

These systems function in dynamic outdoor environments, demanding mechanical gearing, adaptive control strategies, and integrated sensors to ensure efficient propulsion and rider safety. They are typically built on lightweight bicycle or tricycle frames, often made of aluminum or carbon fiber to maximize performance [27]. Most designs feature a gear-shifting system similar to conventional bicycles, allowing riders or assistants to adjust mechanical resistance according to terrain, whether on flat roads, uphill climbs, or downhill sections. The drivetrain is usually chain-driven, though some advanced prototypes employ belt drives for smoother, quieter operation and reduced maintenance.

A standard setup combines a multi-speed rear cassette with front chainrings, providing a wide range of gear ratios. Lower gears (with higher mechanical advantage) are typically used for starting or ascending inclines, as they reduce the torque demand on electrically stimulated muscles. Conversely, higher gears enable greater speeds on flat terrain but require more muscular effort. In adaptive tricycles, gear shifters are generally positioned within easy reach of the rider's hands, ensuring accessibility. For individuals with severe impairments, automatic gear-shifting systems can be integrated, further enhancing usability and safety in real-world conditions.

Types of Non-static FES-Cycling Equipment

Tricycles (Trikes)

Three-wheeled FES-adapted cycles are the most popular option, as they provide enhanced stability, reducing the risk of falls and making them ideal for individuals with limited balance or severe neurological impairments (e.g., spinal cord injury) (Fig. 3.11).

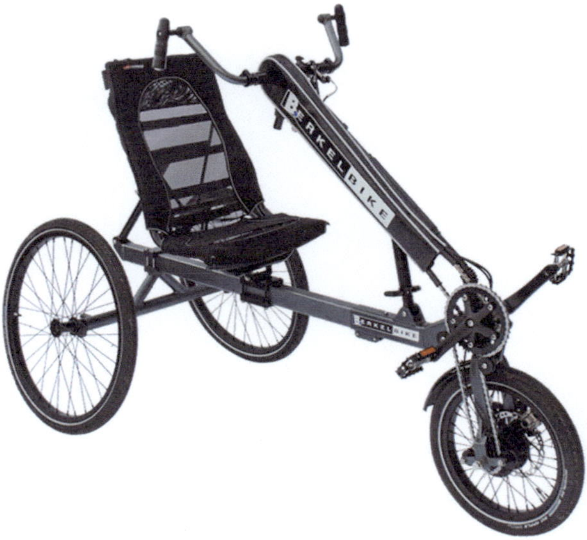

Fig. 3.11 Example of a Trike FES-cycling with one front wheel. (Source: https://activelinx.co.uk/gear/berkelbike-pro/)

Bicycles
Two-wheeled bicycles equipped with FES systems are used by individuals with greater motor control and balance. These setups are often customized for fitness and sports.

Resistance Generation

In non-static FES-cycling there is no fixed resistance unit as in stationary ergometers; instead, resistance comes from road friction, aerodynamics, gradient (uphill/downhill) and gear ratio [28]. Many systems incorporate gearing and lightweight frames to optimize mechanical efficiency for riders with limited muscle output. Additionally, some systems integrate an auxiliary hub motor or mid-drive motor to assist when muscle fatigue occurs or during uphill cycling.

Challenges

There are some challenges for FES-cycling in non-static devices: (1) Synchronization in dynamic environments: maintaining real-time synchronization between stimulation and pedal position outdoors can be challenging due to variable cadence and terrain. (2) Battery life and portability: extended outdoor use requires efficient power management for both the stimulator and sensor systems. (3) Safety: outdoor conditions introduce risks such as falls, collisions, and weather-related issues, requiring robust braking systems and stable design.

Conclusion

FES-cycling is a technology-intensive rehabilitation modality that depends on the precise interaction of its core components: stimulation units, electrodes, sensors, control algorithms, and ergometer systems. These technical developments are fundamental to enhancing the performance and reliability of FES-cycling across therapeutic and functional applications.

References

1. Frazão M, de Gomes Figueiredo T, Cipriano G Jr. Should we use the functional electrical stimulation-cycling exercise in clinical practice? Physiological and clinical effects systematic review with meta-analysis. Arch Phys Med Rehabil. 2025;106(3):404–23.
2. Functional HL, Stimulation E. J Korean Acad Rehabil Medi. 2001;25(1):1–11.
3. González-Graniel E, Mercado-Gutierrez JA, Martínez-Díaz S, Castro-Liera I, Santillan-Mendez IM, Yanez-Suarez O, Quiñones-Uriostegui I, Rodríguez-Reyes G. Sensing and control strategies used in FES systems aimed at assistance and rehabilitation of foot drop: a systematic literature review. J Pers Med. 2024;14(8):874.
4. Cousin C, Duenas V, Dixon W. FES cycling and closed-loop feedback control for rehabilitative human–robot interaction. Robotics. 2021;10(2):61.
5. Thierry Keller AK. Electrodes for transcutaneous (surface) electrical stimulation. J Autom Control. 2008;18(2):35–45.
6. Ivanic R, Novotny I, Rehacek V, Tvarozek V, Weis M. Thin film non-symmetric microelectrode array for impedance monitoring of human skin. Thin Solid Films. 2003;433(1–2):332–6.
7. Patriciu A, Yoshida K, Struijk JJ, DeMonte TP, Joy ML, Stodkilde-Jorgensen H. Current density imaging and electrically induced skin burns under surface electrodes. IEEE Trans Biomed Eng. 2005;52:2024–31.
8. Flodin J, Juthberg R, Ackermann PW. Effects of electrode size and placement on comfort and efficiency during low-intensity neuromuscular electrical stimulation of quadriceps, hamstrings and gluteal muscles. BMC Sports Sci Med Rehabil. 2022;14(11)
9. Chizmadzhev YA, Indenbom AV, Kuzmin PI, Galichenko SV, Weaver JC, Potts RO. Electrical properties of skin at moderate voltages: contribution of appendageal macropores. Biophys J. 1998;74:843–56.
10. Reilly RB, Antoni H, Chilbert MA. Applied bioelectricity from electrical stimulation to electropathology. New York: Springer; 1998.
11. Cope DK. The edge effect for planar electrodes. J Electroanal Chem. 1997;439(1):7–27.
12. Alon G, Kantor G, Ho HS. Effects of electrode size on basic excitatory responses and on selected stimulus parameters. J Orthop Sports Phys Ther. 1994;20:29–35.
13. Duenas VH, Cousin CA, Parikh A, Freeborn P, Fox EJ, Dixon WE. Motorized and functional electrical stimulation induced cycling via switched repetitive learning control. EEE Trans Control Syst Technol. 2019;27(4):1468–79.
14. Chang C-H, Casas J, Sanyal AK, Duenas VH. Motorized FES-cycling and closed-loop nonlinear control for power tracking using a finite-time stable torque algorithm. Front Control Eng. 2022;3:910126.
15. Frazão M, de Lima Martins F, Cipriano G Jr. Recumbent FES-cycling exercise improves muscle performance and ambulation capacity in hospitalized patients: a randomized controlled trial. Artif Organs. 2025;

16. Sijobert B, Le Guillou R, Fattal C, Azevedo Coste C. FES-induced cycling in complete SCI: a simpler control method based on inertial sensors. Sensors. 2019;19(19):4268.
17. Figueiredo T, Frazão M, Werlang LA, Kunz A, Peltz M, Furtado VC, Júnior EB, Júnior JM, Silva RM, Sobral Filho DC. Safety and feasibility of a functional electrical stimulation cycling-based muscular dysfunction diagnostic method in mechanically ventilated patients. Artif Organs. 2024;48(7):713–22.
18. Leung KW, Tong RK, Wang X, Lee GT, Pang PM, Wai HW, Leung HC. The effectiveness of Functional Electrical Stimulation (FES) in on-off mode for enhancing the cycling performance of team Phoenix at 2016 Cybathlon. Eur J Transl Myol. 2017;27(4):7132.
19. Schmoll M, Le Guillou R, Fattal C, Azevedo CC. OIDA: an optimal interval detection algorithm for automatized determination of stimulation patterns for FES-cycling in individuals with SCI. J Neuroeng Rehabil. 2022;19:39.
20. Chen CC, He Z-C, Hsueh YH. An EMG feedback control Functional Electrical Stimulation cycling system. J Sign Process Syst. 2011;64(64):195–203.
21. Wang X, Leung KW, Fang Y, Chen S, Tong RKY. Design of functional electrical stimulation cycling system for lower-limb rehabilitation of stroke patients. In: 40th annual international conference of the IEEE engineering in medicine and biology society (EMBC); 2018. p. 2337–40.
22. Sun M, Cheng F, Wang T, et al. Modeling and control of functional electrical stimulation cycling training system. Sci Rep. 2025;15:6452.
23. de Sousa ACA, Font-Llagunes JM. Predictive framework for electrical stimulation cycling in spinal cord injury. IFAC-PapersOnLine. 2024;58(24):332–7.
24. Arnin J, Yamsa-Ard T, Triponyuwasin P, Wongsawat Y. Development of practical functional electrical stimulation cycling systems based on an electromyography study of the Cybathlon 2016. Eur J Transl Myol. 2017;27(4):7111.
25. Sanna N, Nossa R, Biffi E, Guanziroli E, Diella E, Ferrante S, Molteni F, Peruzzo D, Casali N, Mastropietro A, Rizzo G, Tarabini M, Pedrocchi A, Ambrosini E. Evaluating the health and fitness benefits of a 6-month FES-cycling program on a recumbent trike for individuals with motor complete SCI: a pilot study. J Neuroeng Rehabil. 2025;22(1):55.
26. Hamdan PNF, Hamzaid NA, Abd Razak NA, Hasnan N. Contributions of the Cybathlon championship to the literature on functional electrical stimulation cycling among individuals with spinal cord injury: a bibliometric review. J Sport Health Sci. 2022;11(6):671–80.
27. Metani A, Popović-Maneski L, Mateo S, Lemahieu L, Bergeron V. Functional electrical stimulation cycling strategies tested during preparation for the first Cybathlon competition – a practical report from team ENS de Lyon. Eur J Transl Myol. 2017;27(4):7110.
28. Coelho-Magalhães T, Fachin-Martins E, Silva A, Azevedo Coste C, Resende-Martins H. Development of a high-power capacity open source electrical stimulation system to enhance research into FES-assisted devices: validation of FES cycling. Sensors. 2022;22(2):531.

Physiological Bases of FES-Cycling Therapy: Metabolic, Cardiovascular, and Ventilatory Responses

4

Murillo Frazão and Gerson Cipriano Jr

Introduction

Functional Electrical Stimulation (FES) cycling is a rehabilitation technique that combines electrical stimulation with cycling to induce muscle contractions, offering potential benefits for individuals with various conditions such as ICU-acquired weakness, multiple sclerosis, and spinal cord injuries. This modality impacts the body physiologically, particularly in metabolic, cardiovascular, and ventilatory domains. Just below it is provided a summary of the main FES-cycling exercise responses. However, the following sections explore these physiological impacts in detail.

Metabolic Responses

Metabolically, FES-cycling enhances oxygen uptake (VO_2) and energy expenditure significantly more than passive cycling or neuromuscular electrical stimulation (NMES) alone, with increases of 97% and 102%, respectively, indicating a substantial metabolic demand [1]. In individuals with multiple sclerosis, FES-cycling combined with voluntary cycling resulted in higher VO_2 values compared to voluntary cycling alone, suggesting an enhanced aerobic response [2]. For spinal cord injury patients, FES-cycling can activate paralyzed muscles, allowing training in both aerobic and anaerobic zones, as indicated by changes in the respiratory exchange ratio (RER) [3].

M. Frazão (✉)
Lauro Wanderley University Hospital – EBSERH/UFPB, João Pessoa, PB, Brazil
e-mail: murillo.frazao@gmail.com

G. Cipriano Jr
Physical Therapy Department, University of Brasilia – UNB, Brasilia, DF, Brazil

M. Frazão (ed.), *Functional Electrical Stimulation Cycling in Clinical Practice*,
https://doi.org/10.1007/978-3-032-23937-2_4

Cardiovascular Responses

The FES-cycling increases cardiac output by 21% and enhances the arterial-mixed venous oxygen content difference by 60%, demonstrating improved cardiovascular efficiency compared to NMES and passive cycling [1]. FES-cycling has been shown to train both aerobic and anaerobic systems in patients with spinal cord injuries, as indicated by changes in the respiratory exchange ratio (RER) over time, suggesting improved cardiovascular and pulmonary function [4]. In a sample with multiple sclerosis, FES-cycling elicited a heart rate of approximately 76.4% of peak HR, indicating moderate to vigorous intensity [5].

Ventilatory Responses

Ventilatory responses are also heightened during FES-cycling, with minute ventilation increasing by 115%, which is more pronounced than during NMES or passive cycling [1]. In a study involving spinal cord injury patients, FES-cycling training led to changes in ventilation ratios (VE/VO_2 and VE/VCO_2), indicating improved ventilatory efficiency over time [3]. In children with cerebral palsy, FES-assisted cycling led to higher cycling cadences, although the achievements in peak VO_2 and heart rate were not significantly different from those in a control group, indicating that higher training intensities might be necessary for significant ventilatory improvements [6]. Overall, FES-cycling provides a robust stimulus for enhancing metabolic, cardiovascular, and ventilatory functions, making it a valuable rehabilitation tool for individuals with various conditions, including ICU-acquired weakness, multiple sclerosis, and spinal cord injuries.

Basic Exercise Physiology

Fundamental Principles of Exercise Physiology

Exercise physiology is a multifaceted scientific discipline that examines how physical activity influences the physiological responses and adaptations of the human body. It involves a comprehensive understanding of various physiological systems, including cardiovascular, respiratory, musculoskeletal, and neuromuscular systems, which are all engaged during exercise to optimize performance and health outcomes [7]. Fundamental principles of exercise physiology include the body's and chronic adaptations to physical activity, such as cardiovascular remodeling and enhanced respiratory efficiency, but most importantly, peripheral muscle adaptation, which is crucial for meeting increased metabolic demands during high-intensity or high-volume exercise [8].

Cardiopulmonary exercise testing (CPET) is a key tool in this field, measuring variables like oxygen uptake (VO_2) and lactate threshold to assess aerobic capacity and guide individualized training and health interventions. Moreover, exercise physiology emphasizes the importance of individual differences, suggesting that variations in body type and health status can significantly influence exercise effectiveness and outcomes [9].

Definition of Physical Exercise and Its Phases (Aerobic and Anaerobic)

Physical exercise encompasses activities where muscles generate force, utilizing aerobic and anaerobic exercises [10]. Aerobic exercise depends on the oxidative synthesis of adenosine triphosphate (ATP), entailing oxygen consumption and carbon dioxide production, which are closely connected to pulmonary oxygen uptake and carbon dioxide release. This exercise type promotes cardiovascular fitness through prolonged activities where oxidative phosphorylation dominates [11]. Conversely, anaerobic exercise includes high-intensity efforts independent of oxygen, such as resistance training, leveraging glycolysis and the phosphagen system for swift energy delivery over brief periods [12]. The metabolic responses vary between modes: aerobic exercises utilize a broader range of substrates and more fatty acids, whereas anaerobic exercises increase purine turnover and glycolytic activity. These distinctions are pivotal for tailoring exercise prescriptions to enhance health, aid rehabilitation, and boost exercise performance.

Muscular and Neuromuscular Responses During Exercise

Muscular and neuromuscular responses to exercise encompass a range of complex physiological adaptations. Skeletal muscle responds to diverse stimuli by modifying contractile proteins and mitochondrial functions, which are essential for enhancing strength and endurance [13]. Various types of muscle contractions—such as isometric, concentric, and eccentric—differently influence neuromuscular fatigue and muscle damage. Notably, eccentric contractions are associated with the most significant prolonged force loss and muscle soreness [14]. Moreover, the intensity of exercise dictates neuromuscular responses, with higher intensities affecting muscle fibers directly, while lower intensities involve more significant central nervous system engagement [15]. These insights highlight the critical need for customized training regimens to optimize muscular and neuromuscular responses and enhance overall health outcomes.

Effects of Exercise on Metabolism, Cardiovascular Function, and Respiration

Exercise physiology explores the comprehensive effects of physical activity on metabolism, cardiovascular function, and respiration, encompassing both immediate responses and long-term adaptations. Cardiovascular adaptations to exercise include increased cardiac output and enhanced blood flow to active muscles, improving oxygen supply and waste removal [16]. These changes are supported by the heart to undergo structural and functional remodeling, increasing efficiency. Metabolically, physical activity initiates a series of cellular events that ramp up energy production via aerobic and anaerobic pathways, which is crucial for muscle performance. Oxygen consumption (VO_2) is pivotal in gauging exercise capacity, reflecting the body's oxygen use during intense activities. Regular training reduces myocardial oxygen consumption both at rest and during exercise, increasing cardiac function during high-intensity activities [17]. Respiratory adaptations enhance blood pH regulation, which is vital during heightened metabolic activity. These physiological adjustments highlight the role of exercise in health promotion and disease prevention, supporting the "Exercise is Medicine" initiative [7].

Relationship Between Electrical Stimulation and Physical Exercise

The interplay between electrical stimulation and physical exercise offers unique advantages for various health contexts. Electrical stimulation helps individuals with physical limitations by enhancing muscle activation, aiding recovery, improving glucose uptake, and boosting venous return to lower thrombotic risks [18]. Additionally, electrical stimulation combats muscle atrophy and boosts strength, which is useful for those unable to participate in active training [19]. These findings demonstrate electrical stimulation capability to augment or replace traditional exercise, offering customized benefits for diverse health needs.

Internal and External Power Development

Total power output is the sum of the internal and external power (Fig. 4.1) and all metabolic, cardiovascular, and ventilatory responses during FES-cycling exercise depends on it.

Development of Internal Power

Internal power is the amount of energy used by active muscles during a "zero load" exercise. It can be defined as the power generated to overcome inertial and gravitational forces related to the movement of lower limbs during cycling [20].

During FES-cycling, the internal power can vary according to the amount of motor unit recruitment and the cycling cadence. Higher electrical stimulus intensity promotes higher muscle recruitment, developing higher internal power. The muscle contraction induced by electrical stimulation will make a propulsive movement of the legs pushing/pulling the crank, however, with no load resisting to this movement. A higher cycling cadence will require a higher number of muscle contractions per period of time, as well as a higher movement velocity.

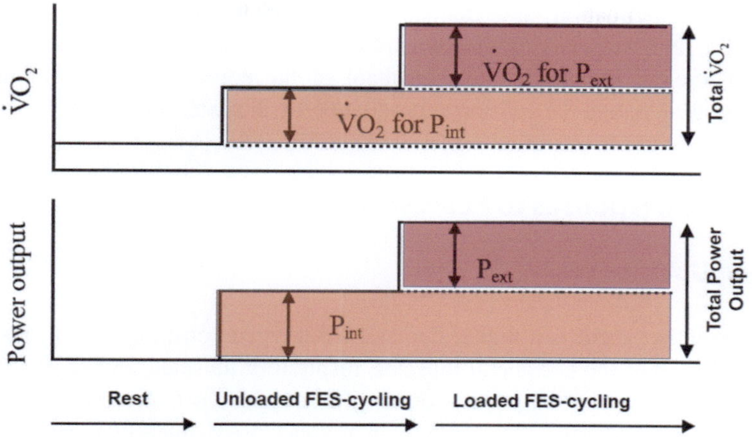

Fig. 4.1 Illustration of internal (Pint), external (Pext) and total power output (Ptot) and oxygen uptake (VO_2) for Pint and Pext. (Tokui and Hirakoba [20])

Development of External Power

The external power is the amount of energy used by active muscles during an external loaded exercise. It can be defined as the sum of joint powers, each calculated as the product of the joint (net) moment and angular velocity. This definition of external power is closely related to the mean external power as applied to exercise physiology: the sum of joint powers reflects all mechanical power, which, in principle, can be used to fulfill a certain task [21]. In other words, it is the power generated to overcome the workload produced by the ergometer during the cycling exercise.

Beyond the amount of motor unit recruitment and the cycling cadence, the external power is also dependent on the mechanical work generated during FES-cycling. At this time, the muscle contraction induced by electrical stimulation will make a propulsive movement of the legs, pushing/pulling the crank against a resistive load. Eighty-five percent of the power generated is during the crank-pushing movement, and the other 15% is during the pulling movement of the opposite leg [22].

In stationary ergometers, the workload can be produced in different ways, according to exercise modality. During an isokinetic exercise, the equipment motor will maintain the cycling cadence. Therefore, the power output will be proportional to the propulsive movement of the legs pushing/pulling the crank. Higher electrically stimulated muscle contraction will induce higher resistance (power output) of the equipment motor. During an isopower exercise, the equipment motor will maintain the power set by adjusting the resistance according to the cycling cadence. As the power is a result of force times angular velocity, during lower cycling cadences, the equipment motor will increase the resistance. During higher cycling cadences, the equipment motor will decrease the resistance.

In non-stationary ergometers, the workload will be a resultant of the ergometer gear combination, ergometer design (wheels size, axis distance, cyclist positions, etc.), ground inclination, and characteristics (asphalt, rubber, grass, sand, etc.). Frequently, non-stationary ergometers are adapted to stationary ergometers. In this situation, the workload will be a resultant of the ergometer gear combination, ergometer design, and the resistance production by the external device.

Metabolic Responses to FES-Cycling

Oxygen Uptake (VO_2)

During exercise, there is a higher demand for oxygen consumption to satisfy the increased work of the peripheral muscles, respiratory muscles, and heart at higher ventilatory and cardiac output responses. The oxygen cost of work performance depends on the work rate. VO_2 normally increases close to linearly as external work (power output) increases [23].

FES-cycling exercise is a more intense stimulus modality than other comparative therapeutic modalities. There is a high certainty of evidence that FES-cycling induces higher oxygen consumption with a clinically important difference. Higher VO_2 differences are especially greater when FES-cycling is compared to passive cycling (without FES) (Fig. 4.2). However, it is also higher when compared to isolated electrical stimulation (without cycling) or associated with an arm crank [24]. FES-cycling reaches a higher oxygen consumption because it generates higher external power [1].

Carbonic Gas Production (VCO_2)

There is a high certainty of evidence that FES-cycling induces higher carbonic gas production with a clinically important difference compared to other therapeutic modalities [24]. Contrary to physiological voluntary muscle contraction, motor unit recruitment during electrical stimulation reflects a nonselective, spatially fixed, and temporally synchronous pattern. Muscle fibers are recruited without obvious sequencing related to fiber types [25]. Therefore, functional electrical stimulation promotes type I and II fiber contraction in all exercise intensities [26]. This

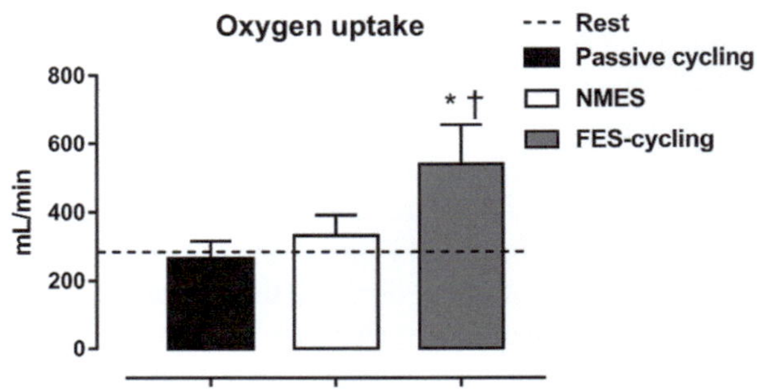

Fig. 4.2 Oxygen uptake between comparative therapeutic modalities. NMES: neuromuscular electrical stimulation. * higher than passive cycling. † higher than NMES. (Adapted from Frazão et al. [1])

counter-physiological recruitment pattern has a great metabolic impact because type II has more glycolytic activity and enzymatic profile.

Lactic acid is produced during glycolytic pathway utilization. The H^+ produced in the cell as lactate must be immediately buffered upon its formation. However, because HCO_3^- is a volatile buffer, the resulting H_2CO_3 does not remain in the cell but leaves its formation as CO_2, thereby removing H^+ from the intracellular environment [27]. This "extra "CO_2 is the main reason for higher CO_2 production during FES-cycling [1].

Lactate Production

There is a high certainty of evidence that FES-cycling induces higher lactate production, with a clinically important difference compared to other therapeutic modalities [24] (Fig. 4.3). It suggests greater metabolic stress, exercise intensity, and glycolytic fiber recruitment.

As well as extra CO_2 production, lactate production also comes from the buffering of lactic acid. There are three mechanisms resulting in great glycolytic fiber recruitment: nonselective recruitment pattern of electrical stimulation, high-intensity electrical stimulation, and high muscle tension production induced by the workload.

Energy Expenditure

As FES-cycling promotes external work, it produces high energy expenditure. Such level of exercise intensity/muscle recruitment affects aerobic/anaerobic

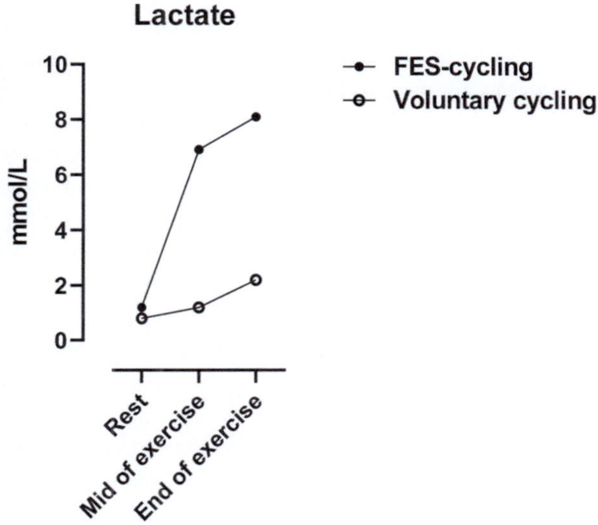

Fig. 4.3 Example of lactate production pattern during FES-cycling

balance metabolism. Commonly, the respiratory exchange ratio is higher than 1.0, suggesting that the proportion of carbohydrate utilization in the bioenergetics and metabolic process during FES-cycling is higher than lipid utilization.

There is a linear relationship between work rate and energy expenditure. The Fenn effect states that the energy liberated is equal to the energy cost of isometric force production plus the work done. The total amount of energy released varies with the work performed [28]. In normal cycling, about 90% of all variance in energy expenditure can be explained by work rate, with only about 10% being explained by cycling cadence [29].

Ettema and Loras, 2009 [29].

It is important to emphasize that the metabolic efficiency during FES-cycling is lower than voluntary cycling [30]. It ranges from 30% to 50% of the metabolic efficiency of voluntary cycling in the mean. Kjaer et al. [31] bring a very good example of this in their classical study. They studied a group of healthy subjects cycling normally (voluntary) and, following epidural anesthesia, during FES-cycling. The subjects reached similar oxygen consumption in both conditions ($VO_2 = 1.9$ L/min); however, the power output was markedly lower during FES-cycling. The power output was approximately 120 W during volitional cycling and 40 W during FES-cycling. Such metabolic inefficiency is a consequence of two primary features of FES-cycling: unfavorable biomechanics and non-physiological recruitment of muscle fibers [30].

Cardiovascular Responses to FES-Cycling

Heart Rate

There is a moderate certainty of evidence that FES-cycling induces a higher heart rate with a clinically important difference compared to other therapeutic modalities [24]. The heart rate increase is completely dependent on autonomic balance. The autonomic nervous system plays a key role in bringing about the cardiovascular responses to exercise necessitated by the increased metabolic requirements of the active skeletal muscle. The complex interaction of central and peripheral neural control mechanisms evokes a decrease in parasympathetic activity and an increase in sympathetic activity to the heart during exercise [32].

During FES-cycling exercise, the mechano and metaboreceptor activities of the muscles influence cardiac autonomic control. Looking at the mechanoreceptors, a rapid increase in heart rate is evoked during electrically stimulated contractions [33] where peripheral feedback is present, but the parallel activation of somatomotor and cardiovascular centers is missing (when the central command is bypassed, for example).

Williamson et al. [34] observed that passive cycling combined with electrical stimulation evoked an instantaneous shortening of the R–R interval, but only when the movement was initiated within the first one-third of the interval. These findings suggest that heart rate changes elicited by central command can occur at least twice as fast as responses produced by the muscle-heart reflex but that the muscle-heart reflex can play a role in R–R interval shortening if the contraction is initiated early enough in the interval to incorporate this reflex mechanism.

Looking at the metaboreceptors, exercise-induced metabolites accumulate and activate metabolically sensitive skeletal muscle afferents. When muscle metaboreflex activation is evoked during exercise, a notable increase in heart rate is elicited. The muscle metaboreflex activation-mediated increases in heart rate are principally attributable to increased cardiac sympathetic activity, and only following exercise with a large muscle mass (as during FES-cycling) is there a contribution from the partial withdrawal of cardiac parasympathetic tone [35].

Stroke Volume

There is a high certainty of evidence that FES-cycling induces higher stroke volume with a clinically important difference compared to other therapeutic modalities [24]. During FES-cycling, the muscle contraction promoted by electrical stimulation against resistance causes compression of the vessels, followed by vasodilation and conductance improvement. Additionally, greater muscle activity promotes greater pumping of blood (blood return), which is drained from the periphery to the heart, improving stroke volume.

Therefore, the physiological mechanisms for an enhanced stroke volume during FES-cycling exercise may include enhanced diastolic filling due to increases in blood return, left ventricular diameter, and ventricular compliance; enhanced systolic emptying due to increases in myocardial contractility; and decreases in ventricular afterload, or both [36].

Exercise intensity may also be taken into account. At low levels of exertion, an increase in left ventricular filling pressure and end-diastolic volume are important determinants of the stroke volume response through the Starling mechanism. At high levels of exertion, exercise tachycardia is accompanied by a decrease in end-diastolic volume despite a progressive increase in filling pressure, so stroke volume must be maintained by a decrease in end-systolic volume [37].

Cardiac Output

There is a high certainty of evidence that FES-cycling induces higher cardiac output with a clinically important difference compared to other therapeutic modalities [24]. Medrinal et al. [38] demonstrated that cardiac output is especially greater when compared to electrical stimulation or passive cycling/mobilization alone (Fig. 4.4). Cardiac output increase is a physiological adjustment to satisfy the muscles' metabolic demand during FES-cycling exercise. It can reach more than double the

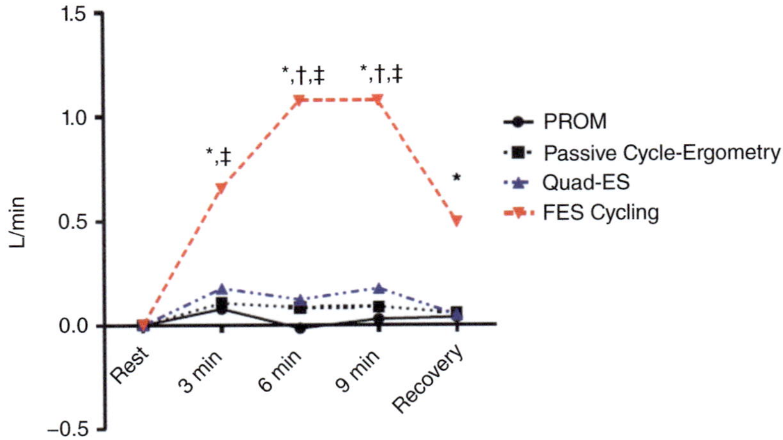

Fig. 4.4 Cardiac output over time for each exercise. Black circles represent a passive range of leg movement (PROM); black squares represent passive cycle-ergometry; blue triangles represent quadriceps electrical stimulation; red triangles represent functional electrical stimulation cycling (FES-Cycling). *Significant difference between PROM and FES-Cycling; †significantly difference between passive cycle-ergometer and FES-Cycling; ‡significantly difference between quadriceps electrical stimulation and FES-Cycling. (Medrinal et al. [38])

baseline (rest) values. It is a result of heart rate and stroke volume increase; however, some studies demonstrate that cardiac output increase is more dependent on the heart rate variance than stroke volume [39, 40].

Blood Pressure

In exercise-induced blood pressure dynamics, the systolic blood pressure typically exhibits a linear increase according to exercise intensity. This hemodynamic pattern also happens during FES-cycling exercise [40]. This rise in systolic blood pressure is a complex interplay of factors that include not only increased cardiac output but also sympathetic activation, changes in vascular resistance, and thermoregulatory responses that collectively increase blood flow to the active musculature [41]. Conversely, diastolic blood pressure is relatively stable during exercise. Some people may even experience a slight decrease. This stability or decrease is primarily due to metabolic vasodilation in the exercising muscles, ensuring adequate oxygen delivery and waste removal [41].

Blood pressure is the result of the product of cardiac output and peripheral vascular resistance. Therefore, the autonomic nervous system plays a central role in the modulation of blood pressure during exercise. High sympathetic activity will increase the heart rate and arterial smooth muscle tone (vasoconstriction) in specific vascular territories, influencing overall blood pressure.

However, it is very important to state that several studies [42–45] demonstrate that FES-cycling exercise does not affect the mean arterial pressure (MAP) in spinal

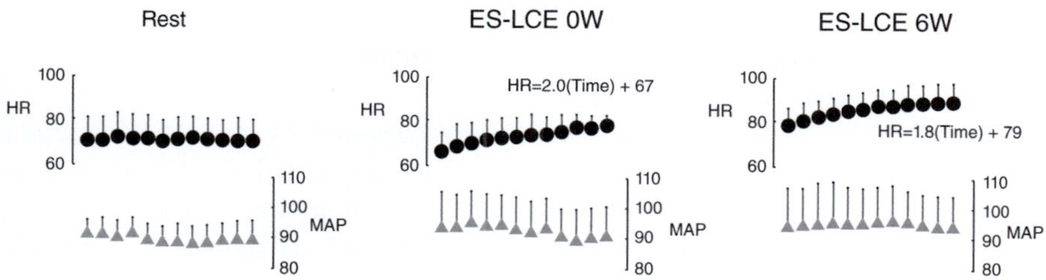

Fig. 4.5 Cardiovascular pattern during two electrical stimulation-induced leg cycling (ES-LCE) intensities in people with paraplegia. *HR* heart rate, *MAP* mean arterial pressure. (Raymond et al. 2002 [42])

cord-injured patients (Fig. 4.5). Hooker et al. [46] showed that this pattern persists even when FES-cycling is associated with arm-crank exercise. There are two plausible hypotheses for this: (1) The plegic muscles are unable to reach the cardiovascular control centers and thereby elicit any reflex change in blood pressure, or (2) There is a drop in diastolic blood pressure that compensates systolic blood pressure increase in the MAP calculation (MAP = systolic blood pressure + 2 × diastolic blood pressure/3). As the studies present only the MAP values, without discrimination of systolic and diastolic blood pressure, the physiological reason remains unclear.

Peripheral Muscle Oxygen Extraction

There is a moderate certainty of evidence that FES-cycling induces higher peripheral muscle oxygen extraction with a clinically important difference compared to other therapeutic modalities [24]. FES-cycling induces a concentric muscle contraction against resistance. As previously mentioned, there is a metabolic response during FES-cycling exercise. Muraki et al. [47] showed a higher deoxyhemoglobin in passive FES-cycling compared to passive cycling. It promotes an intensification in oxygen release by hemoglobin due to greater accumulation of tissue metabolism co-products, as well as increased heat production per unit of muscle (Bohr effect). Furthermore, the muscle contraction plays an important role in muscle oxygen extraction. During muscle contraction, arterioles have greater vasodilatation, irrigating the active muscles with increased muscular blood perfusion [48]. Gojda et al. [49] reported this, demonstrating a 165% increase in leg blood flow index during FES-cycling.

Ventilatory Responses to FES-Cycling

There is a high certainty of evidence that FES-cycling induces higher ventilation with a clinically important difference compared to other therapeutic modalities [24]. The respiratory system is lined with several receptors that directly influence ventilatory behavior. In this context, it is important to highlight the effects of FES-cycling exercise on muscle receptors (mechano and metaboreceptors) and chemical receptors (Fig. 4.6).

The group III muscle afferents are mainly triggered by muscle contraction (mechanoreceptors) [50]. Commonly, the parameters are set to induce a strong muscle contraction during FES-cycling exercise. The group IV afferent discharge increases according to ischemia and the accumulation of metabolites from muscle

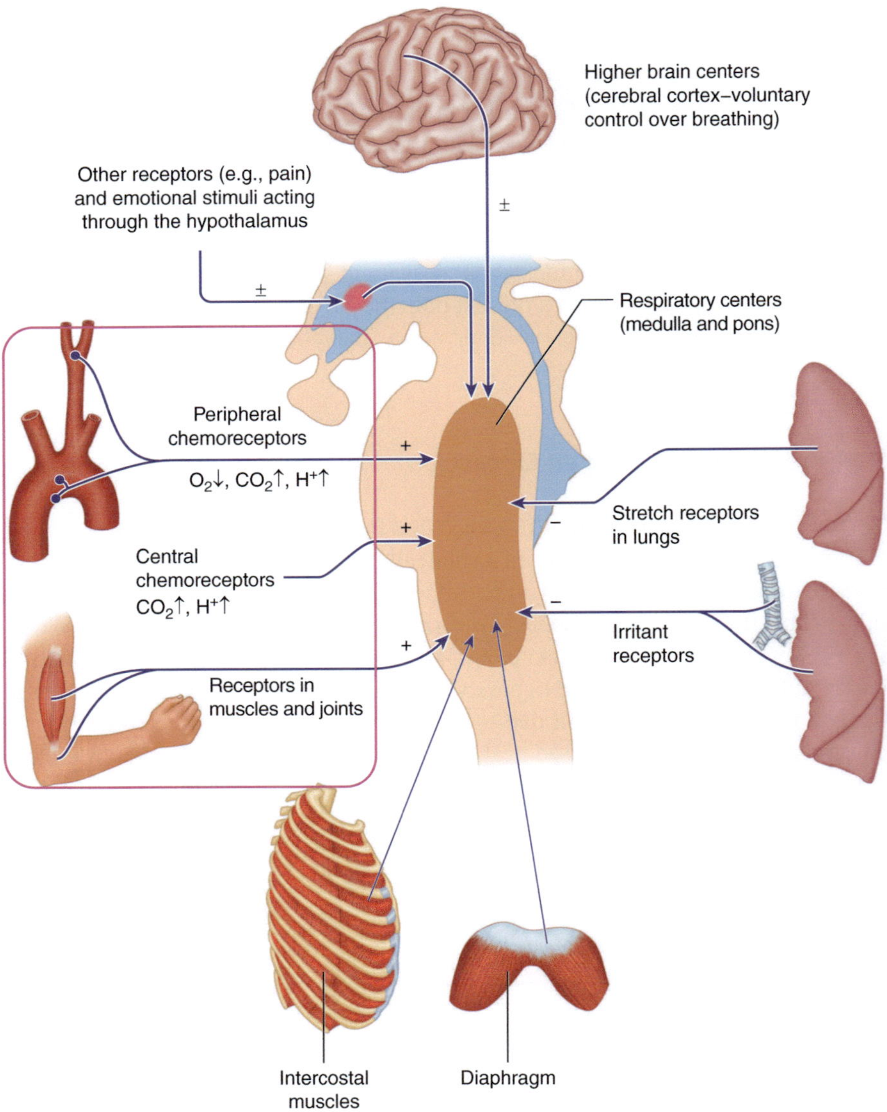

Fig. 4.6 Highlighted are the main receptors activated during FES-cycling exercise

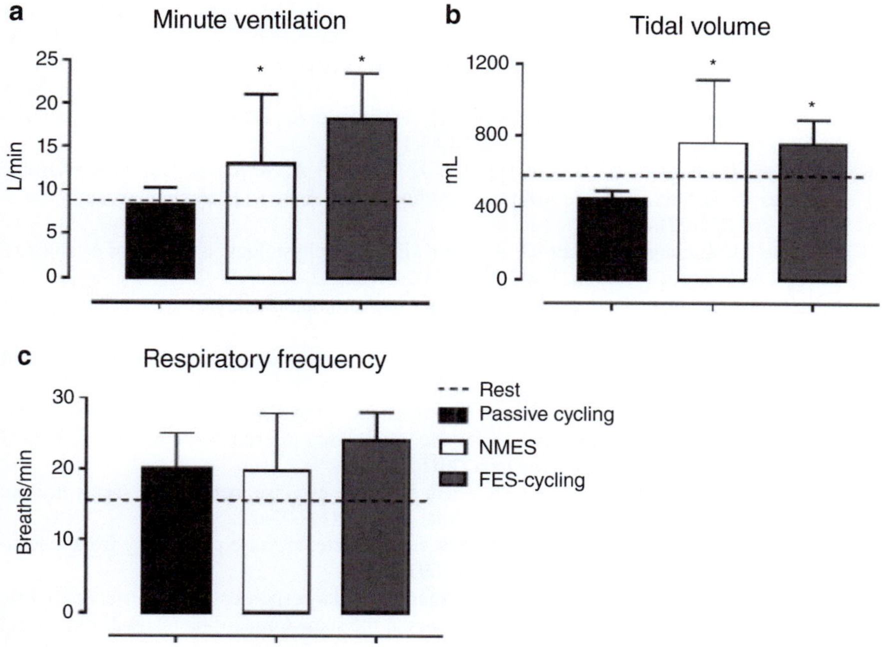

Fig. 4.7 Ventilatory pattern during FES-cycling exercise. Frazão et al. [1]. *NMES* neuromuscular electrical stimulation. * higher than passive cycling

contraction (metaboreceptors) [51]. As previously mentioned, FES-cycling exercise promotes an elevated muscle metabolite accumulation (i.e., lactate) due to high glycolytic metabolic pathway utilization.

The chemoreceptors are extensions of the peripheral nervous system that respond to changes in pH and gas concentrations in arterial blood, playing an important role in controlling breathing. The ventilatory response during exercise is closely related to the determinants of $PaCO_2$ [52]. As FES-cycling increases CO_2 production, central chemoreceptors and carotid bodies are activated [53]. Looking at the breathing pattern, the ventilation is increased due to an increase in tidal volume more than in respiratory frequency during FES-cycling exercise [1] (Fig. 4.7).

References

1. Frazão M, Werlang LA, Azevedo C, Kunz A, Peltz M. Metabolic, ventilatory and cardiovascular responses to FES-cycling: a comparison to NMES and passive cycling. Technol Health Care. 2022;30(4):909–18.
2. Máté S, Corr N, Hackett D, Barnett M, Singh MF, Fornusek C. Functional electrical stimulation combined with voluntary cycling accentuates VO2 response in people with severe multiple sclerosis: a pilot study. Mult Scler Relat Disord. 2024;85:105552.
3. Fodor ANM, Mravcsik M, Klauber A, Cserháti P, Laczko J, Horváth M. Effect of FES controlled cycling training on cardiovascular and pulmonary systems in a spinal cord injured patient. Curr Dir Biomed Eng. 2022;8(3):29–32.

4. Sijobert B, Daubigney A, Fachin-Martins E, Coste CA, Fattal C. Longitudinal feasibility study of a SCI subject one-year training based on sublesional muscles FES assisted cycling. IFESS: International Functional Electrical Stimulation Society; 2017. lirmm-01547869f
5. Edwards TA, Motl RW, Pilutti LA. Cardiorespiratory demand of acute voluntary cycling with functional electrical stimulation in individuals with multiple sclerosis with severe mobility impairment. Appl Physiol Nutr Metab. 2018;43(1):71–6.
6. Sansare A, Harrington AT, Wright H, Alesi J, Behboodi A, Verma K, Lee SCK. Aerobic responses to FES-assisted and volitional cycling in children with cerebral palsy. Sensors (Basel). 2021;21(22):7590.
7. Matthews M, Kanungo S, Baker RJ, Kenter K. Exercise physiology: a review of established concepts and current questions. Physiologia. 2024;4(2):202–12.
8. Sietsema KE, Rossiter HB. Exercise physiology and cardiopulmonary exercise testing. Semin Respir Crit Care Med. 2023;44(5):661–80.
9. Zhu G. Exercise physiology: the scientific foundation for enhancing physical performance and healthy living. Theor Nat Sci. 2024;70:79–84.
10. Knuttgen HG. What is exercise? A primer for practitioners. Phys Sportsmed. 2003;31(3):31–49.
11. Chamari K, Padulo J. Aerobic' and 'anaerobic' terms used in exercise physiology: a critical terminology reflection. Sports Med Open. 2015;1:9.
12. Pellegrino JK, Anthony TG, Gillies PS, Arent SM. The exercise metabolome: acute aerobic and anaerobic signatures. J Int Soc Sports Nutr. 2022;19(1):603–22.
13. Furrer R, Hawley JA, Handschin C. The molecular athlete: exercise physiology from mechanisms to medals. Physiol Rev. 2023;103(3):1693–787.
14. Royer N, Nosaka K, Doguet V, Jubeau M. Neuromuscular responses to isometric, concentric and eccentric contractions of the knee extensors at the same torque-time integral. Eur J Appl Physiol. 2021;122(1):127–39.
15. Brownstein CG, Millet GY, Thomas K. Neuromuscular responses to fatiguing locomotor exercise. Acta Physiol. 2021;231(2):e13533.
16. Scott J, Cameron G, Goodenough A, et al. Exercise physiology. Biological science: exploring the science of life, biomedical edition. Oxford University Press; 2022.
17. Kim AR. Exercise physiology of the cardiovascular system. Ann Cardio Pulm Rehabil. 2022;2:46–51.
18. Ackermann PW, Juthberg R, Flodin J. Unlocking the potential of neuromuscular electrical stimulation: achieving physical activity benefits for all abilities. Front Sports Active Living. 2024;29(6):1507402.
19. Adams V. Is it beneficial to add electromyostimulation to conventional exercise training in heart failure? European journal of. Eur J Prev Cardiol. 2017;24(15):1594–5.
20. Tokui M, Hirakoba K. Estimation of oxygen cost of internal power during cycling exercise with changing pedal rate. J Physiol Anthropol. 2008;27:133–8.
21. de Groot G, Welbergen E, Clijsen L, Clarijs J, Cabri J, Antonis J. Power, muscular work, and external forces in cycling. Ergonomics. 1994;37(1):31–42.
22. Szecsi J, Straube A, Fornusek C. A biomechanical cause of low power production during FES cycling of subjects with SCI. J Neuroeng Rehabil. 2014;11:123.
23. Hansen JE, Casburi R, Cooper DM, Wasserman K. Oxygen uptake as related to work rate increment during cycle ergometer exercise. Eur J Appl Physiol Occup Physiol. 1988;57:140–5.
24. Frazão M, de Gomes Figueiredo T, Cipriano G Jr. Should we use the functional electrical stimulation-cycling exercise in clinical practice? Physiological and clinical effects systematic review with meta-analysis. Arch Phys Med Rehabil. 2024; 22:S0003-9993(24)01057-8
25. Gregory C, Scott Bickel C. Recruitment patterns in human skeletal muscle during electrical stimulation. Phys Ther. 2005;85(4):358–64.
26. Bickel CS, Gregory CM, Dean JC. Motor unit recruitment during neuromuscular electrical stimulation: a critical appraisal. Eur J Appl Physiol. 2011;111(10):2399–407.
27. Wasserman K, Whipp BJ. Excercise physiology in health and disease. Am Rev Respir Dis. 1975;112(2):219–49.
28. Mommaerts WFHM. What is the fenn-effect? Naturwissensvhaflen. 1970;7:326–30.

29. Ettema G, Lorås HW. Efficiency in cycling: a review. Eur J Appl Physiol. 2009;106:1–14.
30. Hunt KJ, Fang J, Saengsuwan J, Grob M, Laubacher M. On the efficiency of FES cycling: a framework and systematic review. Technol Health Care. 2012;20(5):395–422.
31. Kjaer M, Perko G, Secher NH, et al. Cardiovascular and ventilatory responses to electrically induced cycling with complete epidural anaesthesia in humans. Acta Physiol Scand. 1994;151(2):199–207.
32. Fisher JP. Autonomic control of the heart during exercise in humans: role of skeletal muscle afferents. Exp Physiol. 2014;99(2):300–5.
33. McCloskey DI, Mitchell JH. Reflex cardiovascular and respiratory responses originating in exercising muscle. J Physiol. 1972;224(1):173–86.
34. Williamson JW, Nóbrega AC, Winchester PK, Zim S, Mitchell JH. Instantaneous heart rate increase with dynamic exercise: central command and muscle-heart reflex contributions. J Appl Physiol. 1995;78:1273–9.
35. Fisher JP, Adlan AM, Shantsila A, Secher JF, Sørensen H, Secher NH. Muscle metaboreflex and autonomic regulation of heart rate in humans. J Physiol. 2013;591(15):3777–88.
36. Vella CA, Robergs RR. A review of the stroke volume response to upright exercise in healthy subjects. Br J Sports Med. 2005;39(4):190–5.
37. Higginbotham MB, Morris KG, Williams RS, McHale PA, Coleman RE, Cobb FR. Regulation of stroke volume during submaximal and maximal upright exercise in normal man. Circ Res. 1986;58(2):281–91.
38. Clément Medrinal YC, Prieur G, Quesada AR, Bonnevie T, Gravier FE, Lozeron ED, Frenoy E, Contal O, Lamia B. Comparison of exercise intensity during four early rehabilitation techniques in sedated and ventilated patients in ICU: a randomised cross-over trial. Crit Care. 2018;22(1):110.
39. Nash MS, Bilsker MS, Kearney HM, Ramirez IN, Applegate B, Green BA. Effects of electrically-stimulated exercise and passive motion on echocardiographically-derived wall motion and cardiodynamic function in tetraplegic persons. Paraplegia. 1995;33:80–9.
40. Fornusek C, Davis GM. Cardiovascular and metabolic responses during functional electric stimulation cycling at different cadences. Arch Phys Med Rehabil. 2008;89:719–25.
41. Pesova P, Godula BJ, Jiravsky O, et al. Exercise-induced blood pressure dynamics: insights from the general population and the athletic cohort. J Cardiovasc Dev Dis. 2023;10(12):480.
42. Raymond JD, Davis GM, van der Plas M. Cardiovascular responses during submaximal electrical stimulation-induced leg cycling in individuals with paraplegia. Clin Physiol Funct Imaging. 2002;22:92–8.
43. Thomas AJ, Davis GM, Sutton JR. Cardiovascular and metabolic responses to electrical stimulation-induced leg exercise in spinal cord injury. Meth Inf Med. 1997;36:372–5.
44. Kjaer M, Pott F, Mohr T, Linkis P, Tornøe P, Secher NH. Heart rate during exercise with leg vascular occlusion in spinal cord-injured humans. J Appl Physiol. 1999;86:806–11.
45. Hooker SP, Figoni SF, Glaser RM, Rodgers MM, Ezenwa BN, Faghri PD. Physiologic responses to prolonged electrically stimulated leg-cycle exercise in the spinal cord injured. Arch Phys Med Rehabil. 1990;71:863–9.
46. Hooker SP, Figoni SF, Rodger MM, et al. Metabolic and hemodynamic responses to concurrent voluntary arm crank and electrical stimulation leg cycle exercise in quadriplegics. J Rehabil Res Dev. 1992;29(3):1–11.
47. Satoshi Muraki CF, Raymond J, Davis GM. Muscle oxygenation during prolonged electrical stimulation-evoked cycling in paraplegics. Appl Physiol Nutr Metab. 2007;32(3):463–72.
48. Thomas GD, Segel SS. Neural control of muscle blood flow during exercise. J Appl Physiol. 2004;97(2):731–8.
49. Gojda J, Waldauf P, Hrusková N, et al. Lactate production without hypoxia in skeletal muscle during electrical cycling: crossover study of femoral venous-arterial differences in healthy volunteers. PLoS One. 2019;14:e0200228.
50. Kaufman MP, Longhurst JC, Rybicki KJ, Wallach JH, Mitchell JH. Effects of static muscular contraction on impulse activity of groups III and IV afferents in cats. J Appl Physiol Respir Environ Exerc Physiol. 1983;55(1):105–12.

51. Kaufman MP, Rybicki KJ. Discharge properties of group III and IV muscle afferents: their responses to mechanical and metabolic stimuli. Circ Res. 1987;6(4):I60–165.
52. Whipp BJ, Ward SA, Wassermann K. Ventilatory responses to exercise and their control in man. Am Rev Respir Dis. 1984;129:S17–20.
53. Lahiri S, Forster RE 2nd. CO2-H(+) sensing peripheral and central chemoreception. Int J Biochem Cell Biol. 2003;35(10):1413–35.

5 Functional Assessment Based on FES-Cycling Technology

Murillo Frazão, Thainá de Gomes Figueiredo, Rafael Michel de Macedo, and Juliana Goulart Prata Oliveira Milani

Introduction

FES-cycling may offer objective parameters to assess functional capacity. This technology can be used to evaluate neuromuscular efficiency, muscle performance, muscle synergy, cardiopulmonary capacity, and cardiorespiratory fitness. The results of these assessments are very useful in determining from athletic performance to disease severity and progression. It is also useful to outlining therapeutic/training strategies and measuring their effects.

Adjusting FES-cycling parameters based on functional evaluation results is crucial for optimizing treatment outcomes. Each patient's condition, response to therapy, and overall functional capabilities can vary widely, meaning a

M. Frazão (✉)
Lauro Wanderley University Hospital – EBSERH/UFPB, João Pessoa, PB, Brazil
e-mail: murillo.frazao@gmail.com

T. de Gomes Figueiredo
Oswaldo Crus University Hospital, UPE, Recife, PE, Brazil

Agamenon Magalhães Hospital, Recife, PE, Brazil

Tiradentes University, Recife, PE, Brazil
e-mail: thaina.gfigueiredo@upe.br

R. M. de Macedo
Agamenon Magalhães Hospital, Recife, PE, Brazil

Costantini Cardiologic Hospital, Curitiba, PR, Brazil
e-mail: rafael.macedo@hospitalcostantini.com.br

J. G. P. O. Milani
Faculty of Rehabilitation Sciences, Rehabilitation Research Center (REVAL), Hasselt University, Hasselt, Belgium

Graduate Programme in Health Sciences and Technologies, University of Brasilia (UnB), Brasilia, DF, Brazil
e-mail: juliana@medicinadoexercicio.com

M. Frazão (ed.), *Functional Electrical Stimulation Cycling in Clinical Practice*, https://doi.org/10.1007/978-3-032-23937-2_5

one-size-fits-all approach to electrical stimulation may not be effective. Functional evaluations, which assess a patient's strength, mobility, and muscle function, provide valuable insights into their current physical state. By tailoring the FES-cycling parameters—such as work load, pulse width, frequency, intensity, and electrode placement—according to these results, clinicians can ensure that the therapy targets the specific muscles or muscle groups that need strengthening or rehabilitation. This personalized approach can improve the efficacy of the treatment, promote faster recovery, and prevent unnecessary strain on healthy tissues.

Moreover, adjusting electrical stimulation parameters based on functional evaluation helps to ensure the patient's safety and comfort during therapy. Some individuals may be more sensitive to certain stimulation intensities or frequencies, and others might need a gradual increase in intensity to avoid overexertion or discomfort. By continuously monitoring the patient's response to electrical stimulation in conjunction with functional evaluations, clinicians can fine-tune the settings to match the patient's tolerance and progress. This dynamic approach allows for a more precise, responsive treatment plan that aligns with the patient's evolving needs, ensuring that the therapy is both effective and well-tolerated over time.

Additionally, evaluating the efficacy of the intervention is a corner stone for therapeutic success. Monitoring a patient's response to a treatment based on FES-cycling is crucial for ensuring both the safety and effectiveness of the intervention. FES-cycling exercise can be a highly beneficial form of treatment, aiding in the management of a variety of conditions such as cardiovascular diseases, diabetes, obesity, and musculoskeletal disorders. However, each patient responds differently to exercise, and understanding these individual responses is key to optimizing outcomes.

Regular monitoring provides valuable insights into how well the patient is progressing toward their treatment goals. Tracking improvements in strength, endurance, mobility, or overall fitness helps to assess whether the prescribed exercise program is achieving the desired therapeutic outcomes. If progress is slower than expected, modifications can be made to the plan, ensuring the patient remains on the path toward recovery or improved health.

Key Functional Outcomes in FES-Cycling Assessment

Muscle Strength and Power

Several techniques are available for detecting muscle weakness. Maximal voluntary strength and power assessment are common methods, but it relies on the patient's voluntary effort and may be not feasible in some specific situations (i.e., spinal cord injury, hospitalized patients, hemiplegic patients, etc.). Beyond the therapeutic uses, FES-cycling is a promising non-volitional evaluation method for detecting muscle weakness. Objectively, the equipment provides an electrical stimulus and measures the muscle's mechanical response. Strength (torque) must be reported in newton meter (Nm) and power output in watts (W). By stimulating the lower limb muscles,

FES-cycling provides valuable data on the capacity of muscles to generate force under functional, dynamic conditions, closely resembling real-world activities.

It offers an alternative to traditional assessments, especially in cases where patients have diminished voluntary control or consciousness. The method also enables clinicians to monitor changes in muscle performance over time, aiding in the development of personalized rehabilitation plans. As FES-cycling can engage a large number of muscles simultaneously, it provides a comprehensive evaluation of both strength and power, making it a valuable tool in the management of muscle dysfunction, particularly in critically ill or rehabilitation patients.

A common approach involves the use of torque sensors installed on the pedals or the bicycle's crankshaft. These devices capture the force exerted by the muscles during each pedaling cycle, enabling a detailed analysis of power output and movement efficiency [1, 2] (Fig. 5.1).

Another technique employed is isokinetic dynamometry, which evaluates muscle strength and power during movements performed at a constant velocity [3]. In the context of FES-cycling, isokinetic dynamometers can be used to measure the torque produced by electrically stimulated muscles throughout the pedaling motion. This assessment provides detailed information on muscle performance across different joint angles, aiding in the identification of potential deficiencies and the prescription of targeted rehabilitation programs. Torque information is generated by the servo motor drive (Fig. 5.2).

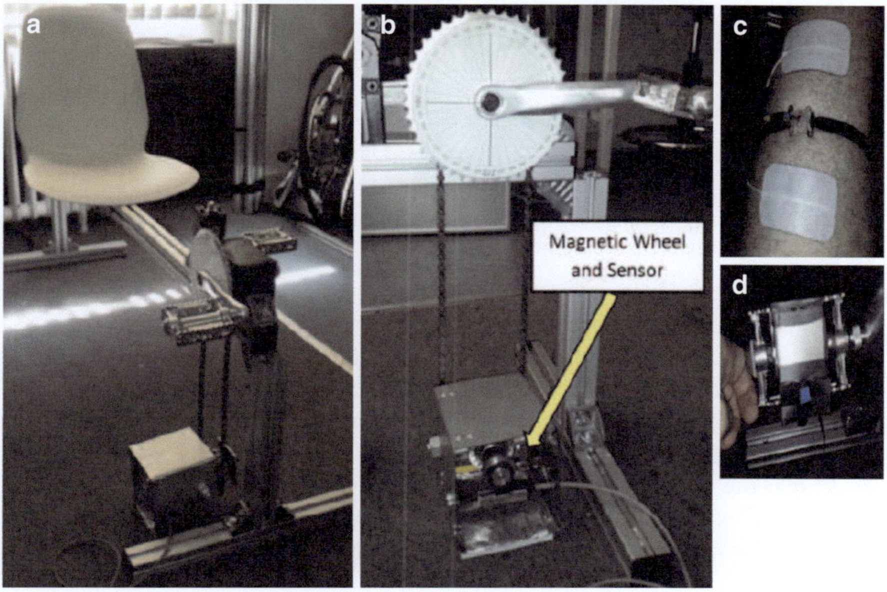

Fig. 5.1 (**a**) Recumbent bicycle rig and (**b**) the crank angle encoder box with the magnetic wheel and sensor mounted. (**c**) Arrangement of FES electrodes (white pads) and mechanomyographic probe (transparent plastic held by black elastic band) and the Velcro strapping attachment of a force sensitive resistor. (**d**) Pedal sensors. (Woods et al. [2])

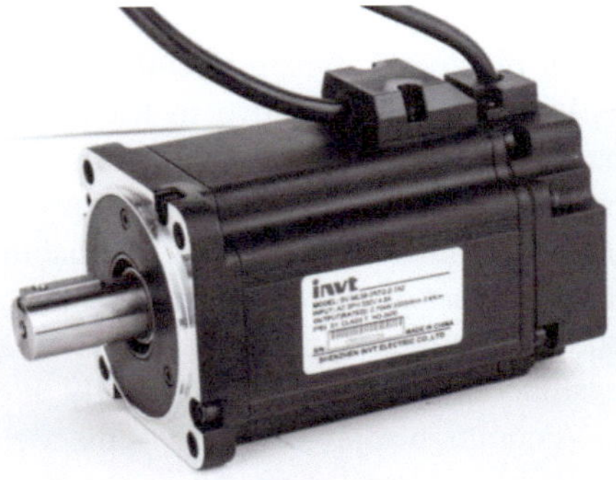

Fig. 5.2 An example of servo motor used in commercial FES-cycling equipment. (https://www.kalatec.com.br/servo-motor-750w/)

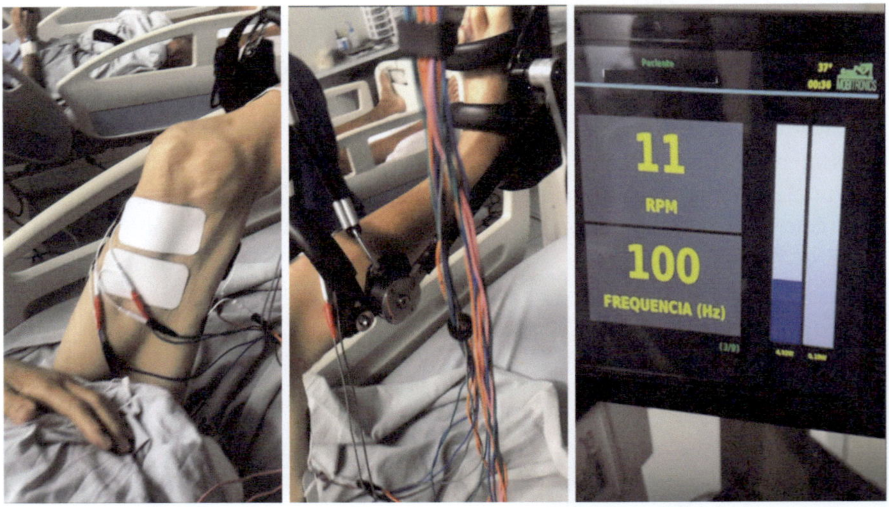

Fig. 5.3 FES-cycling-based muscular performance assessment. The screen shows the left leg power output. (Source: Prepared by the authors)

The servo motor has an auto tuning which provides a specific electrical charge to maintain the programmed rotation. The torque calculation is based on the variance of electrical charge applied to maintain the rotation. The servo motor drive also provides the angular velocity. The power output values are achieved by mathematical calculation (torque times angular velocity) [4]. Figures 5.3 and 5.4 bring examples of real-life muscle performance measurements.

Figure 5.5 brings an example of torque and power output measurement in three different pulse frequency and cycling cadence, maintaining a fixed pulse width and intensity:

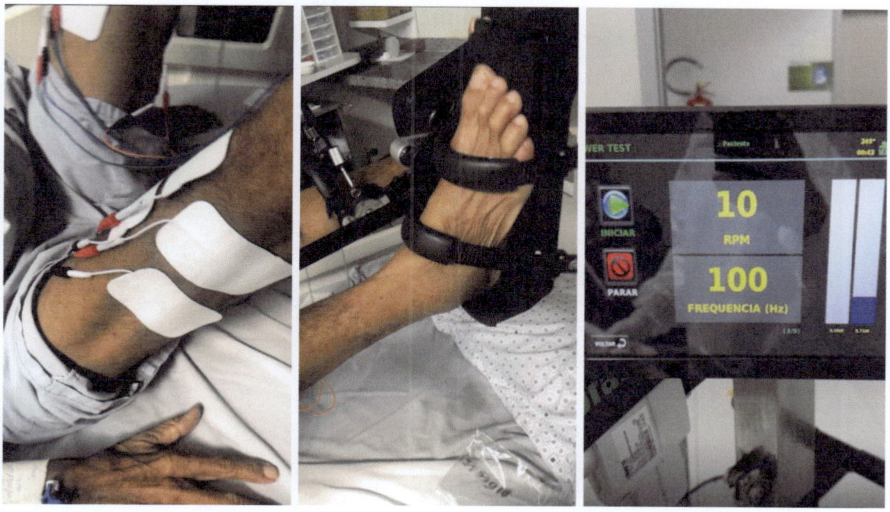

Fig. 5.4 FES-cycling-based muscular performance assessment. The screen shows the right leg power output. (Source: Prepared by the authors)

Muscle Synergy

The loss of lower limb strength and motor coordination is among the most common deficits leading to long-term disability after a stroke and other neurological conditions [5]. These patients often experience muscle weakness, abnormal muscle activity, and disrupted intermuscular coordination. These factors are key contributors to asymmetrical movements and changes in locomotor function [6].

Muscle synergies analysis can provide a deep understanding of motor impairment caused by the disease and of changes after rehabilitation [7]. The analysis of leg cycling can be done during FES-cycling, and also during voluntary cycling without FES.

During FES-cycling, it is performed an electromechanical analysis. In simple words, the torque/power output is measured during the electrical stimulation (Fig. 5.6). If there is asymmetry, there will be a large difference in muscle performance for the same electrical stimulation load in both limbs. Additionally, it is possible to measure the electromechanical delay existing between the stimulation input and the onset of muscle force [8] (Fig. 5.7).

During voluntary cycling without FES, it is performed a neuromechanical analysis. In this type of evaluation, an electromyography (EMG) equipment must be synchronized with the cycle ergometer. In this case, it will be evaluated the muscle activity (EMG) and the muscle performance (torque/power output) (Fig. 5.8).

Looking for the muscle performance analysis, the methods can vary according the equipment's models. The equipment can measure the torque/power output may demand additional devices or not (Fig. 5.9). I the first case, torque information is generated by the servo motor drive (details in muscle strength and power section).

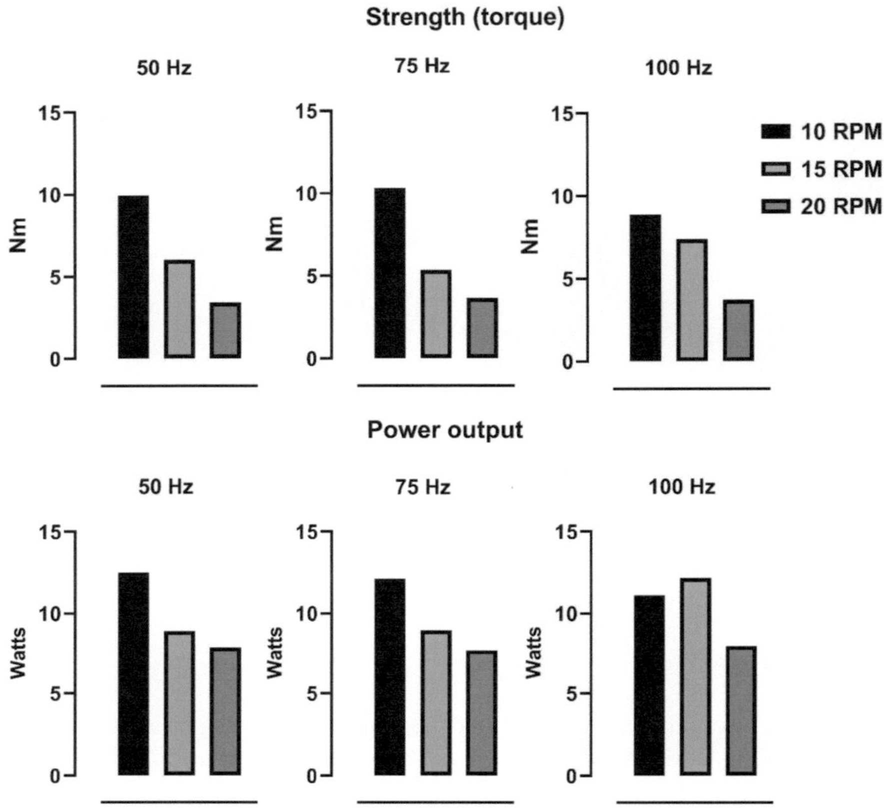

Fig. 5.5 Example of torque and power variation at different pulse frequency and cycling cadence, maintaining a fixed pulse width and intensity. *RPM* rotation per minute. (Source: Prepared by the authors)

In the second case, devices, mounted between the crank and each pedal, are necessary to measure the force produced. Each measuring device is based on a two-sensor system which measured the magnetic field variations (Hall effect) as a result of the displacement of a small sensor from a magnet. It is also equipped with accelerometers to measure the crank angle.

Muscle Efficiency

Oxygen cost and stimulation cost may be used to assess the muscle efficiency during FES-cycling. While oxygen cost is related to metabolic efficiency, stimulation cost measures the neuromuscular efficiency. The oxygen cost can be calculated as the ratio of the change in the rate of oxygen uptake to the change in mechanical work rate [9]. It can be reported in milliliters/minute/watt (mL/min/W). For example, if during an evaluation a patient presented 400 mL oxygen

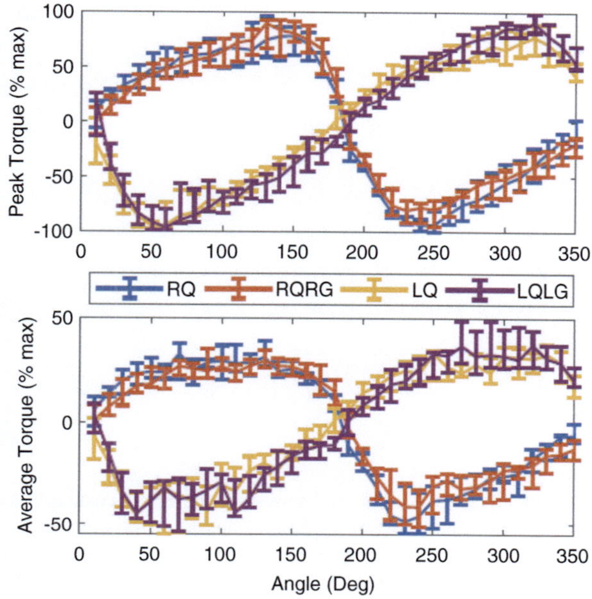

Fig. 5.6 Torque measurements for each electrical stimulation muscle combination (i.e., right quadriceps (RQ), right quadriceps and gluteal (RQRG), left quadriceps (LQ), and left quadriceps and gluteal (LQLG) muscle groups). The 0 degree crank angle corresponds to the crank being horizontal with the ground and the right leg extended. (Allen et al. [8])

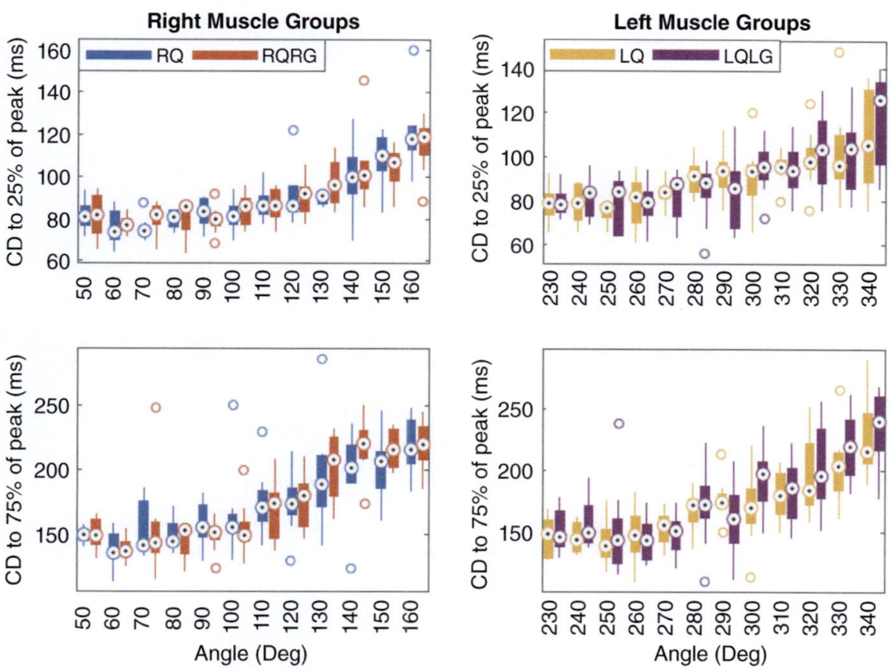

Fig. 5.7 Box plots of the contraction delay (CD) measurements for each muscle combination (i.e., right quadriceps (RQ), right quadriceps and gluteal (RQRG), left quadriceps (LQ), and left quadriceps and gluteal (LQLG) muscle groups). The 0 degree crank angle corresponds to the crank being horizontal with the ground and the right leg extended. (Allen et al. [8])

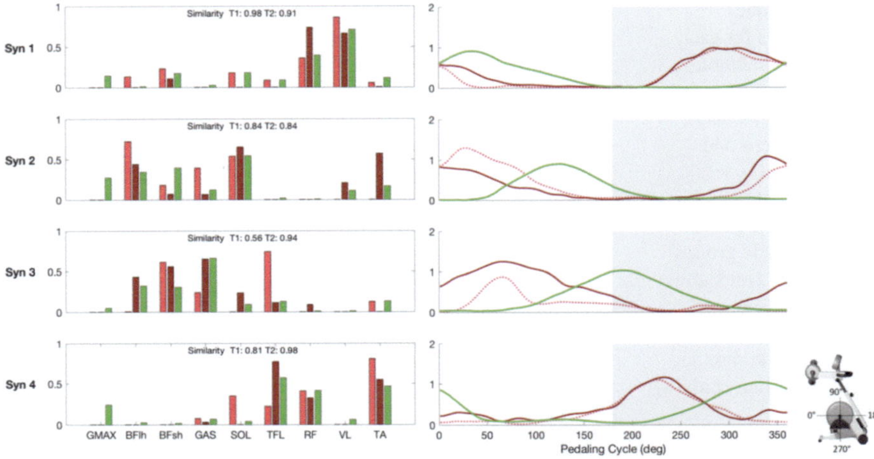

Fig. 5.8 Synergy weights and activation coefficients examples of four synergies analysis. Muscle synergies extracted before (light red) and after the training (dark red) are compared to healthy (green). The grey area represents the knee flexion phase. Gluteus Maximus (Gmax), Biceps Femoris long head (BFlh), Biceps Femoris short head (BFsh), Gastrocnemius Medialis (GAS), Soleus (SOL), Tensor Fasciae Latae (TFL), Rectus Femoris (RF), Vastus Lateralis (VL), and Tibialis Anterior (TA). (Ambrosini et al. [7])

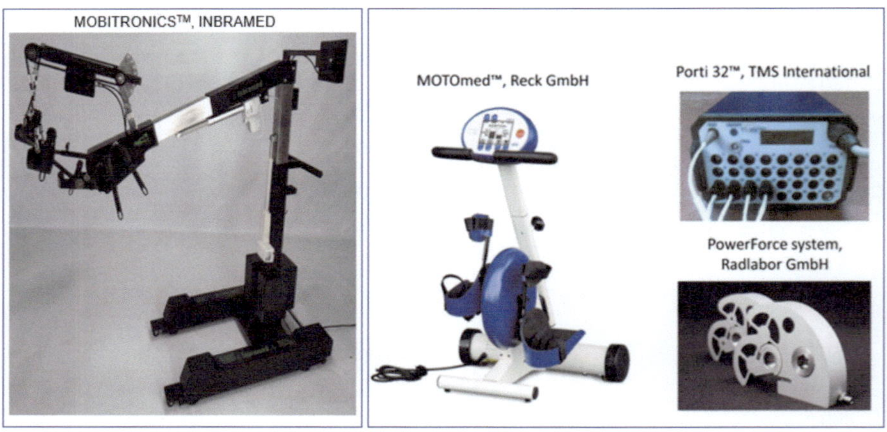

Fig. 5.9 Examples of FES-cycling equipment's for muscle synergy/performance measurement. It may demand additional devices (right pictures) or not (left picture). (Source: Prepared by the authors)

uptake during 0 W and increased the VO_2 to 600 mL at 10 W of power, the oxygen cost was 20 mL/min/W (calculations: [600–400]/10). Oxygen cost will be better discussed ahead.

Stimulation cost is the total electrical charge delivery rate per watt of output power for the stimulated muscle groups during exercise [9]. The charge for each individual stimulation pulse is obtained from the product of instantaneous pulse width and intensity. The stimulation cost must be reported in microcoulomb/watt (μC/W). For example, if during an evaluation a patient required 500 μs pulse width and 80 mA to generate 10 W of power, the stimulation cost will be 4000 μC/W ([500 × 80] /10). Higher values indicate lower neuromuscular efficiency. It provides a useful, easily computed, and experimentally verified means of evaluating the performance of the stimulation patterns employed in FES-cycling. The stimulation cost is a benchmark measure in FES-cycling assessment. This variable has a wide use in clinical practice. For example, it can be used for test a novel controller algorithm for real-time adaptation of the stimulation pattern for race competition [10] (Fig. 5.10), as well as establishing survival prognosis in critically ill patients [4] (Fig. 5.11).

Cardiorespiratory Fitness (VO_2)

Cardiorespiratory fitness (CRF) is a key indicator of health in both clinical and non-clinical populations, with low levels of CRF linked to a higher risk of morbidity and mortality [11, 12]. FES-cycling offers a compelling approach to assessing CRF in individuals with limited voluntary mobility (such as those with spinal cord injuries, critical illnesses, or severe motor impairments). By electrically stimulating the lower limb muscles to induce cycling, it elicits sufficient physiological stress to produce measurable responses, enabling an objective evaluation of aerobic capacity without relying on voluntary effort (Hunt KJ 2013 [13, 14]).

The cardiopulmonary exercise test (CPET), conceptualized through the classic Wasserman gears, provides an integrated assessment of the cardiovascular, respiratory, and muscular systems (Figs. 5.12 and 5.15). When combined with FES-cycling, CPET—which integrates a traditional exercise test with expired gas and ventilation analyses [16, 17]—allows for the direct assessment of oxygen uptake (VO_2), the primary indicator of CRF [12]. Additionally, it enables the evaluation of other key variables, including heart rate, power output, work rate, respiratory exchange ratio (RER = carbon dioxide production [VCO_2] /VO_2), and perceived exertion. Figures 5.13 and 5.14 illustrate a schematic and an actual setup of FES-cycling integrated with CPET.

In the context of assessing CRF with FES-cycling, additional key metrics such as oxygen cost and energy cost are used to evaluate exercise efficiency and cardiorespiratory demands [19, 20], particularly in individuals with spinal cord injuries (SCI) [13]. Lower oxygen and energy costs during FES-cycling reflect more efficient cardiovascular and respiratory function, serving as indicators of improved CRF and guiding clinicians and researchers in evaluating and refining protocols to optimize cardiovascular health outcomes [19, 20].

Oxygen cost, commonly expressed in mLO_2/min/W or mLO_2/kg/m, refers to the amount of oxygen consumed per unit of mechanical work during FES-cycling (e.g., per watt or per distance) and serves as an indicator of the metabolic demand required to perform the activity. In this approach, where electrical stimulation induces muscle contractions, oxygen cost provides valuable insight into how efficiently the body

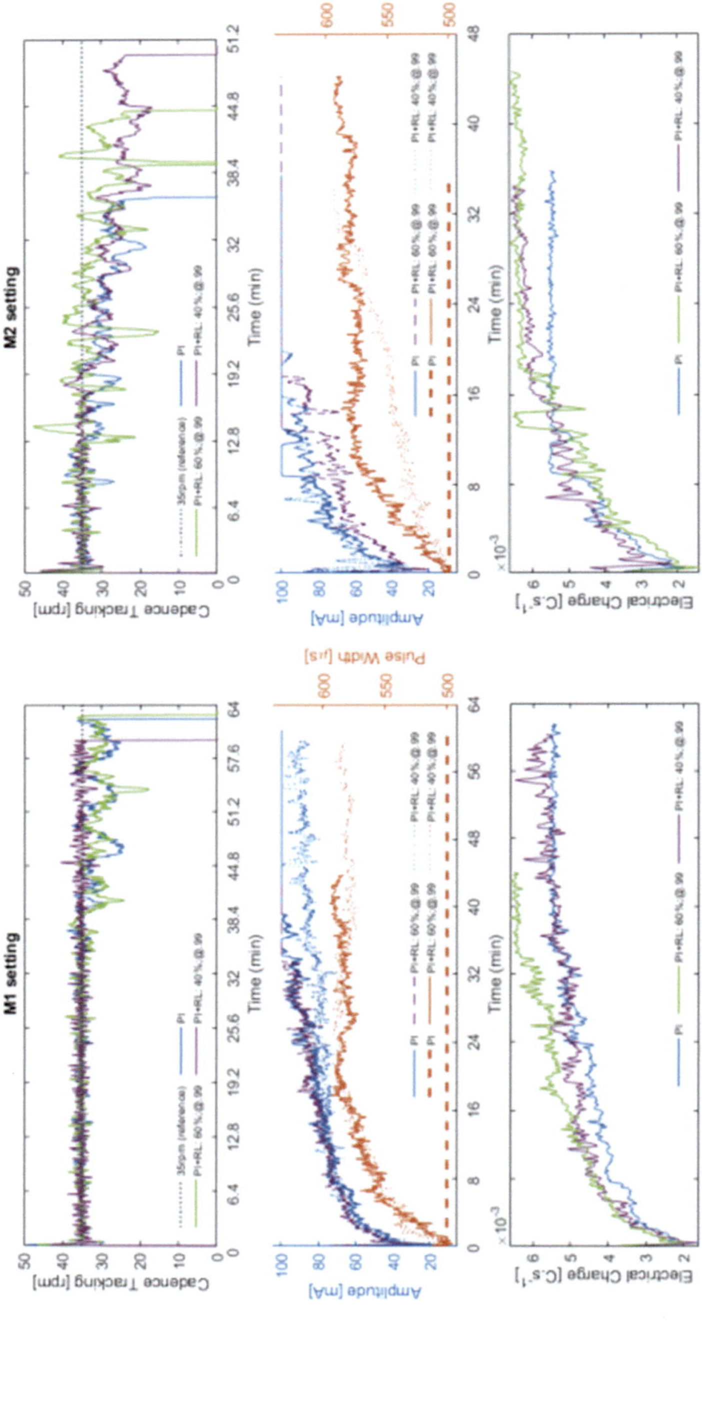

Fig. 5.10 stimulation cost analysis for determine an algorithm performance for FES-cycling race competition. (Coelho-Magalhães et al. [10])

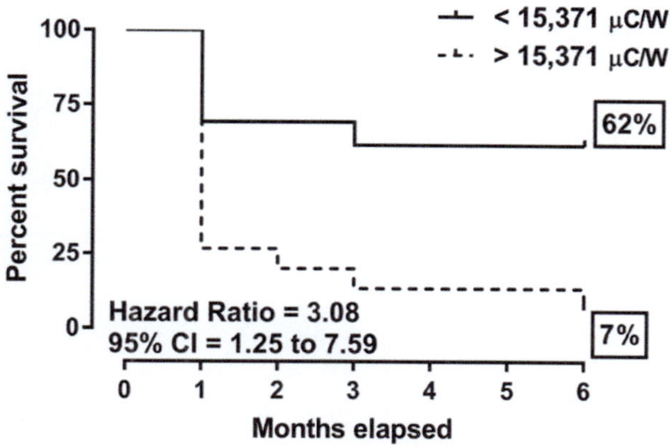

Fig. 5.11 Kaplan–Meier survival curve for stimulation cost in mechanically ventilated patients. Higher values indicate worst prognosis. CI, confidence interval; μC/W, microcoulombs per watt. (Figueiredo et al. [4])

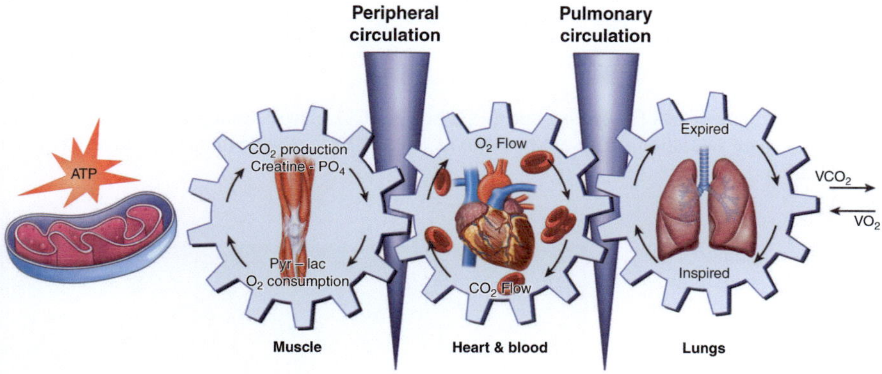

Fig. 5.12 Wasserman's model: physiological gears of oxygen uptake, transport, and metabolism during exercise. ATP, adenosine triphosphate; CO_2, carbon dioxide; O_2, oxygen; VCO_2, carbon dioxide output; VO_2, oxygen uptake. (Ferguson et al. [15])

utilizes oxygen to generate movement [20]. Evidence suggests that different muscle activation patterns during constant-power FES-cycling lead to varying oxygen costs [20], underscoring the importance of protocol selection in promoting more efficient oxygen utilization.

Energy cost reflects the total energy expenditure during FES-cycling, encompassing both aerobic and anaerobic contributions [19, 21], and can be estimated using Weir's equation [22], which calculates energy expenditure from VO_2 and VCO_2 as follows: $(3.941 \times VO_2) + (1.106 \times VCO_2)$, with both gases measured in liters per minute. In a 16-week randomized controlled trial, Farkas et al. (2021) found that individuals with SCI who engaged in regular FES-cycling showed significant gains in CRF and energy expenditure, with improved energy cost efficiency contributing to enhanced overall fitness over time [19].

Further important parameters in FES-cycling employed to assess exercise efficiency and cardiorespiratory demands include metabolic cost and metabolic

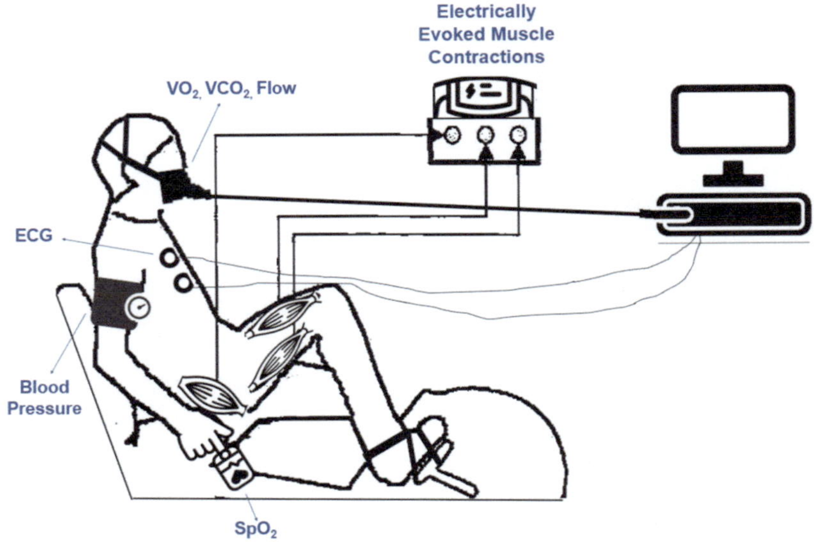

Fig. 5.13 Schematic of FES-cycling and CPET setup. ECG, electrocardiogram; SpO_2, peripheral capillary oxygen saturation; VCO_2, carbon dioxide output; VO_2, oxygen uptake. (Source: Prepared by the authors)

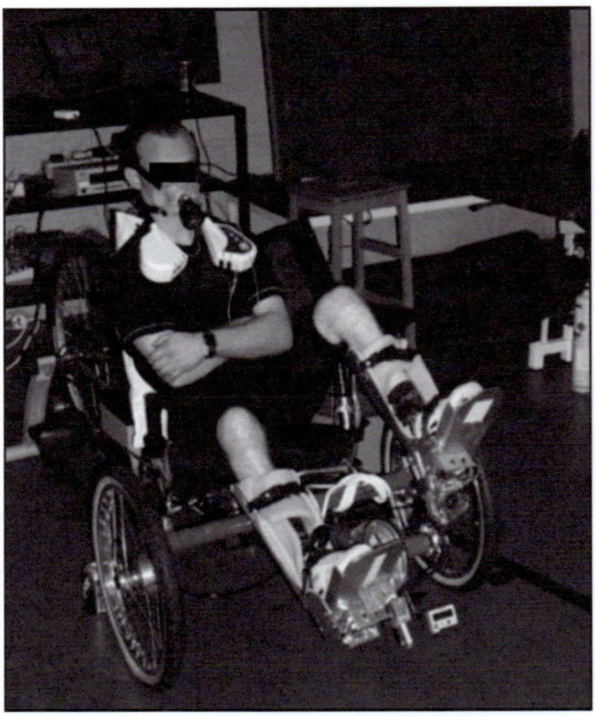

Fig. 5.14 Example of a FES-cycling setup with stimulation equipment and a CPET system. (Hunt et al. [18])

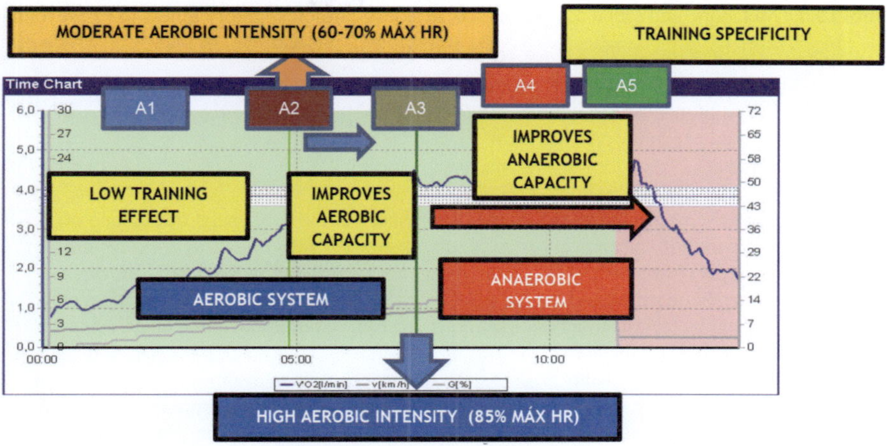

Fig. 5.15 Distribution of intensity based on heart rate. (Source: Prepared by the authors)

efficiency. *Metabolic cost* reflects the internal energy expenditure of the body, estimated from oxygen uptake (VO_2) and the corresponding substrate utilization [21, 23]. *Metabolic efficiency*, typically expressed as a percentage, is the ratio between the mechanical useful work produced during FES-cycling—which is the external power measured at the cranks (torque × angular velocity)—and the metabolic energy cost required to generate this output (derived from oxygen consumption during steady-state aerobic exercise) [9, 14]. Hence, a higher metabolic efficiency indicates that more mechanical work is produced for a given metabolic cost.

It is calculated as [9]:

$$\text{Metabolic Efficiency} = \eta = \text{Useful work done} / \text{Metabolic energy cost}^{*}100\%.$$

Table 5.1 provides a summary of the metabolic and efficiency parameters pertinent to the evaluation of CRF during FES-cycling.

Notably, studies have shown that FES-cycling can elicit moderate to vigorous intensity levels. For example, individuals with multiple sclerosis reached about 63.5% of their VO_2peak during sessions, demonstrating substantial aerobic engagement and indicating that active FES-cycling provides a sufficient stimulus to enhance CRF [24]. Then, some protocols incorporate exercise testing with ventilatory thresholds and VO_2peak measurements adapted to the patient's capacity, providing valuable guidance for planning effective cardiorespiratory rehabilitation.

Additionally, assessing mechanical output through measures such as work rate and power output during FES-cycling provides objective information about exercise intensity, while subjective indicators like the rating of perceived exertion (RPE) offer valuable complementary insights.

A recent systematic review confirmed that FES-cycling exercise yields significant benefits across multiple health and fitness-related outcomes in individuals with spinal cord injury, including improvements in CRF, muscle health, power output, and other physiological parameters [25].

Table 5.1 Metabolic and efficiency parameters to assess cardiorespiratory fitness in FES-cycling

Variable	Definition	Units	Primary application
Oxygen cost	Oxygen consumed per unit of mechanical output (e.g., per watt or per meter)	mLO_2/min/W or mLO_2/kg/m	Assesses aerobic economy (oxygen efficiency). "H*ow much oxygen is used"*
Energy cost	Total energy expended per unit of mechanical output (from all metabolic pathways)	J/W or kcal/km	Assesses the total energetic demand of exercise. *"How much energy is actually used to produce movement"*—the direct energy spent to generate mechanical work
Metabolic cost	Total metabolic energy expended by the body, often estimated from oxygen uptake and caloric equivalents	kcal or J	Reflects overall metabolic load during exercise. *"How much total metabolic energy the body uses to perform the exercise"*—the overall energy expenditure from metabolic processes (including oxygen consumption and substrate use)
Metabolic efficiency	Ratio of mechanical work output to metabolic energy input; indicates how effectively energy is converted to work	%	Assesses energy conversion efficiency during exercise. "*How well that energy is converted into movement"*

Therefore, the assessment of CRF allows for precise adjustment of exercise intensity by modifying stimulation parameters such as pulse width, frequency, and intensity. This approach enables the tailoring of protocols to the individual, ensuring both clinical relevance and safety.

Cardiovascular Performance (Heart Rate, Stroke Volume, Cardiac Output, Blood Lactate and Peripheral Oxigenation)

Although FES relies on artificial stimulation, it generates a physiological muscle contraction. This contraction creates an internal training load that is proportional to the intensity of effective muscle recruitment, the duration of each contraction, and the total exercise time [26].

The internal training load generated is proportional to the prescribed external load. Depending on the training specificity, its effects can be localized—enhancing neuromuscular fitness—or systemic—improving cardiorespiratory fitness [27].

To improve physical fitness, external load stimuli must induce a degree of overload that is progressively increased over time. Table 5.2 presents the conceptual definitions related to the body's physiological responses to physical training stimuli [27].

FES-cycling enables neuromuscular electrical stimulation to be applied to specific motor points, generating coordinated muscle contractions that produce pedaling on a cycle ergometer. This activity induces mechanical strain and localized muscle stress, while also contributing to cardiovascular effects through enhanced

Table 5.2 Conceptual definitions related to organic responses to physical stimuli [27]

Term	Definition
Training load	Training load is the term used by sports scientists, coaches, physical therapists, athletes and patients as an elaborated variable of a stimulus that will generate a desired training response Training load accommodates a variety of metrics that can be described as external or internal, depending on whether the measurable aspect in question is internal or external to the individual
External training load	It implicitly refers to the external training load performed by an individual. The external load was defined as the physical work prescribed in the training and/or treatment plan. Consequently, the term external load accommodates quantification and prescription in a variety of ways, allowing the use of a wide range of external load measures and metrics. Some common measures of external load include GPS -derived units (e.g., speed, accelerations, etc.) and resistance level
Internal training load	Internal load usually refers to the psycophysiological stress experienced by an individual. It can be measured by specific metrics such as heart rate and blood lactate. However, measurements of these variables must be correlated with corresponding variables, for example: heart rate is a valid measure of internal load for cardiovascular cycle training, but not so much for muscular strength training
Psycho-physiological load	Refers to the physicophysiological stress experienced by an individual in response to a given external load. The most common physicophysiological measure is the rate of perceived exertion (RPE)
Mechanical load	Refers to the forces experienced by specific tissues or biological structures and may be external or internal, originating form, for example, collision with an opponent or muscle pulling on bone. Mechanical loading is the stimulus that results in the mechanical loading responses (stress and deformation)
Stress	Stress is defined as the force per unit area and develops within a structure/tissue in response to externally applied mechanical loads (force). Strain is descriptive of the internal forces that neighboring particles of a given material exert on each other. Stress can be characterized as normal (force perpendicular to a plane) or shear (force parallel to a plane). Normal stress can be tensile or compressive, depending on the mode of loading
Strain	Refers to the amount of deformation expressed as a normalized change in shape or size. Two basic types of strain exist: Normal strain, which is related to the change in length, and shear strain, which is related to the change in angle

venous return and joint mobilization—particularly in the knee. Additionally, FES-cycling promotes physiological responses such as increased heart rate, stroke volume, and cardiac output [28].

Heart Rate

Heart rate during FES-cycling exercise increases proportionally to the applied training load. Figure 5.15 illustrates the monitoring of intensity distribution, which can be used to prescribe training zones based on heart rate during cycling sessions.

Exercise prescription using FES-cycling primarily promotes training at level A1. This approach is especially beneficial for patients with low functional capacity and limited tolerance to high-intensity exercise. The modest increase in heart rate observed with FES-cycling is due to the neuromuscular nature of the stimulus. However, it is important to note that, compared to passive pedaling, the addition of FES significantly enhances heart rate response [28].

Training intensity can be monitored through continuous electrocardiographic tracing or with portable devices such as heart rate monitors or fingertip pulse oximeters.

Stroke Volume

During FES-cycling exercise, an increase in stroke volume is typically observed, primarily as a result of enhanced preload. When performed during a CPET analysis, this hemodynamic response can be indirectly assessed through oxygen pulse variable. Figure 5.16 presents the oxygen pulse curve obtained via metabolic gas analysis.

It is important to emphasize that a decline in stroke volume during exercise may signal myocardial ischemia—even prior to ST-segment changes detectable on electrocardiographic tracing. Furthermore, patients with heart failure, particularly those with reduced ejection fraction, commonly exhibit diminished stroke volume and reduced tolerance to physical exertion. Notably, when compared to passive pedaling, the inclusion of FES has been shown to enhance stroke volume, demonstrating its added physiological benefit [28].

In patients with cardiomyopathy, FES-cycling does not appear to increase stroke volume. However, in individuals with normal ventricular function, the pedaling motion induced by FES suggests a potential for gradual increases in stroke volume. Figure 5.16 illustrates the oxygen pulse curve obtained through metabolic gas analysis [29].

Cardiac Output

Conceptually, the increase in cardiac output induced by FES-cycling parallels the mechanisms behind stroke volume enhancement. This increase is proportional to

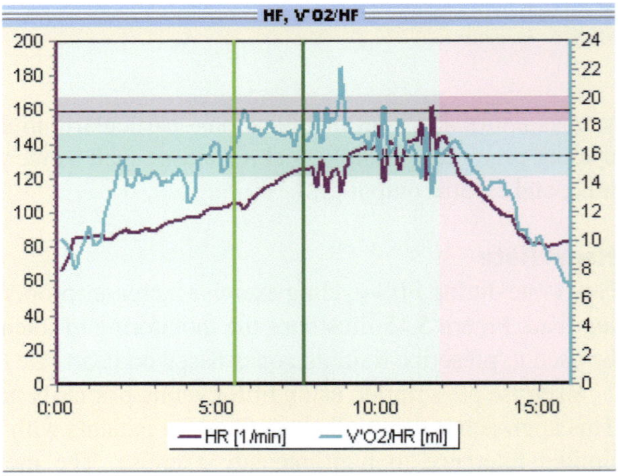

Fig. 5.16 Oxygen pulse graph obtained through metabolic gas analysis. (Source: The authors)

the internal training load, which depends on factors such as the intensity of electrical stimulation, exercise duration, patient's physical condition, and presence of underlying cardiovascular diseases. Patients with low functional capacity generally exhibit reduced peripheral oxygen consumption. An individual's exercise capacity is directly related to their functional status; for example, athletes can mobilize higher cardiac output, sometimes accompanied by increased cardiac chamber dimensions. Studies have demonstrated that FES-cycling can effectively increase cardiac output both in healthy individuals and in patients with spinal cord injury [29].

There are several techniques that can be used non-invasively to monitor cardiac output during a FES-cycling exercise assessment. Among these, the following stand out: 1. Transthoracic echocardiogram, which can be performed during physical exertion. This method allows the assessment of cardiac output and myocardial contractility; 2. Non-invasive cardiac output monitors: A) Nexfin: Uses continuous blood pressure technology to estimate cardiac output; B) Finometer: uses continuous blood pressure technology to estimate cardiac output. It is important to consider that the accuracy and reliability of these methods may vary depending on the operator's skill and the specific technology used. Furthermore, compared to passive pedaling, the addition of FES has been shown to significantly increase cardiac output [13].

Blood Lactate

Lactate levels can be measured by collecting a venous blood sample or by obtaining a drop of blood from the patient's fingertip or earlobe. Portable devices allow analysis by applying the blood drop to a specialized test strip (Fig. 5.17). Lactate values

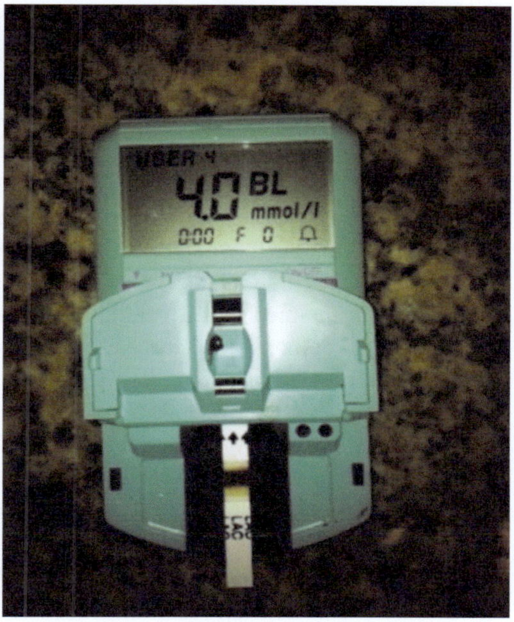

Fig. 5.17 Portable device for blood lactate analysis. (Source: The authors)

below 4.0 mmol/L indicate that the activity is predominantly supported by the aerobic energy system. Values above this threshold suggest that the activity relies primarily on the lactic or anaerobic energy system [26].

To guide exercise prescription based on the lactate threshold, an incremental load test with blood lactate measurements at each stage is recommended. This field test is commonly used in physical training and rehabilitation settings. It is important to note that previous studies have shown that when large muscle groups are electrically stimulated, synaptic fatigue may occur before metabolic fatigue. As a result, patients may experience functional impairment in maintaining movements even in the absence of metabolic changes such as lactic acidosis [26].

Peripheral Oxygenation

Peripheral muscle oxygen extraction results vary depending on the analysis method used. Analysis based on arterial-mixed venous oxygen content difference demonstrated a clinically significant advantage for FES-cycling. However, Near-Infrared Spectroscopy (NIRS) analysis did not reveal a clear superiority of FES-cycling. Still, a clinically relevant trend favoring FES-cycling over passive cycling was observed.

NIRS enables non-invasive monitoring of tissue oxygenation and oxygen extraction, including in the brain. This technique uses near-infrared light to assess interactions with hemoglobin, providing indicators of oxygen saturation and extraction [30].

Ventilatory Capacity

Integrating FES-cycling with ventilatory assessment offers a valuable approach to evaluating ventilatory capacity in diverse clinical populations, particularly in individuals with limited mobility or impaired pulmonary function [13, 24, 31–33]. By enabling controlled exercise through electrically evoked muscle contractions, FES-cycling combined with a non-invasive respiratory monitoring system (with or without gas exchange analysis) allows for the assessment of ventilatory responses to exercise, including minute ventilation (VE), tidal volume, and breathing frequency, even in patients unable to voluntarily perform traditional aerobic exercise. Evidence supports its use in individuals with spinal cord injuries, neuromuscular diseases, and those requiring mechanical ventilation, for instance [3, 24, 32].

Frazão et al. demonstrated in healthy individuals that this combined approach effectively stimulates and assesses ventilatory capacity during exercise, as evidenced by significant increases in VE by 115 ± 26%, tidal volume by 46 ± 20 mL, and respiratory frequency, surpassing the responses observed with neuromuscular electrical stimulation (NMES) alone and passive cycling (Fig. 5.18 [28].

From a physiological perspective, the ventilatory response during exercise is primarily governed by factors that regulate arterial carbon dioxide levels ($PaCO_2$), including the rate of muscular metabolism and the activation of central respiratory control mechanisms [34]. In this context, FES-cycling has the potential to enhance

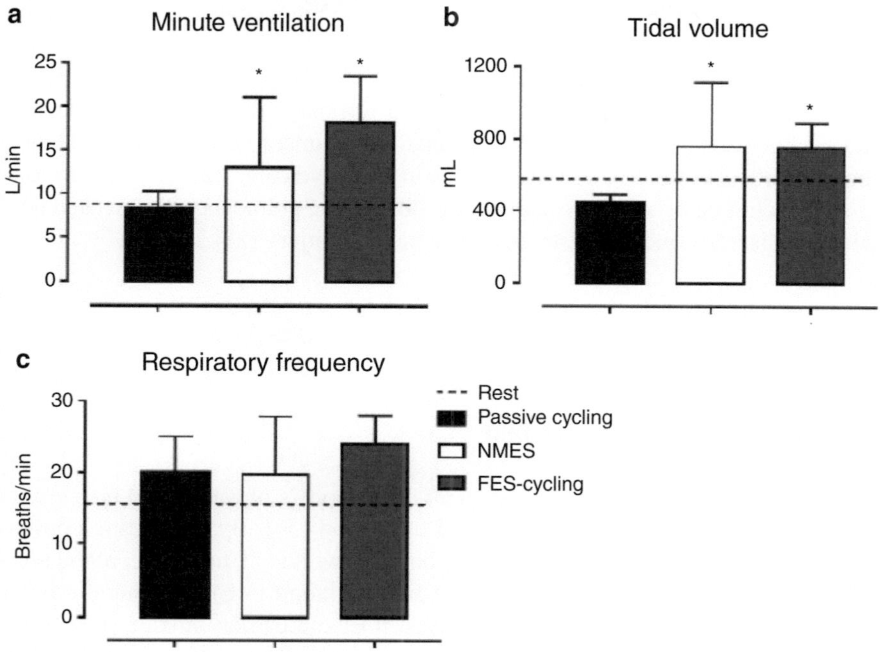

Fig. 5.18 Ventilatory responses during FES-cycling compared to passive cycling and NMES in healthy individuals. NMES, neuromuscular electrical stimulation. *$P < 0.05$ compared to rest. (Frazão et al. [28])

ventilatory activity by increasing CO_2 production, which may stimulate central chemoreceptors and carotid bodies, thereby leading to elevated VE through increases in both tidal volume and respiratory frequency [35]. Importantly, stimulation of proprioceptors, muscle spindles, and possibly nociceptors contributes to the early ventilatory response during FES-cycling, as evidenced by an immediate increase in VE following limb movement, preceding any significant metabolic changes [28]. Although protocols were performed at the highest comfortably tolerated intensity, the influence of pain on ventilation cannot be ruled out [28].

Furthermore, the measurement of VE, combined with gas analysis (as performed in CPET), also allows for the evaluation of important ventilatory efficiency parameters, such as the ventilatory equivalent for oxygen (VE/VO_2) and for carbon dioxide (VE/VCO_2). These ratios represent the volume of air required to extract 1 liter of oxygen and to eliminate 1 liter of carbon dioxide, respectively [16, 17, 31]. Lower values of VE/VO_2 and VE/VCO_2 indicate better ventilatory efficiency, meaning less air ventilation is needed to achieve gas exchange, whereas higher values may reflect ventilatory inefficiency often observed in pulmonary or cardiac conditions. Therefore, the applicability of FES-cycling assessment for this purpose in certain patient populations, such as those with chronic obstructive pulmonary disease, could become a valuable tool for pulmonary rehabilitation in this and related conditions [31].

A systematic review encompassing 52 studies demonstrated that FES-cycling leads to statistically and clinically significant improvements across multiple domains of physical fitness, including ventilatory parameters [33]. Thus, assessing ventilatory parameters alongside other physiological responses during FES-cycling provides valuable insights to guide and individualize treatment across a range of clinical conditions, including critically ill patients in intensive care, cardiopulmonary diseases like chronic heart failure and chronic obstructive pulmonary disease, and neurological disorders including stroke and spinal cord injury [28].

Other Methods of Functional Assessment Used for Measuring FES-Cycling Therapy Results

Cardiopulmonary Exercise Test

The CPET offers an integrated assessment of the body's physiological response to exertion, including oxygen transport and utilization [36]. By integrating conventional exercise test parameters (electrocardiogram, workload, heart rate, blood pressure, and symptoms) with measurements of ventilation (VE), peripheral oxygen saturation, and expired gas analysis (oxygen [O_2] and carbon dioxide [CO_2]), the method provides a comprehensive assessment of clinical, hemodynamic, electrocardiographic, and ventilatory responses [16, 17, 37–39]. Thus, it stands out as a valuable and cost-effective tool for gathering clinically relevant variables, supporting its widespread use in both clinical practice and research, for assessing CRF, stratifying risk, and guiding personalized, phenotype-based exercise prescription [16, 17, 39].

Methodologically, CPET uses two systems—electrocardiographic recording and measurement of ventilation with expired gases (VO_2 and VCO_2)—with gas analysis performed either breath-by-breath or via a mixing chamber. The treadmill and cycle ergometer are the most common ergometers [17, 38]. In summary, the test requires the participant to perform exercise with gradually increasing intensity until volitional exhaustion or the appearance of limiting symptoms and/or signs [38].

Ramp protocols (with gradual, continuous load increases) are preferred over stepwise protocols for more accurate assessment of exercise capacity [16, 17, 38]. The ramp slope should be tailored to the individual's estimated tolerance to ensure a test duration between 8 and 12 minutes, yielding valid and reproducible results [16, 17, 38]. Inadequate load progression can underestimate true maximal capacity, as VO_{2peak} validity declines with protocols that are too short or too long [16, 40].

The main variables and their interrelationships are systematically summarized in the nine-panel display proposed by Wasserman and colleagues [17, 41, 42] which enables a reliable and structured interpretation, allowing for optimized presentation of CPET results. Figure 5.19 illustrates one of the panel arrangements that is widely adopted and commonly included in CPET software-generated reports. Panels are numbered 1 to 9, arranged top-to-bottom and left-to-right. Panels 1–3 present cardiovascular and oxygen transport data; Panels 4, 6, and 7 address pulmonary gas exchange and ventilation/perfusion mismatch; Panels 5 and 9 show ventilatory

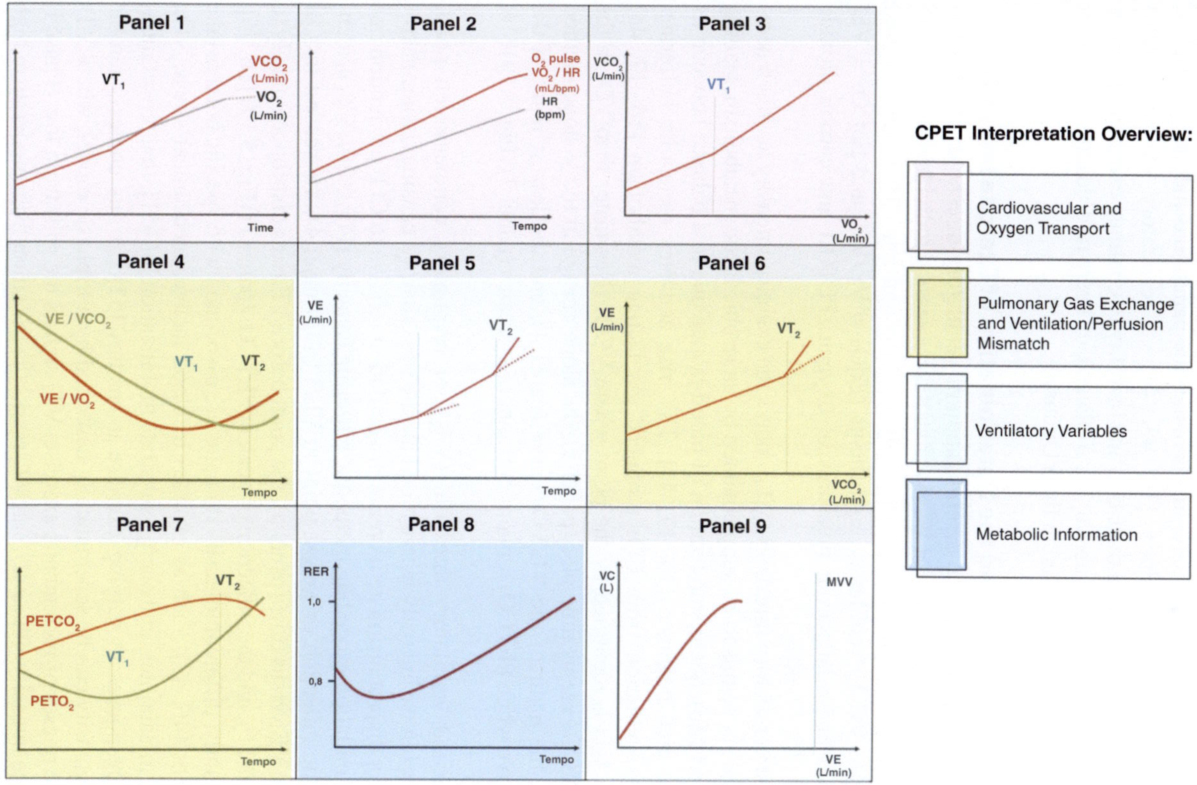

Fig. 5.19 9-panel plot in CPET: interpretation Overview And Threshold Identification. *CPET* cardiopulmonary exercise test, *HRpeak* peak heart rate, *MVV* maximum voluntary ventilation, $PETCO_2$ end-tidal carbon dioxide partial pressure, $PETO_2$ end-tidal oxygen partial pressure, *RER* respiratory exchange ratio, VCO_2 carbon dioxide output, *VE* ventilation, VO_2 oxygen uptake, VT_1 first ventilatory threshold, VT_2 second ventilatory threshold. (Source: Prepared by the authors)

variables; and Panel 8 displays metabolic information via the RER (VCO_2/VO_2), which reflects exercise intensity. It is important to note that, although a suggested layout exists, the specific arrangement of the charts may vary.

Moreover, for accurate interpretation and application of the test, it is essential that the professional is able to identify whether the patient has met the criteria for maximal effort, which include [16, 43, 44]: a respiratory exchange ratio (RER) ≥ 1.10; clear signs of exhaustion and inability to continue exercising; a Borg rating of perceived exertion above 17; a plateau in heart rate despite increasing exercise intensity; and a plateau in the VO_2 curve.

Ventilatory Thresholds and the Determination of Exercise Intensity

Figure 5.19 also illustrates the determination of ventilatory thresholds (VTs) from CPET data. The identification of VTs is crucial for assessing individual responses to incremental exercise and requires the analysis of the multiple CPET panels, based on VE, VO_2, VCO_2, ventilatory equivalents ($EqO_2 = VE/VO_2$ and $EqCO_2 = VE/VCO_2$), and end-tidal partial pressures of oxygen ($PETO_2$) and carbon dioxide ($PETCO_2$) [16, 17, 45].

The first ventilatory threshold (VT_1) marks the exercise intensity at which aerobic metabolism begins to be supplemented by anaerobic lactic metabolism, leading to a rise and subsequent stabilization of blood lactate due to a balance between its production and clearance [16, 17, 45]. This rise activates metabolic buffering, increasing ventilation from CO_2 produced via lactate metabolism [16, 17, 45] (Fig. 5.2). VT_1 is identified by the point where VCO_2 rises faster than VO_2 in the VO_2 and VCO_2 versus time plot (panel 1), the slope change in the V-slope method (panel 3), the nadir of the VE/VO_2 curve (panel 4), and the lowest point of the $PETO_2$ curve while $PETCO_2$ remains constant or increases (panel 7) (Fig. 5.19) [16, 17, 45].

The second ventilatory threshold (VT_2), or respiratory compensation point, marks the exercise intensity where blood lactate rises sharply, causing tissue anaerobiosis and a disproportionate increase in ventilation relative to CO_2 production due to H^+ accumulation exceeding metabolic buffering capacity (Fig. 5.20). VT_2 is identified by the inflection or lowest point in VE/VCO_2 (panel 4), the second loss of linearity in VE versus time (panel 5), the point before VE rises disproportionately to VCO_2 (panel 6), and the inflection or peak in $PETCO_2$ (panel 7) (Fig. 5.19) [16, 45].

Importantly, different intensity domains are associated with specific homeostatic disturbances [46, 47], such as changes in blood lactate, mechanical stress, VO_2, heart rate, metabolites, and energy substrate mobilization [46–51], that reflect intramuscular responses to varying exercise intensities [52]. In this context, aerobic exercise intensity can be schematically described by a triphasic model, where VTs mark three phases of incremental exercise: VT_1 signals the shift from low (Phase I) to moderate intensity (Phase II), and VT_2 marks the transition from moderate to high intensity (Phase III) [17, 39, 45]. Figure 5.20 summarizes the physiological responses to incremental exercise based on this model, including a schematic representation of the underlying metabolic processes.

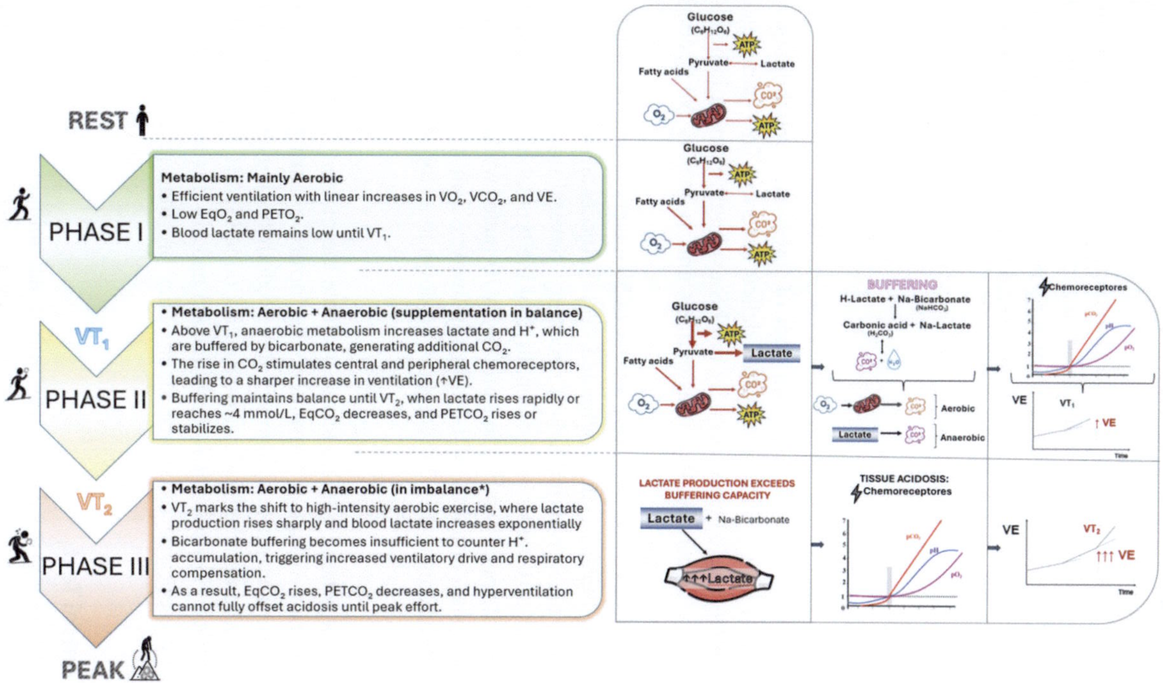

Fig. 5.20 Triphasic model of aerobic exercise intensity: physiological and metabolic overview. *ATP* adenosine triphosphate, *CO_2* carbon dioxide, *H* hydrogen ion (H^+), *$EqVCO_2$* ventilatory carbon dioxide equivalent, *EqO_2* ventilatory oxygen equivalent, *H_2O* water; Na, sodium ion (Na^+), *O_2* Oxygen, *pCO_2* partial pressure of carbon dioxide, *pH* potential of hydrogen, *pO_2* partial pressure of oxygen, *VE* ventilation, *VCO_2* carbon dioxide output, *VT_1* first ventilatory threshold, *VT_2* second ventilatory threshold, *$PETO_2$* partial pressure of end-tidal oxygen, *$PETCO_2$* end-tidal partial pressure of carbon dioxide. The variation in arrow thickness indicates fluctuations in contributions from different energy pathways. *The term “imbalance” refers to lactate production exceeding its breakdown/removal rate (Source: Prepared by the authors)

Hence, CPET is widely regarded as the gold standard for determining exercise intensity, with threshold-based method recommended for its ability to accurately quantify intensity by capturing the body's physiological responses to exercise—particularly oxygen transport and utilization—thus allowing for a more individualized, phenotype-based approach [17, 36, 39, 45, 53, 54].

Of note, VTs determination may be constrained by interobserver variability and practical challenges, especially in elderly, deconditioned, or chronic heart failure patients, and in those with comorbidities such as advanced pulmonary or peripheral arterial disease, or marked muscle weakness from surgery or cancer cachexia [17, 36, 39, 55]. Nonetheless, when evaluated by experienced professionals, the coefficient of variation is relatively low [17, 40, 53].

Mobility

Gait Speed

Restoration of walking is considered the main goal of lower limb rehabilitation, with gait speed regarded as a reliable marker of deficit severity. This parameter measurement is frequently evaluated, especially in FES-cycling treatment in hemiparetic patients [56–58]. Generally, the measurement unit is meters per second (m/s) and can be assessed by different ways:

The gait speed can be measured by timing a walk of 50 meters with a stopwatch, being regarded as zero if the test is not completed [59]. Subjects are asked to walk at a self-selected speed, using walking aids if necessary. Several times this test is chosen because a 50-meter distance is representative of the typical indoor walking need of patients. The gait speed can be measured by a 10-meter walking test also. The walking course consists of a total of 14 m in a hallway: a 2-m warm-up, 10 m used for the speed measurement, and 2 m for slowing down to a stop [60].

Motricity Index

The motricity index is a general clinical test to evaluate the mobility of the ankle, knee, and hip joints during voluntary movements performed against gravity or an external resistance [59]. The method involves the strength testing of six muscle actions using a modification of the Medical Research Council (MRC) system [61]. The muscle actions (ankle dorsiflexion, knee extension and hip flexion) are graded based on movement present and resistance taken. They are then given weighted scores (Table 5.3):

Upright Motor Control Test

The upright motor control test is used to assess functional abilities of the impaired leg during single-limb standing. Voluntary control of the hip, knee, and ankle of the involved lower extremity is tested with the subject standing. Extension is graded on a three-point scale according to the patient's ability to extend the knee from a flexed position while in single-limb stance. Completing the full range of extension is graded as strong 3; just supporting body weight on the flexed knee is a moderate

Table 5.3 Scoring of lower extremity muscle action strength using the Motricity Index

Score	Muscle action performance
0	No movement
9	Palpable contraction, but no movement
14	Movement, but not full range or against gravity
19	Movement, full range against gravity, not against resistance
25	Movement against resistance, weaker than contralateral side
33	Normal strength

grade 2; and inability to bear full weight on a flexed knee is graded as weak 1. Flexors are graded on a two-point scale: strong 3 and weak 1, based on the completion of a rapid change of flexion at each joint. The "moderate" grade 2 is omitted because according to Toman [62] it provided no additional information to that of grade 1. Each patient's hip, knee, and ankle scores is summed to provide an individual score with a maximum of 18.

Left, Knee extension: this test involves knee extension in control of body weight during single-limb stance. The patient bends both knees to approximately 30° and then lifts the unaffected leg off the ground. Knee extension grades: strong, straightens the flexed knee to full extension; moderate, supports body weight on the flexed knee; weak, unable to support body weight on the flexed knee. Right, Knee flexion: this test involves knee flexion of the unloaded leg during single-limb stance. The patient stands as straight as possible and brings the knee and foot on the affected side up toward the chest as high and as fast as possible, repeated three times. Knee flexor grades: strong, joint flexes more than 60°; weak, joint flexes less than 60° or cannot complete three efforts in 10 seconds [63]. Perry et al. [63].

Gross Motor Function

The mobility and gross motor skills of people with cerebral palsy can be measured by gross motor function measurement (GMFM) and/or Gross Motor Function Classification System (GMFCS).

The GMFCS looks at movements like sitting and walking. It provides a clear description of someone's current motor function, and an idea of what equipment or mobility aids a child or adult may need in the future, like crutches, a walker, or a wheelchair. It is graded in five levels [64] (Fig. 5.21).

Physical Function in Intensive Care Test Score (PFIT-S)

The PFIT-s is a battery of tests used to measure endurance, strength, cardiovascular capacity, and functional level in hospitalized patients (critically ill) [65]. The tasks performed are the level of assistance from sit to stand; step cadence (steps/minute) and muscle strength. It is scored on a continuous scale of 0 (worst) to 10 (best) (Tables 5.4 and 5.5). The PFIT-s is a safe and inexpensive test of physical function with high clinical utility. It is valid, responsive to change, and predictive of key outcomes.

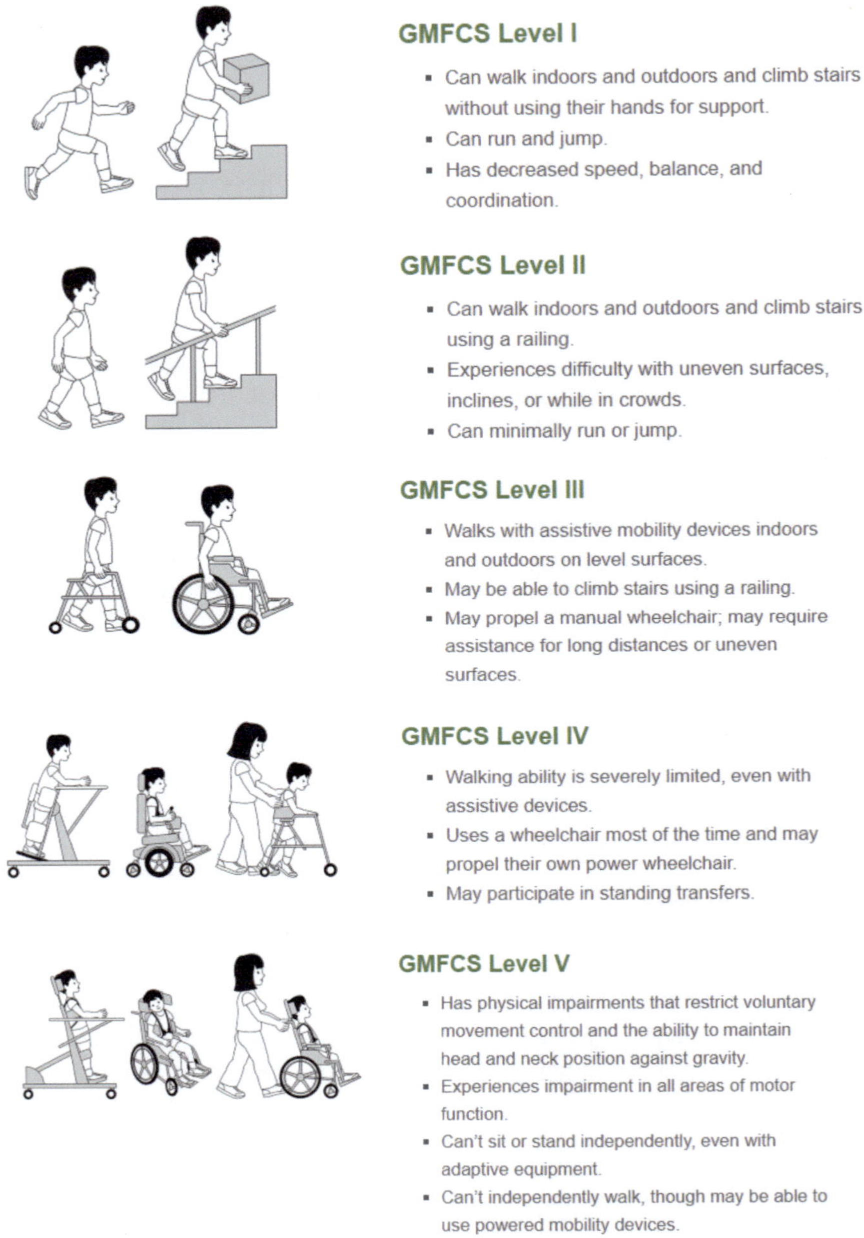

Fig. 5.21 Gross Motor Function Classification System (GMFCS) levels. (Available at: https://cparf.org/what-is-cerebral-palsy/severity-of-cerebral-palsy/gross-motor-function-classification-system-gmfcs/?psafe_param=1&gad_source=1&gclid=Cj0KCQiA19e8BhCVARIsALpFMgFaYISSJLxqiKa4KQYfKOgBJSaFVExh6Z3IwqCBFvJ_cNZMMQqW0KQaAph9EALw_wcB)

Tables 5.4 and 5.5 Original PFIT-s [65].

Classification of Component Scores Used in the Physical Function ICU Test (Scored) (PFIT-s) Ordinal Score

PFIT-s Components			
Assistance	**Cadence (steps/min)**	**Shoulder Strength**[a]	**Knee Strength**[b]
0=unable	0=unable	0=grade 0, 1, or 2	0=grade 0, 1, or 2
1=assist × 2	1=>0–49	1=grade 3	1=grade 3
2=assist × 1	2=50–<80	2=grade 4	2=grade 4
3=no assistance	3=80+	3=grade 5	3=grade 5

[a] Maximum strength of left or right shoulder flexion using the Oxford grading system.
[b] Maximum strength of left or right knee extension using the Oxford grading system.

Ordinal Scores and Equivalent Interval Scores for the Physical Function ICU Test (Scored) (PFIT-s)[a]

Scale	PFIT-s Score												
Ordinal	0	1	2	3	4	5	6	7	8	9	10	11	12
Interval	0	2	3.2	3.9	4.4	4.9	5.4	5.9	6.4	7.1	7.9	8.8	10

[a] Algorithm for conversion from ordinal to interval score=5.418 + (1.068 × logit location of ordinal score).

Spasticity

Pedulum Test

The pendulum test provides a straightforward method for assessing spasticity by utilizing gravity to induce the stretch reflex of the knee muscles. In this test, the lower leg is dropped from a resting horizontal position, and its oscillatory movement is observed. The patient is instructed to relax, allowing the limb to fall freely while knee angle, joint velocity, and muscle activity are recorded [66]. The test's simplicity, combined with the use of commonly available sensors such as electromyography (EMG) with video, goniometers, or even accessible devices like the Wii remote, has made it an objective and reliable tool for quantifying spasticity in the knee extensors [67] (Fig. 5.22).

Because spasticity is velocity-dependent, the initial and second swings of the pendulum test are considered crucial for detecting it [66]. The maximum angular velocity of the knee occurs during the first flexion oscillation, which is the most sensitive to changes in spasticity in the quadriceps. This first excursion (F1amp) is particularly useful for identifying differences in spasticity. Researchers like Bajd and Vodovnik [66] refined this approach by dividing F1amp by the plateau angle to calculate the relaxation index (RI) [67], which adjusts for changes in muscle length and structure resulting from ongoing spasticity or activity-induced shifts in tonic reflex. Stillman and McMeeken [68] introduced the extension relaxation index (ERI), along with its characteristic amplitude (E1amp), which describes the excursion of the first return extension oscillation. While theoretically sensitive to flexor spasticity, there is limited evidence supporting the use of ERI/E1amp in clinical studies [67].

Ashworth Scale

Ashworth has described a five-point ordinal scale for grading the resistance encountered during such passive muscle stretching [69]. Ashworth's scale grades spasticity as follows: 0 = normal muscle tone; 1 = slight increase in muscle tone, "catch" when

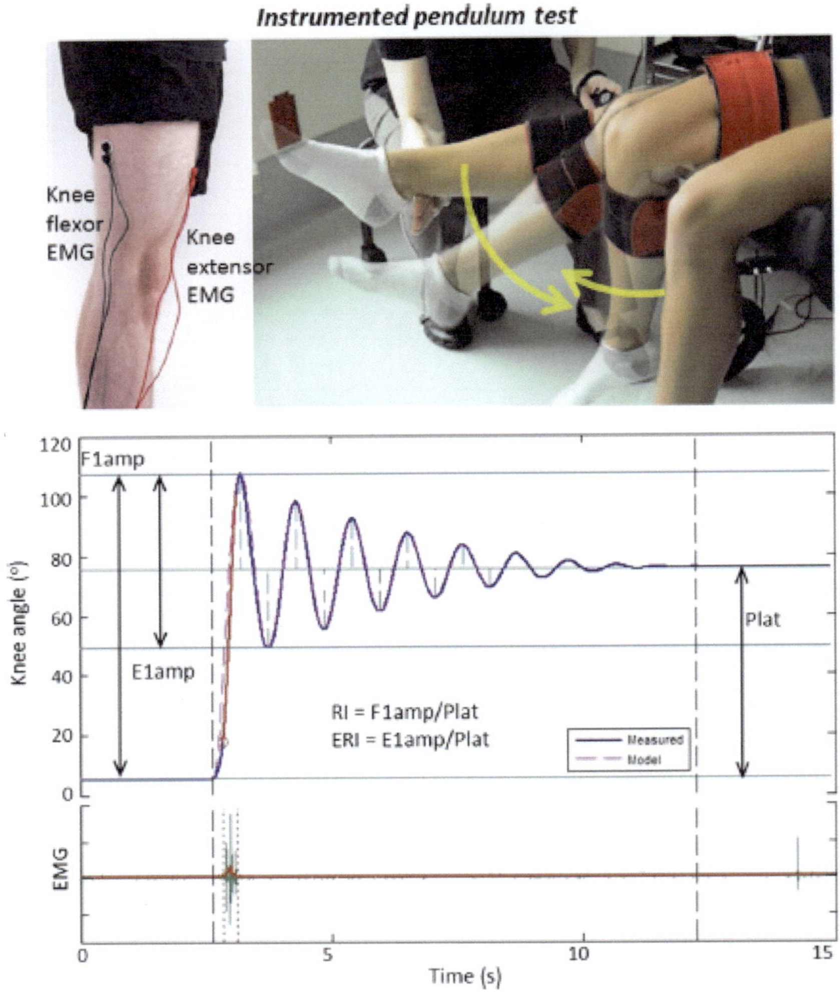

Fig. 5.22 BioTone™ toolkit for lower-extremity assessment of spasticity using the pendulum test. Top: Electromyographic (EMG) electrodes are placed on extensor and flexor muscles and used to ensure muscle relation prior to the start of testing and to monitor involuntary contractions during the test, and fiber-optic goniometer (FOG) system used to measure knee angle during the pendulum test. Bottom: Pendulum test metrics include the plateau angle (Plat), first flexion amplitude (F1amp), and first extension amplitude (E1amp) which are used to compute the relaxation index (RI) and the extension relaxation index (ERI). (Whelan et al. [67])

limb moved; 2 = more marked increase in muscle tone, but limb easily flexed; 3 = considerable increase in muscle tone; and 4 = limb rigid in flexion or extension. As Ashworth's scale assigns grades to a manually determined resistance of muscle to passive stretching, it measures spasticity as defined herein.

The scale, therefore, demonstrates face validity, along with several other characteristics recommended for ordinal scales by MacKenzie and Charlson [70]. However,

Table 5.6 Modified Ashworth scale for grading spasticity

Grade	Description
0	No increase in muscle tone
1	Slight increase in muscle tone, manifested by a catch and release or by minimal resistance at the end of the range of motion when the affected part(s) is moved in flexion or extension
1+	Slight increase in muscle tone, manifested by a catch, followed by minimal resistance throughout the remainder (less than half) of the range of motion (ROM)
2	More marked increase in muscle tone through most of the ROM, but affected part(s) easily moved
3	Considerable increase in muscle tone, passive movement difficult
4	Affected part(s) rigid in flexion or extension

many hemiplegic patients exhibits spasticity levels that are often classified at the lower end of the Ashworth scale, with the grade "1" being too vague. To enhance the scale's precision, a new grade, "1+" made slight adjustments to the definitions (Modified Ashworth Scale) (Table 5.6). These changes have resulted in a scale that aligns more closely with the guidelines set forth by MacKenzie and Charlson, offering a more refined and discrete measure of spasticity compared to the original Ashworth scale.

Technological Tools for Assessment

Cycle Ergometers with Integrated Feedback to Measure Patient Power, Resistance and Progression

Cycle ergometers with integrated feedback are stationary bicycles equipped with sensors and electronic systems that measure and display, in real time, data such as power, resistance, and patient progress. These devices are widely used in rehabilitation, physical therapy, sports training, and medical research, as they allow for detailed monitoring of the user's physical evolution. There are three main aspects for monitoring:

Power Measurement (Pedaling Force)

Power is the amount of energy generated while pedaling. This measurement is expressed in watts (W) and depends on two main factors:

- Force applied to the pedals—The greater the force exerted, the higher the power generated.
- Pedal rotation speed (cadence)—The faster the pedaling, the power can increase, as long as the resistance is maintained.

Cycle ergometers are equipped with strain gauges (tension meters) that detect the force applied to the pedals or servo motors that provides real-time information. Additionally, the rotation of the pedals is recorded to calculate total power.

Resistance Control (Pedaling Difficulty)

Resistance determines how difficult it will be to pedal. It can be adjusted either manually or automatically, depending on the evaluation objectives. If the cycle ergometer is programmed to maintain a fixed power level (isopower), it can increase resistance when the patient reduces the cycling cadence, ensuring that the effort remains balanced.

Feedback and Progress Monitoring

Integrated feedback is one of the major advantages of modern cycle ergometers. It allows both the patient and healthcare professional to track performance in real time.

Key data monitors include:

- Power generated (W)—Indicates the patient's effort.
- Cadence (RPM)—Measures the number of revolutions per minute the patient is pedaling.
- Heart rate—Monitored by sensors on the handlebars or chest straps.
- Training time and distance covered—Used to evaluate endurance.

In addition, these data are stored and compared over time, allowing for the monitoring of patient progress. Some equipment even integrates with virtual reality and interactive games to make training more motivating.

Data Analysis Software

Software used for FES-cycling-based functional assessment plays a vital role in facilitating the evaluation of muscle strength, endurance, and overall functional performance during cycling sessions. These software platforms allow for the precise control and adjustment of electrical stimulation parameters, such as intensity, frequency, and timing, to optimize the effectiveness of the functional assessment. By tracking the patient's muscle response in real time, the software enables clinicians to tailor the stimulation to each individual's needs, providing an accurate reflection of the patient's functional capacity. This helps ensure that the assessment is as objective and consistent as possible, even when the patient cannot voluntarily engage in traditional strength testing.

In addition to controlling stimulation, the software used in FES-cycling-based functional assessments often includes tools for monitoring progress and recording key data points such as pedal power, cycling speed, and muscle activation levels. These metrics are valuable for clinicians to evaluate functional improvements or setbacks over time. Advanced software systems may also incorporate analytical tools that help interpret this data, providing insights into the patient's muscle function and offering recommendations for modifications to the training or assessment protocol. By combining real-time performance monitoring with comprehensive data analysis, FES-cycling software enables a detailed, personalized approach to functional assessment, supporting more effective rehabilitation strategies.

Interpretation of Functional Assessment Results

The results obtained in functional tests and assessments can be interpreted in comparison to reference values or intra-subjects analysis.

When the aim of the evaluation is determining a therapeutic effect (comparison of pre- and post-intervention results to determine the effectiveness of FES-cycling) or disease pattern over the time, intra-subjects analysis must be done. In these situations, the patient will be the reference for himself and multiples (at least two) evaluations are necessary.

When the aim of the evaluation is determining disease severity, the results must be compared to a healthy subjects reference values. An illustrative example of this is the Figueiredo et al. study [4]. A FES-cycling based muscular evaluation method was used to detect muscle disfunction in critically ill mechanically ventilated patients. The critically ill patients were compared to a group of community recruited individuals who reported no cardiopulmonary and/or musculoskeletal morbidity. The patients and healthy subjects were paired by age, sex, and height.

Several variables can be measured during a FES-cycling based evaluation. Currently, mathematical equations for physiological values prediction are rare. However, previous published data of healthy subjects measurements may be used as reference values in daily life clinical practice. For example, Kjaer et al. [71] reported the oxygen uptake (VO_2), ventilation, heart rate, and cardiac output values in healthy young males.

Challenges in Functional Assessment of FES-Cycling

Challenges in Establishing Consistent Standards for Evaluating Different Patients

In general, FES-cycling equipment was originally developed for physical exercise rather than specific assessments. As a result, there are only a limited number of commercial devices designed to perform precise assessments. This presents a challenge in standardizing tests for inter-subject evaluations, as variability in equipment and protocols can impact the reliability and comparability of results. The lack of standardized assessment tools makes it difficult to establish consistent benchmarks for evaluating muscle function across different individuals.

Several factors contribute to this challenge, including differences in the type of electrical stimulation used, variations in cycling protocols, and patient-specific variables such as muscle tone and neurological impairments. These factors can all influence the effectiveness and accuracy of assessments, making it harder to compare results across patients or settings. To address this issue, further development of standardized FES-cycling equipment and protocols is needed to ensure more reliable and reproducible evaluations of muscle strength and function in clinical settings.

Physiological Challenges

In voluntary contractions, motor unit recruitment occurs gradually and selectively, following Henneman's size principle. This principle states that, under normal conditions, type I muscle fibers (oxidative, slow-twitch, and fatigue-resistant) are recruited first, followed by type II fibers (glycolytic, fast-twitch, and fatigue-prone) as force demands increase [72] (Fig. 5.23). This mechanism ensures efficient energy utilization, promoting greater endurance and reducing fatigue accumulation.

In contrast, electrically evoked contractions recruit muscle fibers non-selectively and simultaneously [73]. Since the electrical current directly stimulates peripheral nerves, all available motor units within the stimulation field are activated regardless of their size (Fig. 5.24). As a result, type II fibers (fast-twitch) may be recruited early, generating force rapidly but also leading to a faster onset of fatigue.

During voluntary control, motor units fire asynchronously, meaning that some muscle fibers remain active while others rest, allowing for an efficient distribution of effort and reducing fatigue. Conversely, in electrically induced contractions, all recruited motor units are activated simultaneously and synchronously, without the natural alternation observed in voluntary recruitment. This can result in an initially higher force output but also leads to rapid muscle fatigue, as the recruited fibers do not experience intermittent rest periods [74].

Additionally, in voluntary control, the central nervous system continuously adjusts contraction intensity by progressively recruiting additional motor units and modulating motor neuron firing rates as needed. This enables fine-tuned muscle force regulation and efficient movement control. In electrically induced contractions, however, contraction intensity is dictated by the parameters of the applied current (frequency, intensity, and pulse duration). As a result, muscle activation may be less efficient in terms of motor control, as the external stimulus overrides the natural modulation of the nervous system [74].

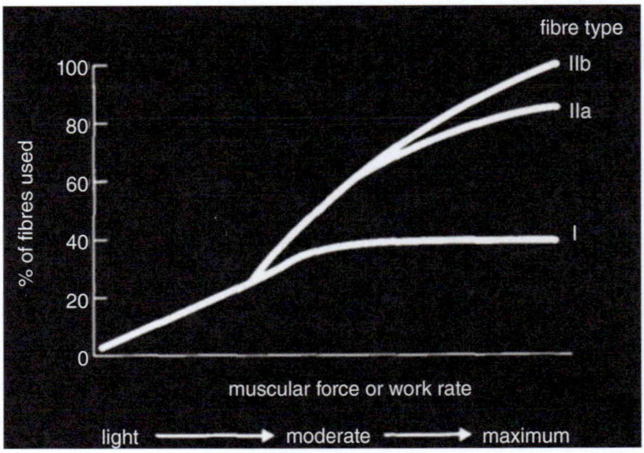

Fig. 5.23 Physiological muscle fibers recruitment according to exercise intensity. (Source: Produced by authors)

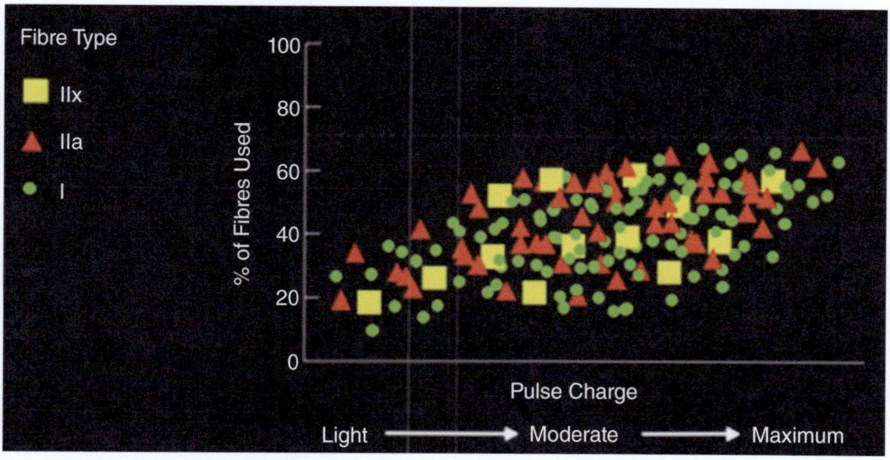

Fig. 5.24 Electrically evoked muscle fibers recruitment according to exercise intensity (Source: Produced by authors)

Conclusion

FES-cycling has emerged as a valuable tool for both rehabilitation and functional assessment, especially in individuals with limited mobility or low exercise tolerance. By integrating electrical stimulation with cycling, this technology allows for safe, repeatable, and quantifiable evaluations of neuromuscular and cardiorespiratory performance. Parameters such as torque, power output, heart rate response, oxygen consumption, stroke volume, and even lactate levels can be monitored, offering clinicians a comprehensive view of a patient's functional capacity.

Moreover, FES-cycling-based assessments provide insights that go beyond traditional passive measures, allowing for the early detection of physiological impairments and more personalized rehabilitation plans. As research continues to support its validity and clinical utility, FES-cycling stands as a promising method not only to promote physical recovery but also to enhance the precision of functional evaluations in diverse patient populations.

References

1. Bakir T, Bonnard B, Gayrard S, Rouot J. Finite Dimensional approximation to muscular response in force-fatigue dynamics using functional electrical stimulation. Automatica. 2022;144(1):hal-03154450v3.
2. Woods B, Subramanian M, Ali Shafti A, Faisal A. Mechanomyography based closed-loop functional electrical stimulation cycling system. In: 7th IEEE international conference on biomedical robotics and biomechatronics (biorob). Enschede; 2018.
3. Figueiredo T, Frazão M, Werlang LA, Kunz A, Peltz M, Furtado VC, Júnior EB, Júnior JM, Silva RM, Sobral Filho DC. Safety and feasibility of a functional electrical stimulation

cycling-based muscular dysfunction diagnostic method in mechanically ventilated patients. Artif Organs. 2024;48(7):713–22.
4. Figueiredo TG, Frazão M, Werlang LA, Peltz M, Sobral Filho DC. Functional electrical stimulation cycling-based muscular evaluation method in mechanically ventilated patients. Artif Organs. 2024;48(3):254–62.
5. Jorgensen H, Nakayama H, Hans R, Olsen T. Recovery of walking function in stroke patients: the Copenagen stroke study. Arch Phys Med Rehabil. 1995;76:27–32.
6. Olney SJ, Richards C. Hemiparetic gait following stroke. Part I: characteristics. Gait Posture. 1996;4(1):36–48.
7. Ambrosini E, Parati M, Peri E, et al. Changes in leg cycling muscle synergies after training augmented by functional electrical stimulation in subacute stroke survivors: a pilot study. J Neuroeng Rehabil. 2020;17:35.
8. Allen BC, Stubbs KJ, Dixon WE. Electromechanical delay during functional electrical stimulation induced cycling is a function of lower limb position. Disabil Rehabil Assist Technol. 2023;18(5):491–6.
9. Hunt KJ, Fang J, Saengsuwan J, Grob M, Laubacher M. On the efficiency of FES cycling: a framework and systematic review. Technol Health Care. 2012;20(5):395–422.
10. Coelho-Magalhães T, Azevedo Coste C, Resende-Martins H. A novel functional electrical stimulation-induced cycling controller using reinforcement learning to optimize online muscle activation pattern. Sensors (Basel). 2022;22(23):9126.
11. Lang JJ, Prince SA, Merucci K, et al. Cardiorespiratory fitness is a strong and consistent predictor of morbidity and mortality among adults: an overview of meta-analyses representing over 20.9 million observations from 199 unique cohort studies. Br J Sports Med. 2024;58(10):556–66.
12. Ross R, Blair SN, Arena R, et al. Importance of assessing cardiorespiratory fitness in clinical practice: a case for fitness as a clinical vital sign: a scientific statement from the American Heart Association. Circulation. 2016;134(24):e653–e99.
13. Fornusek C, Gwinn T, Heard R. Cardiorespiratory responses during functional electrical stimulation cycling and electrical stimulation isometric exercise. Spinal Cord. 2014;52(8):635–9.
14. Hunt KJ, Hosmann D, Grob M, Saengsuwan J. Metabolic efficiency of volitional and electrically stimulated cycling in able-bodied subjects. Med Eng Phys. 2013;35(7):919–25.
15. Ferguson C, Girardi M, DeCato TW. Supine vs upright exercise: far-reaching implications for invasive cardiopulmonary exercise test interpretation. Chest. 2024;165(5):1046–8.
16. Carvalho T, Freitas O, Chalela WA, et al. Brazilian guideline for exercise test in the adult population –2024. Arq Bras Cardiol. 2024;121(3):e20240110.
17. D'Ascenzi F, Cavigli L, Pagliaro A, et al. Clinician approach to cardiopulmonary exercise testing for exercise prescription in patients at risk of and with cardiovascular disease. Br J Sports Med. 2022; https://doi.org/10.1136/bjsports-2021-105261.
18. Hunt KJ, Stone B, Negard NO, et al. Control strategies for integration of electric motor assist and functional electrical stimulation in paraplegic cycling: utility for exercise testing and mobile cycling. IEEE Trans Neural Syst Rehabil Eng. 2004;12(1):89–101.
19. Farkas GJ, Stone B, Dolbow DR, Berg AS, Gater DR Jr. Energy expenditure, cardiorespiratory fitness, and body composition following arm cycling or functional electrical stimulation exercises in spinal cord injury: A 16-week randomized controlled trial. Top Spinal Cord Inj Rehabil. 2021;27(1):121–34.
20. Hunt KJ, Ferrario C, Grant S, et al. Comparison of stimulation patterns for FES-cycling using measures of oxygen cost and stimulation cost. Med Eng Phys. 2006;28(7):710–8.
21. Heymsfield SB, Smith B, Dahle J, et al. Resting energy expenditure: from cellular to whole-body level, a mechanistic historical perspective. Obesity (Silver Spring). 2021;29(3):500–11.
22. JB WEIR. New methods for calculating metabolic rate with special reference to protein metabolism. J Physiol. 1949;109(1–2):1–9.
23. Brooks GA, Mercier J. Balance of carbohydrate and lipid utilization during exercise: the "crossover" concept. J Appl Physiol. 1994;76(6):2253–61.

24. Edwards T, Motl RW, Pilutti LA. Cardiorespiratory demand of acute voluntary cycling with functional electrical stimulation in individuals with multiple sclerosis with severe mobility impairment. Appl Physiol Nutr Metab. 2018;43(1):71–6.
25. van der Scheer JW, Goosey-Tolfrey VL, Valentino SE, Davis GM, Ho CH. Functional electrical stimulation cycling exercise after spinal cord injury: a systematic review of health and fitness-related outcomes. J Neuroeng Rehabil. 2021;18(1):99.
26. Macedo RM, Nohama, P. Avaliação da Fadiga Muscular a Partir da Variação de Lactato em Indivíduos Paraplégicos Submetidos à Estimulação Elétrica Neuromuscular. Dissertação (Mestrado em Engenharia Elétrica e Informática Industrial) - Universidade Tecnológica Federal do Paraná; 2004.
27. Kalkhoven JW, Watsford ML, Coutts AJ, Edwards WB, Impellizzeri FM. Training load na injury: causal pathways and future directions. Sports Med. 2021;51(6):1137–50.
28. Frazao M, Werlang LA, Azevedo C, Kunz A, Peltz M. Metabolic, ventilatory and cardiovascular responses to FES-cycling: A comparison to NMES and passive cycling. Technol Health Care. 2022;30(4):909–18.
29. Hamzaid NA, EJ N. Heart rate and blood pressure following functional electrical stimulation evoked activity amongst in patients with spinal cord injury. Neurorehabil Neural Repair. 2018;32:527.
30. Lima A, Bakker J. Near-infrared spectroscopy for monitoring peripheral tissue perfusion in critically ill patients. Rev Bras Ter Intensiva. 2011;23(3):341–51.
31. Medrinal C, Prieur G, Combret Y, et al. Functional electrical stimulation-A new therapeutic approach to enhance exercise intensity in chronic obstructive pulmonary disease patients: A randomized, controlled crossover trial. Arch Phys Med Rehabil. 2018;99(8):1454–61.
32. Qiu S, Alzhab S, Picard G, Taylor JA. Ventilation limits aerobic capacity after functional electrical stimulation row training in high spinal cord injury. Med Sci Sports Exerc. 2016;48(6):1111–8.
33. Frazao MFT, Cipriano G Jr. Should we use the functional electrical stimulation-cycling exercise in clinical practice? Physiological and clinical effects systematic review with meta-analysi. Arch Phys Med Rehabil. 2025;106(3):404–23.
34. Whipp BJ, Ward SA, Wasserman K. Ventilatory responses to exercise and their control in man. Am Rev Respir Dis. 1984;129(2 Pt 2):S17–20.
35. Lahiri S, Forster RE. CO2/H(+) sensing: peripheral and central chemoreception. Int J Biochem Cell Biol. 2003;35(10):1413–35.
36. Davos CH. Do we have to reconsider the guidelines for exercise intensity determination in cardiovascular rehabilitation? Eur J Prev Cardiol. 2019;26(18):1918–20.
37. Guazzi M, Adams V, Conraads V, et al. EACPR/AHA scientific statement. Clinical recommendations for cardiopulmonary exercise testing data assessment in specific patient populations. Circulation. 2012;126(18):2261–74.
38. Herdy AH, Ritt LE, Stein R, et al. Cardiopulmonary exercise test: background, applicability and interpretation. Arq Bras Cardiol. 2016;107(5):467–81.
39. Milani J, Milani M, Verboven K, Cipriano G Jr, Hansen D. Exercise intensity prescription in cardiovascular rehabilitation: bridging the gap between best evidence and clinical practice. Front Cardiovasc Med. 2024;11:1380639.
40. Jamnick NA, Pettitt RW, Granata C, Pyne DB, Bishop DJ. An examination and critique of current methods to determine exercise intensity. Sports Med. 2020;50(10):1729–56.
41. Glaab T, Taube C. Practical guide to cardiopulmonary exercise testing in adults. Respir Res. 2022;23(1):9.
42. D'Ascenzi F, Cavigli L, Pagliaro A, Focardi M, Valente S, Cameli M, et al. Clinician approach to cardiopulmonary exercise testing for exercise prescription in patients at risk of and with cardiovascular disease. Br J Sports Med. 2022;56:1180.
43. Baccanelli G, Tomaselli M, Ferri U, et al. Effects of cardiac rehabilitation on cardiopulmonary test parameters in heart failure: a real world experience. Int J Cardiol Cardiovasc Risk Prev. 2023;17:200178.

44. Marcadet DM, Pavy B, Bosser G, et al. French Society of Cardiology guidelines on exercise tests (part 1): methods and interpretation. Arch Cardiovasc Dis. 2018;111(12):782–90.
45. Hansen D, Abreu A, Ambrosetti M, et al. Exercise intensity assessment and prescription in cardiovascular rehabilitation and beyond: why and how: a position statement from the secondary prevention and rehabilitation section of the European Association of Preventive Cardiology. Eur J Prev Cardiol. 2022;29(1):230–45.
46. Vanhatalo A, Black MI, DiMenna FJ, et al. The mechanistic bases of the power-time relationship: muscle metabolic responses and relationships to muscle fibre type. J Physiol. 2016;594(15):4407–23.
47. Jones AM, Wilkerson D, Fulford J. Muscle [phosphocreatine] dynamics following the onset of exercise in humans: the influence of baseline work-rate. J Physiol. 2008;586(3):889–98.
48. Egan B, Zierath J. Exercise metabolism and the molecular regulation of skeletal muscle adaptation. Cell Metab. 2013;17(2):162–84.
49. Rossiter HB, Ward SA, Kowalchuk JM, Howe FA, Griffiths JR, Whipp BJ. Dynamic asymmetry of phosphocreatine concentration and O(2) uptake between the on- and off-transients of moderate- and high-intensity exercise in humans. J Physiol. 2002;541(3):991–1002.
50. Messonnier LA, Emhoff C, Fattor JA, Horning MA, Carlson TJ, Brooks GA. Lactate kinetics at the lactate threshold in trained and untrained men. J Appl Physiol. 2013;114(11):1593–602.
51. Black MI, Jones AM, Blackwell JR, et al. Muscle metabolic and neuromuscular determinants of fatigue during cycling in different exercise intensity domains. J Appl Physiol. 2017;122(3):446–59.
52. Mann T, Lamberts R, Lambert MI. Methods of prescribing relative exercise intensity: physiological and practical considerations. Sports Med. 2013;43(7):613–25.
53. Anselmi F, Cavigli L, Pagliaro A, et al. The importance of ventilatory thresholds to define aerobic exercise intensity in cardiac patients and healthy subjects. Scand J Med Sci Sports. 2021;31(9):1796–808.
54. Milani J, Milani M, Machado FVC, et al. Accurate prediction equations for ventilatory thresholds in cardiometabolic disease when gas exchange analysis is unavailable: development and validation. Eur J Prev Cardiol. 2024;31(16):1914–24.
55. Marcin T, Eser P, Prescott E, et al. Training intensity and improvements in exercise capacity in elderly patients undergoing European cardiac rehabilitation - the EU-CaRE multicenter cohort study. PLoS One. 2020;15(11):e0242503.
56. Ambrosini E, Ferrante S, Pedrocchi A, Ferrigno G, Molteni F. Cycling induced by electrical stimulation improves motor recovery in postacute hemiparetic patients: a randomized controlled trial. Stroke. 2011;42(4):1068–73.
57. Ambrosini E, Peri E, Nava C, Longoni L, Monticone M, Pedrocchi A, Ferriero G, Ferrante S. A multimodal training with visual biofeedback in subacute stroke survivors: a randomized controlled trial. Eur J Phys Rehabil Med. 2020;56(1):24–33.
58. Ambrosini E, Ferrante S, Ferrigno G, Molteni F, Pedrocchi A. Cycling induced by electrical stimulation improves muscle activation and symmetry during pedaling in hemiparetic patients. IEEE Trans Neural Syst Rehabil Eng. 2012;20(3):320–30.
59. Ferrante S, Pedrocchi A, Ferrigno G, Molteni F. Cycling induced by functional electrical stimulation improves the muscular strength and the motor control of individuals with post-acute stroke. Europa Medicophysica-SIMFER 2007 Award Winner. Eur J Phys Rehabil Med. 2008;44:159–67.
60. Tilson JK, Sullivan KJ, Cen SY, et al. Meaningful gait speed improvement during the first 60 days poststroke: minimal clinically important difference. Phys Ther. 2010;90(2):196–208.
61. Cameron D, Bohannon RW. Criterion validity of lower extremity Motricity index scores. Clin Rehabil. 2000;14(2):208–11.
62. Toman CJ. Upright control as a predictive gait measure in patients with hemiplegia. Los Angeles: University of Southern California; 1983.
63. Perry J, Garrett M, Gronley JK, Mulroy SJ. Classification of walking handicap in the stroke population. Stroke. 1995;26(6):982–9.

64. Palisano R, Rosenbaum P, Walter S, Russell D, Wood E, Galuppi B. Development and reliability of a system to classify gross motor function in children with cerebral palsy. Dev Med Child Neurol. 1997;39(4):214–23.
65. Denehy L, de Morton NA, Skinner EH, Edbrooke L, Haines K, Warrillow S, Berney S. A physical function test for use in the intensive care unit: validity, responsiveness, and predictive utility of the physical function ICU test (scored). Phys Ther. 2013;93(12):1636–45.
66. Bajd T, Vodovnik L. Pendulum testing of spasticity. J Biomed Eng. 1984;6(1):9–16.
67. Whelan A, Sexton A, Jones M, O'Connell C, McGibbon CA. Predictive value of the pendulum test for assessing knee extensor spasticity. J Neuroeng Rehabil. 2018;15(1):68.
68. Stillman B, J MM. A video-based version of the pendulum test: technique and normal response. Arch Phys Med Rehabil. 1995;72(6):166–76.
69. Ashworth A. Preliminary trial of carisoprodal in multiple sclerosis. Practitioner. 1969;192:540–2.
70. MacKenzie CR, Charlson ME. Standards for the use of ordinal scales in clinical trials. Br Med J. 1986;292:40–3.
71. Kjaer M, Perko G. Secher NH cardiovascular and ventilatory responses to electrically induced cycling with complete epidural anaesthesia in humans. Acta Physiol Scand. 1994;151(2):199–207.
72. Henneman E, Somjen G, Carpenter DO. Functional significance of cell size in spinal motoneurons. J Neurophysiol. 1965;28(3):560–80.
73. Bickel CS, Gregory C, Dean JC. Motor unit recruitment during neuromuscular electrical stimulation: a critical appraisal. Eur J Appl Physiol. 2011;111(10):2399–407.
74. Maffiuletti NA. Physiological and methodological considerations for the use of neuromuscular electrical stimulation. Eur J Appl Physiol. 2010;110(2):223–34.

FES-Cycling Clinical Applicability in Neurological Diseases

6

Lara A. Pilutti, Ashwini Sansare, Laurie Magerfleisch, Colleen Connaughton, and Murillo Frazão

Introduction

Neurological diseases are among the most prevalent causes of long-term disability worldwide, affecting millions of individuals across all age groups. Conditions such as spinal cord injury (SCI), stroke, cerebral palsy (CP), and multiple sclerosis (MS) disrupt motor, sensory, and autonomic function, often resulting in paralysis, spasticity, cardiovascular deconditioning, and reduced independence. Rehabilitation is essential to improve recovery, minimize secondary complications, and enhance quality of life. However, conventional physiotherapy and exercise programs are frequently limited by patients' reduced ability to generate voluntary movement, insufficient training intensity, and difficulties in maintaining long-term adherence.

Functional electrical stimulation (FES) offers a strategy to overcome these barriers. By delivering controlled electrical impulses to peripheral nerves and muscles, FES can activate paralyzed or weakened muscle groups. When combined with cycling exercise (FES-cycling), produces rhythmic and task-oriented lower limb movements, even in individuals with severe motor impairments. The technique

L. A. Pilutti
Interdisciplinary School of Health Sciences, Brain and Mind Research Institute, University of Ottawa, Ottawa, ON, Canada

Thomas Edwards, Northern Ontario School of Medicine, Thunder Bay, ON, Canada
e-mail: lpilutti@uottawa.ca

A. Sansare
Texas A&M University, College Station, TX, USA
e-mail: ashwini@tamu.edu

L. Magerfleisch · C. Connaughton
Restorative Therapies, Nottingham, MD, USA
e-mail: laurie@rtiedu.com; connaughton@restorative-therapies.com

M. Frazão (✉)
Lauro Wanderley University Hospital – EBSERH/UFPB, João Pessoa, PB, Brazil
e-mail: murillo.frazao@gmail.com

M. Frazão (ed.), *Functional Electrical Stimulation Cycling in Clinical Practice*,
https://doi.org/10.1007/978-3-032-23937-2_6

simultaneously strengthens muscles, enhances cardiovascular fitness, and delivers proprioceptive input to the central nervous system, supporting neuroplasticity and functional recovery.

This chapter focuses specifically on the role of FES-cycling in several neurological diseases. It reviews the pathophysiological rationale, current evidence from clinical studies, and reported benefits for muscle health, spasticity, cardiovascular performance, and quality of life in each condition. Treatment protocols, safety considerations, and emerging technological advances are also discussed. By integrating current knowledge, this chapter aims to provide clinicians, researchers, and rehabilitation professionals with a practical and evidence-based perspective on the application of FES-cycling across neurological populations.

Spinal Cord Injury

Impact of SCI on the Body

Spinal cord injury (SCI) leads to motor (paralysis/paresis), sensory (hypo/hyper), and autonomic nervous system dysfunctions. However, the pathophysiology of SCI is complex, and not limited to the nervous system. Indeed, several other organs and tissues are also affected by the injury, directly or indirectly, acutely or chronically, which induces numerous health complications [1]. Some of these health complications are attributable to the SCI per se, but many are secondary to the resulting immobility (Fig. 6.1). Particularly common secondary health complications among people with SCI include pain, spasticity, urinary tract infections, bowel and bladder problems, respiratory difficulties, autonomic dysreflexia, and osteoporosis [2]. Consequently, the incidence of pressure ulcers, type 2 diabetes, and cardiovascular disease is greatly increased in this population [2]. To reduce the disability burden of people with SCI, efforts should be directed toward early prevention of these secondary health complications [3].

How SCI Affects Motor Control, Muscle Strength, and Mobility

SCI is a neurologic condition resulting from trauma or nontraumatic etiologies that disrupt motor, sensory, and autonomic pathways [4]. SCI leads to loss of innervation of skeletal muscle, decreased motor function, and significantly reduced load on skeletal muscle, resulting in atrophy [5]. The resulting profound muscle atrophy below the level of lesion has a devastating impact on functional recovery and long-term health.

The acute physiological response to traumatic SCI involves a period of spinal shock, which may take weeks to resolve [6]. Neurogenic shock, part of spinal shock, consists of severe arterial hypotension and bradycardia. The spinal shock's characteristics are sensory deficits, flaccid paralysis, absence of deep tendon reflexes, abolishment of reflex somatic activity, and thermoregulatory disturbances below the

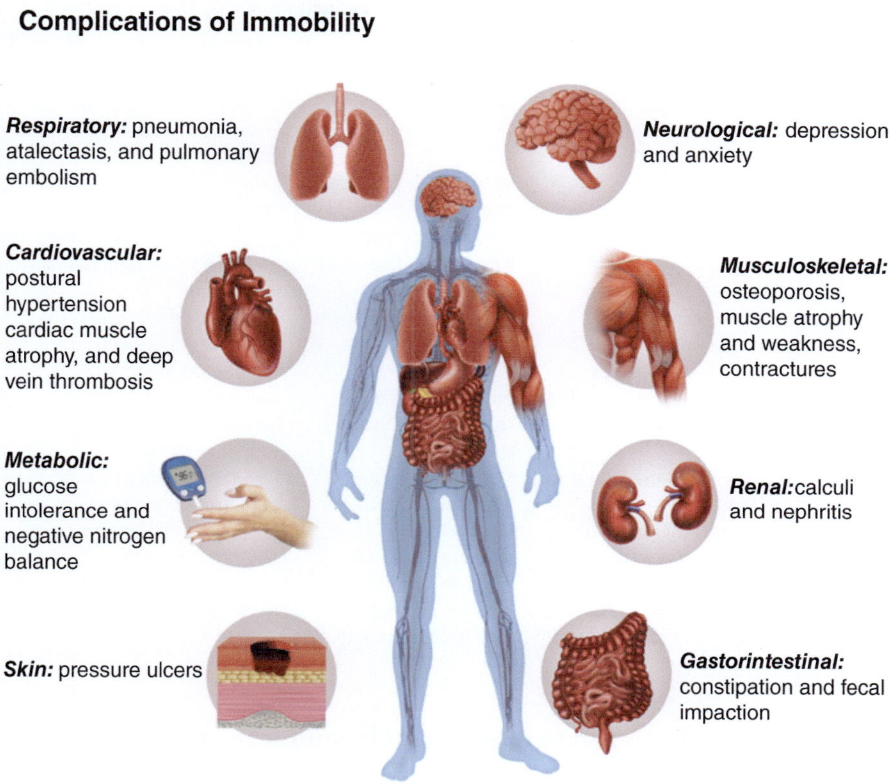

Fig. 6.1 Overview of body systems affected by immobility. (©Restorative Therapies)

level of injury. Autonomic dysreflexia appears during the chronic phase, after spinal shock resolution, and it is a life-threatening syndrome of massive imbalanced reflex sympathetic discharge occurring in patients with SCI above the splanchnic sympathetic outflow (T5-T6) [7].

The combination of flaccid paralysis and decreased activity in the acute period causes rapid atrophy of skeletal muscle tissue [8]. Skeletal muscle atrophy not only hinders the recovery of motor function but is also closely related to many systemic dysfunctions, affecting the prognosis of patients with spinal cord injury [9]. As the main component of human tissue structure, skeletal muscle accounts for about 40% of body mass and, as highly metabolically active tissue, accounts for a large proportion of total body energy expenditure and 70% of glucose utilization [10–12]. In addition to maintaining the homeostasis of exercise, skeletal muscle also plays a number of physiological functions such as support, protection, and respiration [13, 14]. The muscle type most frequently atrophied after SCI is skeletal muscle, manifesting as loss of mass and strength [10], with 18–46% decreases in cross-sectional area (CSA) of skeletal muscle 6 weeks after injury [15–17] (Table 6.1).

Table 6.1 [8, 9] How motor control, strength and mobility are impacted by level of injury

SCI level	Motor control	Muscle strength	Mobility impact
C1–C4	Severely impaired or absent in all limbs. May require ventilator (esp. C1–C3)	Little to no voluntary strength in arms/legs	Completely dependent; electric wheelchair, 24/7 care needed
C5	Partial shoulder/elbow control (can flex elbow)	Weak biceps, no hand/finger control	Limited self-mobility in powered wheelchair
C6	Shoulder/elbow/wrist control (wrist extension possible)	Better upper limb strength, no fine hand control	Some self-care possible; powered or adapted manual wheelchair
C7–C8	Elbow extension (C7), some hand function (C8)	Increasing hand/finger strength	Independent with adaptive tools; can drive with modifications
T1–T6	Normal upper body control	Full upper limb strength, no lower limb strength	Manual wheelchair use; independent upper body function
T7–T12	Full trunk control improves at T9+	Strong core muscles, legs still paralyzed	Can transfer more easily; may use braces for standing
L1–L5	Some hip and knee movement possible	Gradual return of leg strength (improves lower in spine)	May walk with braces, crutches, or walker
S1–S5	Control of hips, legs, bladder, bowel improves	Near-normal leg and foot strength possible	May walk independently with minor assistance

Differentiation Between Complete and Incomplete SCI

SCIs can be complete or incomplete. SCI is considered complete when there is an absence of sensory and motor function in the lowest sacral segments (S4-S5) (i.e., no sacral sparing) [18]. The term incomplete SCI is used when there is preservation of any sensory and/or motor function below the neurological level that includes the lowest sacral segments S4-S5 (i.e., presence of "sacral sparing") [8]. Table 6.2 outlines distinguishing characteristics between the two. Waters et al. [19].

The level of injury in a SCI is defined as the most caudal segment with motor function rated at greater than or equal to 3/5, with pain and temperature preserved [20]. The standard neurological classification of SCI provided by the American Spinal Injury Association (ASIA) assigns grades from A (complete SCI) through E (normal sensory/motor), with B, C, and D representing varying degrees of injury between these extremes [20].

The standard neurological classification of SCI provided by the American Spinal Injury Association (ASIA) assigns grades from A (motor and sensory complete) through E (normal sensory/motor), with B (motor complete, sensory incomplete), C and D (motor and sensory incomplete) representing varying degrees of injury between these extremes [20]. Figure 6.2 provides details on the breakdown of the ASIA Impairment Scale (AIS) classification.

Table 6.2 Differences between complete and incomplete SCI [8, 9, 22]

Characteristic	Complete SCI	Incomplete SCI
Definition	No motor/sensory function in the lowest sacral segments	Some sensory/motor function preserved below injury level
ASIA impairment Scale	AIS A	AIS B, C, D, or E
Sacral sparing	Absent	Present
Motor function	Completely lost below lesion	Absent (AIS B) Partially preserved (AIS C/D) Preserved (AIS E)
Sensory function	Completely lost below lesion	Partially preserved
Reflexes (early phase)	Spinal shock → absent reflexes	May be reduced but often partially present
Spasticity (later phase)	Often develops after weeks	Often present, depending on pathways spared
Muscle atrophy	More pronounced	Less affected
Common causes	Severe trauma, complete cord transection	Trauma, ischemia, tumors, incomplete compression

Application of FES-Cycling

Use of FES-Cycling to Promote Mobility in Patients with SCI

Functional electrical stimulation (FES) combined with cycling exercise (FES-cycling) has shown promise in improving muscle function and health in individuals with SCI [23]. A prospective study in 2015 [24] investigated the effects of FES-cycling on functional recovery, spasticity, gait, and oxygen consumption with walking in ten subjects with chronic (>2 years) incomplete SCI who were able to ambulate at least 10 m without an orthosis. The subjects performed 1 h of FES-cycling three times weekly for 16 weeks. At 6-month follow-up, the subject demonstrated significant improvements in total motor (AIS clinical exam) and Functional Independence Measure (FIM) scores, as well spasticity levels. Oxygen consumption during walking decreased; however temporal spatial gait parameters did not show significant changes. Later [25], 15 patients with SCI (>6 months) underwent evaluation of Functional Independence Measure (FIM), Nottingham Health Profile (NHP), 6-min walk test (6MWT), and 20-m walk test (20MWT) before and after FES-cycling three times weekly for 6 weeks. The subjects were all able to stand and walk with long leg braces or assistive devices prior to intervention. They demonstrated improvements in motor and total scores of FIM, physical mobility subscale of NHP, as well as 6MWT and 20MWT [25].

Stimulation of Paralyzed Muscles to Prevent Muscle Atrophy and Improve Circulation

Muscle Health

Muscle atrophy occurs rapidly after spinal cord injury (SCI), along with increased adipose deposits within the muscle, decreased fiber size, force-generating capacity, and fatigue resistance. People with SCI are also at risk for metabolic syndrome as a

ASIA Imprirment Scale (AIS)

A = Complete. No sensory or motor function is preserved 'in the sacral segments S4-5

B = Sensory Incomplete. Sensory but not motor function is preserved below the neurological level and includes the sacral segments S4-5 (light touch or pin prick at S4-5 or deep anal pressure) AND no motor function is preserved more than three levels below the motor level on either side of the body.

C = Motor Incomplete. Motor function is preserved at the most caudal sacral segments for voluntary anal contraction (VAC) OR the patient meets the criteria for sensory incompleted status (sensory function preserved at the most caudal sacral segments S4-5 by LT, PP or DAP), and has some sparing of motor function more than three levels below the ipsilateral motor level on either side of the body. (This includes key or non-key muscle functions to determine motor incomplete status.) For AIS C – less than half of key muscle functions below the single NLI have a muscle grade ≥ 3.

D = Motor Incomplete. Motor incomplete status as defined above, with at least half (half or move) of key muscle functions below the single NLI having a muscle grade ≥ 3.

E = Normal. If sensation and motor function as tested with the ISNCSCI are graded as normal in all segments, and the patient had prior deficits, then the AIS grade is E. Someone without an initial SCI does not receive an AIS grade.

Using ND: To document the sensory, motor and NLI levels, the ASIA Impairment Scale grade, and/or the zone of partial preservation (ZPP) when they are unable to be determined based on the examination results.

Fig. 6.2 American Spinal Injury Association (ASIA) Impairment Scale (AIS). (Rupp et al. [21])

result of muscle atrophy and decreased activity levels [26]. The effects of FES-cycling on muscle health have been studied for decades, summarized in Table 6.3.

The effects shown in Table 6.3 are not limited to adult subjects. In a study of 30 children [26] that were randomly assigned to FES-cycling, passive cycling or electrical stimulation exercise (non-cycling activity) for 60-min sessions three times weekly for 6 months. Those in the FES-cycling group demonstrated greater changes in strength while the electrical stimulation exercise group demonstrated greater changes in muscle volume.

Table 6.3 Summary of studies examining the effects of FES-cycling on muscle [27]

Reference	Sample	Duration	Intervention	Main result
[28]	N = 17 Complete SCI	6 months	FES-cycling 1-h 3× weekly Low cadence (10 rpm) vs. high cadence (50 rpm)	Low cadence group increased muscle volume by 19%, high cadence group increased by 10%
[29]	N = 8 Complete and incomplete Untrained	6 weeks	FES-cycling 30 min 3× weekly 1 leg on low cadence 10 rpm and the other leg on high cadence 50 rpm Freq = 35 Hz PW = 250 μsec Stim = 140 mA Pedal cadence = 35 rpm	Midthigh girth increases induced By low cadence were significantly greater than those by high cadence ($p = 0.008$). Low cadence also produced greater gains in electrically evoked isometric torque than high cadence after training ($p = 0.023$)
[30]	N = 15 Complete SCI	6 months	FES-cycling 30 min 3× weekly Freq = 30 Hz PW = 350 μsec Stim = up to 130 mA Pedal cadence = 35 rpm	Group trained with FES increased lower extremity muscle volume 1300 cm^3 ($p < 0.001$) while the control group had no change
[31]	N = 45 Complete and Incomplete SCI	29.1 months	FES-CE 50–60 min × 3 times per week Freq = 100 Hz PW = 500 μsec Stim = up to 140 mA Pedal cadence = 50 rpm	FES group had significantly higher anterior (36%; 96.3 cc; $p \leq 0.001$) and posterior (30%; 63.9 cc; $p = 0.005$) thigh compartment muscles than those in the control group Strength in trained muscles of the FES group was significantly greater (quadriceps, $p = 0.006$; hamstrings, $p = 0.011$) than in controls. Quality of life and daily function measures were also significantly higher in FES group.

(continued)

Table 6.3 (continued)

Reference	Sample	Duration	Intervention	Main result
[32]	N = 30 Complete vs incomplete with acute SCI	4 weeks	FES-CE 20 min × 2 times per week Freq = 30 Hz PW = 250 μsec Stim = 10–130 mA Pedal cadence = 15–55 rpm	Greater improvement in circumference in the incomplete group ($p < 0.05$) Those in the incomplete group showed 43.5% increase ($p < 0.001$) in quadriceps femoris muscle and 25% ($p < 0.001$) in gluteus maximus muscle strength by manual muscle testing
[33]	N = 8 Complete and Incomplete thoracic SCI with 6 months FES-cycling	6 weeks	FES-CE 30 min × 3 times per week 1 leg on low cadence 10 rpm and the other leg on high cadence 50 rpm Freq = 35 Hz PW = 250 μsec Stim = 40–140 mA	Both groups reported greater improvement in thigh girth on low cadence side Quadriceps peak torque increased 87% in low cadence side
[34]	N = 10 Complete SCI (acute)	13 weeks	FES-CE 30 min 3x per week Freq = 35 Hz Pedal cadence = 35 rpm 13 weeks	Group trained with FES-CE increased muscle fiber CSA 171% greater than that in the control group ($p = 0.05$)
[35]	N = 1 Complete vs Incomplete SCI	13 weeks	FES-LCE training 1 h × 3 times per week, 40 sessions Freq = 30 Hz PW = 250 μsec Stim = up to 140 mA Pedal cadence = 45 rpm	Both groups had improved knee extension torque 3.8 to 16.9 nm ($p = 0.006$). However, those in incomplete group showed greater improvement
[36]	N = 11 Complete SCI	1 year	FES-cycling 1 h 3–5× weekly Freq = 50 Hz, if rapid fatigue reduced to 20 Hz Pedal cadence = 45–55 rpm	Quadriceps maximal torque increased progressively and significantly throughout training ($p = 0.012$). It had increased by 399% and 673% after 3 and 12 months
[37]	N = 18 Complete and incomplete SCI	8 weeks	FES-CE 30 min × 3 times per week Freq = 30 Hz PW = 300 μsec Stim = 10–130 mA Pedal cadence = 45 rpm	Mild increase in body lean mass after 8 weeks training ($p = 0.03$) Significant increase in both upper and lower limb girth after 4 and 8 weeks of training ($p < 0.05$)

(continued)

Table 6.3 (continued)

Reference	Sample	Duration	Intervention	Main result
[38]	N = 26 Complete SCI	3 months + 6 months	FES-CE 30 min × 3 times per week Pedal cadence = 35–50 rpm FES-IC 1 h × 5 times per week Freq = 60 Hz PW = 375 μsec Stim = up to 140 mA	FES-CE group showed a significant hypertrophy after 6 months on both lower limb and gluteal lean body mass in comparison to FES alone Prevention of atrophy at 3 months Control group lost lean body mass
[23]	6 months	4 Complete Chronic	FES-cycling 30 min 3× weekly Freq = 40 Hz PW = 400–500 μsec Stim = up to 130 mA Pedal cadence = 30–50 rpm	Average increase in muscle volume of 22.3% and 36.7% at 3 and 6 months respectively Compared with baseline. One month post-training, muscle volume remained 23.2% higher than baseline

FES-CE Functional Electrical Stimulation-Cycling Ergometer, *FES-LCE* Functional electrical Stimulation Leg Cycling Ergometer, *FES-IC* Functional Electrical Stimulation Isometric Contraction, *N* Number of participants, *Freq* Frequency, *PW* Pulse Width, *Stim* Stimulation amplitude

Two recent systematic reviews investigated health and fitness-related outcomes of FES-cycling in SCI patients, including muscle and bone health. In 2021 [39], 92 studies encompassing 999 adults with SCI were reviewed showing improvement in muscle health (muscle mass, fiber type composition) in three out of four Level 1–2 and 27 of 32 Level 3–4 studies. Nearly all 35 Level 3–4 studies demonstrated significant improvements in power output and aerobic fitness. The 2023 review [40] looked at the effects FES-supported leg exercises, including FES-cycling, and showed 21 studies using 1–12 months of FES-cycling demonstrated a marginal or significant increase in lower limb and trunk muscle cross-sectional area, as well as improvements in lean body mass, thigh circumference, and leg muscle. The increase in CSA was seen with at least 3 months of FES-cycling.

Circulation/Pressure Injuries

The incidence of pressure ulcers in SCI patients ranges from 20% to 31% annually, with the resulting increased healthcare utilization quadrupling costs compared with SCI patient without pressure injuries [41]. It is estimated that approximately 1–3 million pressure injuries occur per year, and that 20–50% of patients with new SCI will develop at least one hospital-acquired pressure injury during their acute hospitalization [42], with those having complete injury more likely to develop them than those with incomplete injuries [43]. Pressure injuries can lead to other comorbidities such as infection and increased spasticity or autonomic dysreflexia. Annual cost of pressure injuries may exceed $11 million annually [44].

The loss of vasomotor control over skeletal muscle and skin lowers the tone of the vascular bed leading to a reduction in the ability to withstand normal loading conditions [45]. Ischemia and local tissue starvation due to interruptions in microcirculation, as well as muscle atrophy, can increase risk of development of pressure injuries [45].

Nine males with SCI who underwent 6 weeks of lower extremity FES-cycling (30 min 3× weekly for 6 weeks) [46] showed increased femoral artery diameter, peak systolic inflow and mean inflow volumes, and reduced velocity index indicating reduced peripheral resistance. In another study [47] eight males with C5-T6 SCI performed FES-cycling 3 times per week for 8 weeks, with pressure mapping completed before and after the study. Both mean average and maximum seat pressures decreased the intervention. While the changes were not statistically significant there was a strong trend toward a reduction in average and maximal seat pressure. A review of 34 studies [45] evaluating the influence of electrical stimulation, including but not limited to FES-cycling, on risk factors for developing pressure ulcers showed that there is moderate evidence for both short and long-term benefits on outcomes such as ischial tuberosity pressure, muscle volume, circulation, and tissue oxygenation. There is also moderate to high certainty of evidence of clinically important improvements in leg and total lean body mass and power [48] after FES cycle training, which may reduce the risk of pressure injuries.

Evidence supports that the use of FES-cycling after SCI will mitigate muscle atrophy by increasing muscle cross-sectional area, power output, and strength. Studies found that increased arterial blood flow and reduced peripheral resistance were key factors to support the role of FES-cycling in enhancing circulation and vascular function. The combination of these circulatory benefits, along with gains in muscle volume and lean body mass, may reduce the incidence of pressure injuries. This is clinically significant as pressure injuries are a common and costly secondary complication after SCI.

Clinical Benefits

Improvement of Cardiovascular and Metabolic Function

Cardiovascular disturbances are the leading cause of morbidity and mortality in both acute and chronic stages of SCI [6]. Physical activity is essential for maintaining cardiorespiratory fitness, metabolic health, and skeletal muscle mass, with current recommendations for persons with SCI to include moderate- to vigorous-intensity aerobic and strength training activities at least twice per week [49]. The studies discussed here establish the overall cardiovascular benefits of physical activity after SCI, and the crucial role that incorporating FES-cycling into the therapeutic plan of care has in maximizing on the improvements in cardiovascular and metabolic function.

Warburton et al. [50] summarized the strength of the scientific evidence for metabolic and cardiovascular benefits of hybrid exercise reporting that a minimum of 30 min of exercise 3 times per week can achieve health benefits. Specifically, they reported level 1b (very strong) evidence from one RCT and five Level 4 studies that combined both arm-cranking and FES-lower extremity cycling, and FES-rowing training to improve glucose homeostasis, i.e., decreased insulin sensitivity and insulin resistance, and/or improved glucose tolerance. Additionally, Warburton and associates reported that there is level 4 evidence from multiple pre–post studies that improvements in glucose homeostasis are clinically significant for prevention and/or treatment of type II diabetes.

Thirty children with SCI participated in a randomized controlled trial (RCT) to determine the cardiovascular and vascular effects of FES-cycling (ages 5–13 years; C4-T11; AIS A/B/C) [51]. There were 3 groups: (1) FES leg cycling, (2) passive leg cycling, and (3) control group receiving only electrical stimulation, no cycling. Exercise protocol was completed at home under parental supervision with instructions to perform for 1 h 3 times per week for 6 months. Only children in the FES-cycling group showed significant differences in the % increase in VO2peak. No differences were found with resting HR or forced vital capacity (FVC). The electrical stimulation only group showed declines in lipid levels as compared with passive and FES-cycling participants. Figure 6.3 brings an example of FES-cycling exercise in children.

A systematic review from 2021 [52] evaluated the evidence regarding the efficacy of aerobic exercise training in patients with tetraplegia, and its potential for improving health and exercise performance. Of the 75 articles reviewed—none focused solely on tetraplegia, but rather a combination of tetraplegia and paraplegia and with mixed injury levels. The evidence gathered showed that voluntary arm-crank training can increase mean peak power output by 33%. Functional electrical stimulation leg cycling was shown to induce higher peak cardiac output and stroke volume than arm-crank exercise. A range of peak oxygen uptake (VO2peak) values

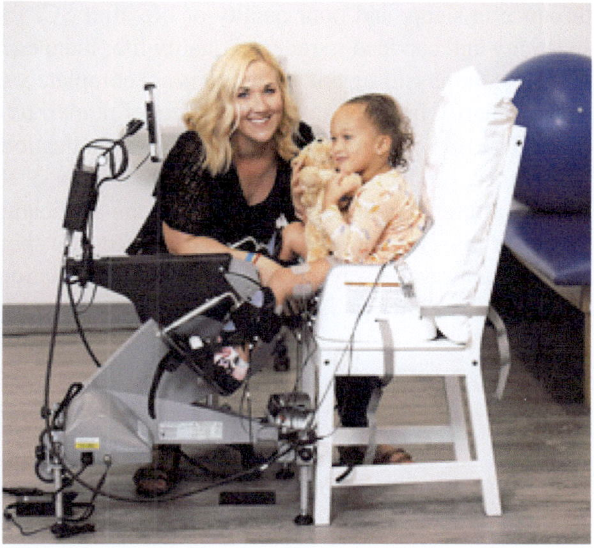

Fig. 6.3 Pictured is the RT300 Lower Extremity FES Cycle with a pediatric patient demonstrating adaptations for smaller body size. (©Restorative Therapies)

have been reported (0.57–1.32 L/min). Both VO2peak and cardiac output may be enhanced via increased muscle pump in the legs and venous return to the heart. Hybrid exercise (arm-crank and functional electrical stimulation leg cycling) can result in greater peak oxygen uptake and cardiovascular responses.

While it has been identified that more investigation is needed to solidify the intensity and dosage of FES-cycling to establish long-term health benefits, there are promising results of a positive effect in the SCI population for improvement in cardiovascular function. There is clinically significant data to show that aerobic exercise alone does not provide these direct results in patients with SCI. When combined with FES-cycling, there are positive influences on VO_2 peak, cardiac output, and stroke volume. Emerging research is indicating that the use of hybrid exercise (arm crank exercise and FES leg cycling) provides better outcomes than FES leg cycling alone. In particular, hybrid cycling has been shown to improve glucose homeostasis which lowers the risk for type II diabetes [50]. Improving metabolic function post SCI is essential for decreasing the risk of secondary complications. The data presented above will guide clinicians in selecting this therapeutic modality for their patients.

Reduction of Spasticity and Improvement in Motor Control

Spasticity is a common consequence of SCI, estimated to affect up to 93% of people living with SCI in the community (Table 6.4) [53]. Of those, about 35% report spasticity to be problematic, meaning it either limits function and/or requires pharmaceutical or medical management. Spasticity tends to develop within the first 6–12 months after injury and is more likely to affect those with higher and complete injuries [54]. Some manifestations of spasticity can be beneficial, such as in standing or transfers, and in preserving skeletal muscle mass [55], but it can also impact activities of daily living, completion of hygiene activities, lead to limited joint mobility and contractures, difficulty with skin integrity, postural abnormalities, disturbance in sleep, and poor quality of life after SCI [54]. Pain often accompanies spasticity and can lead to reduced quality life, independence and function [56].

The pathophysiology of spasticity is not completely understood but is believed to arise primarily from the loss of the effect of numerous descending inhibitory pathways. The upper motor lesion disrupts communication between the brain and the spinal cord, producing a state of net disinhibition of the spinal reflexes [57]. The sensory afferent feedback generated from the application of FES leads to reduction of spastic muscle contraction through its effects on spinal reflex excitability [54].

There are several ways to apply electrical stimulation to modulate tone and spasticity [59], as shown in Table 6.5.

Table 6.4 Risk of developing spasticity after SCI [54, 58]

Cervical		Thoracic	
AIS A	AIS B-D	AIS A	AIS B-D
93%	78%	72%	73%

Table 6.5 Application of electrical stimulation for spasticity/tone modulation [59–61]

Muscle(s) stimulated	Mechanism
Motor-level stimulation of the spastic muscle	Evoked potential travels antidromically along the motor axon to activate Renshaw cells (recurrent inhibition). The Ib afferent is also activated providing autogenic inhibition of the spastic muscle via the Ib interneuron
Motor-level stimulation of the antagonist muscle	Activate the Ia interneuron to reciprocally inhibit the spastic muscle
Reciprocal motor-level stimulation of the spastic and antagonist muscles	Evokes the combined effects of reciprocal, autogenic and recurrent inhibition
Sensory (TENS) level stimulation of the spastic muscle	Hypothesized to modulate spinal circuits via indirect effect on afferents to increase presynaptic inhibition of the hyperactive stretch reflex May reduce painful stimuli that provoke spasticity below level of injury

TENS transcutaneous electrical neuromuscular stimulation

Two systematic reviews of studies using FES-cycling for spasticity management reported that overall, FES-cycling was shown to have a positive impact on spasticity immediately after FES-cycling [62], with sustained effects reported at 6-month follow-up in moderate to high quality studies that included 45–60-min FES-cycling sessions, three times a week for 16 weeks [54]. A meta-analysis of eight studies encompassing 99 subjects with SCI [63] concluded that spasticity decreased significantly (MAS) in favor of FES-cycling and walking ability. Lower limbs muscle strength (LEMS) also improved significantly in favor or FES-cycling. More than 20 training sessions were needed to decrease spasticity significantly.

All the reviews noted that stimulation parameters and dosage varied among the studies and because of the variability in study design, methodology, and subject heterogeneity, recommendations cannot be given [64]. However, Table 6.6 shows examples of ranges of parameters used.

Bone Health

After SCI, there is a rapid loss of bone density that has been reported to last from 1 to 3 years, with as much as 50% of bone mineral density (BMD) lost within this time [66]. The most rapid loss occurs in the distal femur and proximal tibia [67]. Although studies assessing the effects of FES-cycling on bone health in SCI tend to focus on chronic cases, bone loss is most significant in the first 6 months after injury and may be associated with higher femur fracture rates, indicating early intervention may be efficacious [68]. Table 6.7 summarizes evidence related to the effects for FES-cycling on bone health in adults and children with SCI.

After SCI, there is a significant loss in BMD, especially affecting the distal femur and proximal tibia. It is critical to provide early intervention as bone loss correlates to increased fracture risk. With FES-cycling, there is potential to delay loss of and even increase BMD with recommendations to initiate early and use long duration, high intensity protocols. Although conclusions could not be drawn about the most

Table 6.6 Ranges of parameters used in studies supporting FES-cycling for spasticity management [61, 65]

	FES/NMES	Sensory/TENS
Pulse width (μsec)	300–350 (64) 300 (65) 50–600 (54)	100–250 300
Frequency (Hz)	20–30 (64) 35(65) 20–100, most 20–30 (54)	99–100 100
Amplitude (mA)	>100 (64) 300% motor threshold [65] 0–140, most >100 (54)	Below motor threshold/tingling No more than 20

NMES neuromuscular electrical stimulation, *TENS* transcutaneous electrical nerve stimulation

Table 6.7 Studies examining the effects of FES-cycling on bone health in SCI

Reference	Sample	Duration	Intervention	Main result
[69]	N = 37	12 weeks	FES-CE and FES-KE 30 min × 3 times per week Freq = 35 Hz PW = 375 μsec Stim = mA Pedal cadence = 50 rpm 6 kE/min/leg for 36 Exercise sessions	FES intervention Promoted bone density ($p < 0.001$)
[70]	N = 10	12 months 3× weekly followed by 6 months 1x weekly	FES-CE 30 min × 3 times per week Freq = ND PW = ND Stim = up to 130 mA Pedal cadence = ND	After 12 months of training, the BMD of the proximal tibia had increased 10% ($p < 0.05$). After 6 months of reduced training, the BMD in the proximal tibia no longer differed from the BMD before training ($p > 0.05$). No BMD increase ($p > 0.05$) in the lumbar spine and femoral neck
[71]	N = 19 Complete acute	6 months	FES-CE 30 min × 3 times per week Freq = 30, 50, 60 Hz PW = 300–400 μsec Stim = up to 140 mA Pedal cadence = 35–50 rpm	Marginal attenuation reduction in tibial cortical BMD was reported and this was linearly related to the initial BMD and age but unrelated to the degree of immobilization and injury level
[72]	N = 15	6 months	30 min × 5 times per week Freq = 20 Hz PW = 300 μsec Stim = up to 120 mA Pedal cadence = not reported	BMD of the distal femur and proximal tibia increased by 11.13 ± 0.8%, and 12.92 ± 2.24%, respectively ($p < 0.05$)

(continued)

Table 6.7 (continued)

Reference	Sample	Duration	Intervention	Main result
[73]	N = 1 Complete	12 months	FES-CE 60 min × 5 times per week Freq = 50 Hz PW = 300 μsec Stim = up to 140 mA Pedal cadence = 50 rpm	BMD increased by 3.9% after the training
[74]	N = 12	Initially: 14 + 7 weeks of FES for muscle conditioning, Followed by 60 min per session For average of 3.7 + 0.6; FES-cycling sessions/ Week, for 12 months.	FES-cycling 30 min × 3 times per week Freq = 50 Hz PW = up to 500 μsec Stim = to tolerance Pedal cadence = 45–50 rpm	Significant increase ($p \leq 0.05$) in BMD of the bones and muscle CSA of the thigh ($p = 0.003$) was reported
[68]	N = 12	3 months (then 3 months without training)	FES-CE 30 min × 3 times per week Freq = 20 Hz PW = 300 μsec Stim = ND Pedal cadence = ND	Partial attenuation ($p < 0.01$)) of BMD loss of only distal femur in the early stage of training was Observed At 3 months post-FES-cycling, there was no difference between the intervention and control groups
[28]	N = 17	6 months	30 min × 3 times per week Freq = 33 Hz PW = 250 μsec Stim = up to 140 mA Pedal cadence = 20 or 50 rpm	Increase bone volume (10% and 19% for the 2 groups) and general improved bone health were reported
[75]	N = 30 Pediatric	6 months	60 min × 3 times per week Freq = 33 Hz PW = 150–300 μsec Stim = up to 140 mA Pedal cadence = 50 rpm	The FES-cycling group demonstrated increases in hip, distal femur and proximal tibia bone mineral density of 32.4, 6.62 and 10.3% respectively. The passive cycling group showed a 29.2% increase at the hip, but no change at the femur or tibia, while the electrical stimulation exercise group showed no change at the hip or distal femur, and a loss of 7.06% at the proximal tibia

BMD Bone mineral density, *CE* cycle ergometry, *Freq* Frequency, *KE* FES knee extension, *N* number of subjects, *ND* not described, *N* Number of participants, *PW* Pulse Width, *Stim* Stimulation amplitude

optimal stimulation parameters to use, most studies used a frequency of 20–35 Hz and a pulse width of 200–400 msec. Further research is needed to solidify the optimal stimulation and therapy parameters as well as dosage. Evidence indicates that FES-cycling is instrumental in supporting bone health in individuals with SCI.

Pain

Chronic pain is common in patients with spinal cord injury (SCI) and can negatively affect quality of life. Nociceptive pain, arising from tissue damage from trauma, inflammation, disuse, or spasms/contractures related to spasticity, occurs in about 60% of SCI patients. Thirty to 40% experience neuropathic pain related to damage to neural tissues [76]. Sixteen patients with complete or incomplete SCI performed FES-cycling two times daily, 5 days a week for 6 weeks. The 45-min sessions included stimulation of muscles of the knee, hip/trunk extensors and hip/trunk ab/adductors using a stimulation frequency of 50 Hz, pulse width of 500 msec and amplitude no more than 140 mA. Statistically significant changes in numerical rating scale (NRS), Multidimensional Pain Inventory for SCI (MPI-SCI) and the 36-item Short Form Survey (SF-36) and dorsal laser-evoked potentials (LEP). Three patients had high pain relief, six moderate, and five mild pain relief after the FES-cycling training, suggesting this modality is capable of causing pain reduction [76].

Treatment Protocols

The evidence indicates that FES-cycling could help counteract the loss of muscle mass after SCI, which may reduce risk of pressure injuries and increase resting metabolic rates. Although conclusions cannot be drawn regarding optimal stimulation parameters, on average study protocols utilized a pulse width of 300, frequency of 35 Hz and amplitude of 140 mA with FES-cycling for 30 min, 3 times weeks for around 16 weeks [39].

Studies that demonstrated statistically significant changes in muscle spasticity used frequencies of 20–50 Hz, amplitudes of 10–140 mA, and pulse widths of 75–500 μsec [54]. The high-quality studies that showed statistically significant improvement used frequencies of 20–30 Hz, amplitudes of 10–140 mA, and pulse widths of 250 μsec. Long- term effects on spasticity were evident in moderate- to high-quality studies where FES-cycling was conducted for 60 min, three times per week, for 16 weeks [54].

Although the available evidence investigating the benefits of FES-cycling on muscle size and strength is compelling [27], there is insufficient quantity and quality evidence to draw conclusions regarding the specific parameter of FES-cycling that may optimally increase muscle strength, mass, and circumference. However, it can be safely concluded that an effective training session would spend for 45–60 min, 3 times a week for at least 4 weeks to see changes in muscle size and strength [27].

There are over 40 years of work in SCI research focused on the effects of FES-cycling on health and fitness-related outcomes. The evidence is clear that FES-cycling will affect positive changes on metabolic health, bone density, spasticity

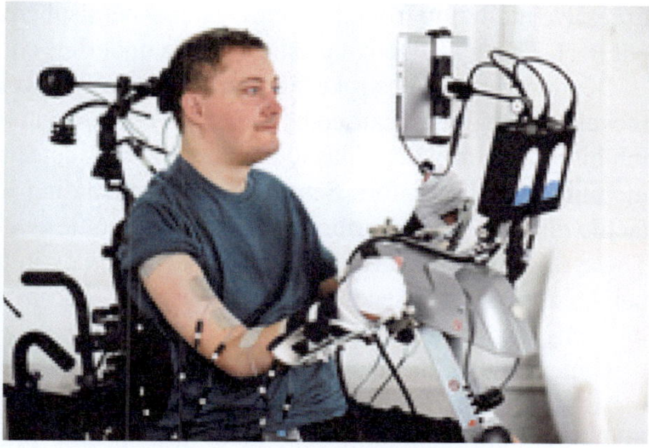

Fig. 6.4 Example of an individual with SCI set-up for upper extremity FES-cycling. Note that the pedals used help offweight the forearm for improved support of the shoulder, in addition to stimulation for subluxation correction. (©Restorative Therapies)

reduction, and muscle mass in individuals with SCI—all leading to decreased risk of pressure injury and other aforementioned secondary complications. It is important to note that as a physical intervention, cessation of therapy leads to reversal of benefits [74]. Although much research has been performed using FES to promote functional mobility and recovery of the lower extremity after SCI, evidence on the effects of FES-cycling on the upper extremities is severely lacking (Fig. 6.4 brings an example of upper extremities exercise). However, it is reasonable to extrapolate that outcomes such as improved/maintenance of range of motion, reduction in muscle atrophy, circulatory benefits, and decreased spasticity would also apply to upper extremity FES-cycling. Dosing recommendations support the need for life-long access to FES-cycling, for example as a home-based intervention, to support individuals with SCI in limiting their risks for secondary health complications.

Stroke

Pathophysiology and Impact on the Nervous System

Stroke can be broadly divided into ischemic and hemorrhagic subtypes. Ischemic strokes, which account for 80–85% of cases, result from arterial occlusion due to thrombus or embolus formation, leading to hypoperfusion and infarction of brain tissue [77]. Hemorrhagic strokes occur less frequently and involve rupture of intracerebral vessels or aneurysms, resulting in bleeding into surrounding brain parenchyma [78]. Despite different etiologies, both types of stroke share a final pathway of energy depletion, excitotoxicity, oxidative stress, inflammation, and neuronal apoptosis [79].

Damage to the corticospinal tract is one of the main contributors to motor deficits observed after stroke. Lesions in this pathway lead to contralateral hemiplegia or hemiparesis, impairing voluntary motor control [80]. Furthermore, interhemispheric imbalance, characterized by reduced excitability of the lesioned hemisphere and excessive inhibition from the contralesional hemisphere, further disrupts motor output [81]. This maladaptive plasticity often underlies chronic motor impairments.

Beyond weakness, stroke survivors frequently develop spasticity and abnormal movement synergies, caused by increased reflex excitability and loss of descending inhibitory control [82]. Spastic hypertonia contributes to gait dysfunction, reduced mobility, and discomfort. Sensory deficits, including impaired proprioception and tactile discrimination, further exacerbate difficulties with balance and coordination. These combined impairments increase dependency in activities of daily living and heighten the risk of secondary complications such as falls, cardiovascular deconditioning, and depression [83].

Understanding the neurophysiological basis of these deficits is crucial for designing effective interventions. By targeting muscle activation, promoting reciprocal inhibition, and facilitating repetitive, task-specific practice, FES-cycling offers a rehabilitation strategy that directly addresses the consequences of corticospinal damage and abnormal reflex control in stroke survivors.

Motor Control, Hemiplegia, and Functional Limitations

Motor deficits following stroke represent the most common and disabling sequelae, typically manifesting as unilateral weakness or paralysis (hemiparesis or hemiplegia). Approximately 80% of stroke survivors experience motor impairments in the acute phase, and for many, these persist chronically [84]. Such impairments involve reduced voluntary muscle activation, altered recruitment of motor units, and abnormal muscle synergies that interfere with functional movements [85].

Weakness is often accompanied by spasticity, defined as a velocity-dependent increase in muscle tone due to hyperexcitability of the stretch reflex [86]. Spasticity affects up to 40% of stroke survivors within the first year and is associated with pain, reduced range of motion, and impaired walking ability [87]. In addition, abnormal co-contraction of agonist and antagonist muscles limits fluid motor execution and contributes to inefficient gait patterns.

Beyond motor control, deficits in coordination and endurance are common. Stroke survivors frequently demonstrate decreased aerobic capacity, reduced muscle endurance, and impaired balance, all of which increase fall risk and limit participation in daily activities [88]. The consequences of immobility further exacerbate disability, leading to muscle atrophy, cardiovascular deconditioning, and metabolic dysfunction [89].

Traditional rehabilitation approaches, such as physiotherapy and occupational therapy, emphasize task-specific training, strengthening, and mobility exercises to restore function. Although effective for many, conventional interventions often fail to fully address severe weakness or promote adequate intensity and repetition of practice (factors crucial for neuroplasticity) [90]. Consequently, adjunctive therapies like functional electrical stimulation have been introduced to enhance recovery by enabling repetitive, patterned muscle activation even in patients with profound paresis [91].

Application of FES-Cycling in Stroke Rehabilitation

FES-cycling allows patients with minimal or no voluntary motor control to engage in active cycling exercise, which is otherwise impossible through voluntary effort alone. In stroke rehabilitation, FES-cycling offers several advantages. First, it promotes bilateral and symmetrical lower limb activation, reducing learned non-use of the paretic side and encouraging interlimb coordination [92]. Second, the repetitive and rhythmic nature of cycling provides high-intensity, task-oriented practice that is strongly associated with cortical reorganization and motor recovery [93]. Third, FES-cycling provides a cardiovascular workout that enhances aerobic capacity and reduces risk factors for recurrent stroke, such as sedentary behavior and metabolic dysfunction.

Another key aspect is the ability of FES-cycling to deliver quantifiable, reproducible training loads. Parameters such as pedaling speed, resistance, and stimulation intensity can be systematically adjusted to ensure progression and individualized prescription. Importantly, the technology can be adapted across the recovery continuum (from acute inpatient settings to chronic outpatient rehabilitation and, more recently, home-based programs).

From a neurophysiological perspective, FES-cycling enhances afferent input from muscle spindles and Golgi tendon organs, which may contribute to neuroplastic changes in the motor cortex. The intervention can also modulate spinal reflex pathways, reducing hyperreflexia and spasticity while facilitating reciprocal inhibition of antagonistic muscles [94]. These mechanisms can explain why FES-cycling has been associated not only with improvements in muscle strength and endurance but also with better motor control and reduced abnormal tone in stroke survivors [95, 96].

Clinical Benefits of FES-Cycling in Stroke

A growing body of evidence supports the use of FES-cycling in stroke rehabilitation, with documented benefits in muscle strength, spasticity reduction, gait performance, cardiovascular fitness, and overall functional independence. Importantly, improvements have been reported in both subacute and chronic stroke populations, suggesting applicability across different stages of recovery [97].

Muscle Strength and Endurance

FES-cycling provides an effective method for counteracting disuse atrophy and improving muscular endurance. Regular sessions stimulate hypertrophy of the quadriceps and hamstrings, leading to increased torque production and improved fatigue resistance. Randomized controlled trials have shown significant gains in lower-limb strength in stroke survivors receiving FES-cycling compared to conventional therapy alone [92]. These adaptations are particularly important, as muscle weakness correlates with walking ability and independence in daily life.

Spasticity Reduction

Spasticity is a major contributor to functional disability in stroke survivors. It has been demonstrated that FES-cycling reduces hypertonia [95, 98]. The reduction in spasticity is thought to result from repeated activation of reciprocal inhibition pathways and modulation of spinal reflex excitability [94], as well as improvement in blood flow. Clinically, decreased spasticity translates into greater comfort, easier limb handling for caregivers, and improved potential for voluntary movement [99].

Gait and Functional Recovery

One of the ultimate goals of stroke rehabilitation is restoration of walking. By improving paretic limb strength, interlimb coordination, and cardiovascular endurance, FES-cycling has been shown to facilitate improvements in gait performance [100]. Studies report increased functional ambulation capacity, walking speed, distance, and symmetry in individuals undergoing FES-cycling interventions [92, 101]. Integration of FES-cycling with conventional gait training yields additive benefits, likely due to enhanced motor relearning and cortical reorganization.

Cardiovascular and Metabolic Health

Stroke survivors are at heightened risk for recurrent vascular events, largely due to reduced physical activity and underlying comorbidities. FES-cycling elicits cardiovascular adaptations such as increased peak oxygen uptake, stroke volume, and heart rate [48]. FES-cycling physical training improves aerobic capacity [102] and can enhance glucose regulation, and lipid metabolism. These effects are clinically relevant, as enhanced cardiorespiratory fitness is directly associated with reduced mortality and morbidity in post-stroke populations [89].

Quality of Life and Participation

Beyond physiological benefits, FES-cycling can contribute to psychological well-being and social participation. It is expected that patients improve confidence, present greater independence in mobility, and enhanced motivation to engage in rehabilitation. The ability to participate in meaningful physical activity, despite severe motor impairment, is a critical factor in long-term rehabilitation success [103].

Treatment Protocols and Practical Considerations

FES-cycling protocols for stroke rehabilitation vary considerably across studies in terms of stimulation parameters, session duration, frequency, and length of treatment programs. Despite this variability, several common principles can be identified. Most interventions involve sessions lasting 30–60 min, performed 3–5 times per week, over a 4–12 week period. The quadriceps, hamstrings, and gluteal muscles are the most frequently stimulated, though some protocols also include the tibialis anterior to assist ankle dorsiflexion during the pedaling cycle.

Stimulation settings typically employ frequencies between 20 and 50 Hz, pulse widths of 200–400 μs, and intensities titrated to patient tolerance (usually within

30–120 mA). Resistance on the ergometer can be gradually increased as voluntary contribution improves, allowing progression of training intensity. Importantly, hybrid modes combining voluntary effort with electrical stimulation appear to yield superior outcomes compared to passive stimulation alone.

Patient selection is an important consideration. FES-cycling has been successfully applied in both subacute and chronic stroke populations, but greater gains are often observed when introduced earlier in the recovery phase [92]. Contraindications include uncontrolled epilepsy, unstable cardiac conditions, skin lesions at electrode sites, and presence of certain implanted devices [94].

Safety and tolerability are generally excellent. Adverse effects are rare and usually limited to mild skin irritation at electrode sites. Importantly, adherence rates are high, reflecting good patient acceptance and motivation. Advances in portable FES-cycling devices now enable community- and home-based use, further enhancing accessibility and continuity of therapy.

The studies summarized in Table 6.8 demonstrate that FES-cycling is feasible and beneficial across different stages of stroke recovery, from the early post-acute period to chronic stroke populations. Despite variability in stimulation settings,

Table 6.8 Summary of clinical trials of FES-cycling in stroke rehabilitation

References	Sample (n)	Stroke stage	Duration and frequency	Stimulation parameters	Main outcomes
[100]	12	Subacute–chronic	20 sessions, 5×/week, 4 weeks	Quadriceps/hamstrings/gluteals, 20–35 Hz, 300 μs	↑ Muscle activation, ↑ pedaling symmetry
[92]	30	Post-acute	25 sessions, 5×/week, 5 weeks	Quadriceps/hamstrings/gluteals, 30 Hz, 300 μs	↑ Motor recovery, ↑ cycling symmetry
[101]	22	Acute–subacute (7 days–6 months)	20 sessions, 5×/week, 4 weeks	Quadriceps/hamstrings/gluteals, 20–40 Hz, 200–300 μs	↑ Muscle strength, ↑ walking ability
[96]	18	Post-acute	15 sessions, 3×/week, 5 weeks	Quadriceps/hamstrings, 25–35 Hz, 200–300 μs	↑ Strength, ↑ motor control (cycling performance)
[102]	20	Chronic (>6 months)	30 sessions, 3×/week, 10 weeks	Quadriceps/hamstrings/gluteals, 35 Hz, 250 μs	↑ VO_2 peak, ↑ endurance, ↑ power output
[95]	14	Chronic	24 sessions, 3×/week, 8 weeks	Quadriceps/hamstrings, 30 Hz, 300 μs	↑ Postural control, ↑ balance measures
[98]	15	Chronic	Single session	Quadriceps/hamstrings, 30 Hz, 300 μs	↓ Hypertonia, acute spasticity reduction

sample sizes, and treatment durations, consistent improvements have been reported in muscle strength, pedaling symmetry, postural control, aerobic capacity, and spasticity reduction. Importantly, even short-term interventions, such as single sessions, yielded measurable decreases in hypertonia, while longer programs enhanced functional outcomes like walking distance, balance, and motor recovery. These findings suggest that while protocols are not yet standardized, FES-cycling provides a safe, adaptable, and effective adjunct to conventional rehabilitation across the stroke continuum.

Cerebral Palsy

Impact of Cerebral Palsy on the Nervous System

Cerebral palsy (CP) occurs due to a non-progressive injury in the developing fetal or infant brain, affecting the development of movement and posture. It is the most common motor disability in children, with global prevalence of approximately 1.5 to 4 per 1000 live births. Depending on the location of the injury, CP can be classified as spastic, ataxic, or dyskinetic. Spastic CP is associated with an injury to the corticospinal tract and is characterized by short and weak muscles, spasticity, and impaired selective motor control. Ataxic CP is associated with a cerebellar injury and presents with impaired balance and coordination while dyskinetic CP is associated with an injury to basal ganglia and symptoms of involuntary muscle contractions during purposeful movements [104]. However, many children have mixed clinical presentations of more than one type. Given that spastic CP is the most common type, affecting about 80% of those diagnosed with CP [105], most research and consequently, the rest of the chapter, is focused on individuals with spastic presentation.

Need for Novel Interventions to Promote Physical Activity in CP

Altered muscle activation patterns and spasticity cause abnormal forces at the joints, leading to bony deformities and muscle contractures. These impairments, in turn, lead to decreased independence and a lack of physical activity in children with CP. Children with CP participate in less physical activity and are sedentary for twice the maximum recommended limit [106, 107]. One major cause of decline in physical function is the disparity that occurs when muscle strength gains are not commensurate to gains in body size or weight. This disparity is often exacerbated by the surgical procedures and other procedures such as serial casting and Botulinum toxin injections that reduce spasticity but in doing so, unmask muscle weakness by either putting the muscle at unfavorable lengths for generating force or by forced periods of prolonged immobility required by corrective procedures [108–112]. Thus, as children with CP mature, they have marked difficulties in maintaining and improving strength, fitness, and functional ability.

Issues with Cycling as an Exercise for Children with CP

Cycling has been proposed as a feasible method of exercising in children with CP because it does not require the strength and postural control that exercises in upright standing or walking position require. Cycling provides a potential means of improving strength and cardiorespiratory fitness and maintaining joint range of motion while performing an activity that can be performed outside of a rehabilitation setting with family and their peers using an adapted cycle. Further, it allows them to exercise in a relatively safe position that is easier to attain and maintain, particularly for individuals with Gross Motor Function Classification System Levels III and IV, that need assistive devices and/or wheelchair for mobility.

However, children with CP may not have the strength or selective motor control to cycle at therapeutically beneficial levels. Children with CP cycle with greater transverse and frontal plane motion at the hip and knee, increased duration of muscle activity and increased co-contraction of agonist and antagonist muscle at the knee and ankle [113, 114], and show altered forces in the form of increased pulling away from the pedal during flexion phase and decreased pushing into the pedal during extension phase [115]. The result is a non-smooth, irregular, and asymmetric crank rotation [116]. All these issues make it difficult to attain heart rates and cycling intensities necessary to achieve musculoskeletal changes and cardiorespiratory training effects and hence, additional means are necessary to improve cycling ability and biomechanics in this population.

Functional Electrical Stimulation Assisted Cycling in Children with CP

Functional electrical stimulation (FES)-assisted cycling in children with CP was a novel translational approach derived from prior work on individuals with spinal cord injury that showed improved body composition and blood glucose control [117], quadriceps muscle strength [118], reduced spastic muscle tone [16, 119], and muscle endurance [120]. While FES has traditionally been used with muscle strengthening exercises and during walking in several studies, it's use during cycling has been explored only more recently in one case study [121] and three RCTs [122–124].

FES was applied either during cycling alone or in addition to interventions targeted at improving range of motion, strength, and balance. The muscles targeted in these protocols range from either a single muscle bilaterally, such as quadriceps or a combination of several muscles such as gluteal muscles, quadriceps, hamstrings, gastrocsoleus, and tibialis anterior. The duration of the training protocols ranges from 4 to 12 weeks, with a frequency of three to five 30-min sessions a week. The FES frequency used was between 30 and 50 Hz, with a pulse width of 250 μsec. The intensity for FES was either to participant tolerance or in the range of 40–100 mA.

Clinical Benefits of FES-Assisted Cycling

FES-assisted cycling has shown to significantly improve motor function in children with CP, as measured by Gross Motor Function Measure as well as participant-reported improvement in function via The Canadian Occupational Performance Measure [121, 123]. Further, children with CP showed increased walking distance and speed on functional measures such as 6 min Walk test and Timed Up and Go test, respectively [121, 124]. FES assistance also helped children attain higher cycling cadence and help retain these gains in cadence 8 weeks after cessation of the FES training protocol [122]. Finally, there was also reduced spasticity in children with CP following FES-assisted cycling training. While muscle strength was not directly measured in the above studies, participants in the FES-assisted cycling group showed higher cycling power output and higher cycling resistance compared to the control group, indicating that FES-assisted cycling may have beneficial effects on lower limb strength.

Prior work on stationary cycling without FES assistance in children with CP has had mixed results on motor function [125–127]. Thus, one of the reasons for the improvements seen in studies using FES-assistance with cycling may be attributed to the incorporation of FES, resulting in appropriately timed muscle contractions that enable the children to reach higher cycling intensities. Some of these studies also used automatic motor assistance during cycling that allowed participants to reach higher cycling speed volitionally but provided assistance if their cycling speed fell below a certain threshold, thus providing some periods of active recovery and preventing fatigue [122, 123]. Lastly, the World Health Organization's International Classification of Function, Health, and Disability (ICF) model stresses the importance of incorporating a child's social and environmental needs into rehabilitation programs. Cycling provides an excellent means of not only addressing the structure and function components of ICF but also encouraging participation in a physical activity that can be done with family and their peers. Children with CP are more likely to participate in a physical activity if it lets them "fit in" and may be discouraged if the motor tasks are too challenging or make their disability stand out. FES-assistance, by enabling faster cycling speeds, may motivate children to participate in a physical activity with higher confidence and self-esteem. This will not only help in addressing the physical but also social development of children with CP, wherein they can engage in an enjoyable activity that is not viewed as "exercise" and thus increase their compliance in a physical activity program.

Special Considerations with Using FES-Assisted Cycling in Children with CP

A critical consideration while combining FES with cycling particularly for the pediatric population is participant tolerance to FES. Typically, children with CP are able to tolerate higher intensities of FES stimulation when applied to larger muscle groups such as quadriceps rather than smaller muscles such as tibialis anterior or gastrocsoleus. It is also not uncommon for children to refuse application of FES on their gluteal muscles due to embarrassment and/or discomfort. In such cases, it is advisable to incorporate acclimatization sessions where participants and their parents can familiarize themselves with the equipment, trial FES at lower stimulation intensities, smaller pulse width and frequencies in larger muscle groups and then move on to smaller muscles such those at the leg and feet. Training parents to place the electrodes on gluteal region may also make the children more comfortable with FES application at this region.

Challenges and Future Directions in Clinical Application of FES-Assisted Cycling in Children with CP

Despite the benefits, the use of FES in clinical practice in pediatric populations is low. The most commonly cited barriers and challenges include lack of appropriate adaptive equipment and resources (cycles adapted for use with pediatric patient populations, stimulators etc.), lack of knowledge and training regarding using FES, and therapist perceptions or preference for other treatment options [128]. For example, despite evidence to the contrary, some physical therapists perceived FES to be an inappropriate intervention for young children. Further, a one-size-fits-all approach to prescribing FES parameters for children may not be feasible as the frequency and duration of FES sessions may depend on several factors, such as the type of CP (spastic or ataxic or dyskinetic, hemiplegic or diplegic), age, GMFCS level, socioeconomic status, resources and environment (family, transportation, funds). Guidelines that help physical and occupational therapists select and adapt the FES parameters and aid in clinical decision making are critical to promote the use of FES-assisted cycling in pediatric population. Another barrier that is unique to application of FES to the pediatric population is parental apprehension [129]. Offering parents familiarization sessions with FES prior to initiating an FES intervention can help alleviate parental anxiety about the use of FES. Overall, providing greater opportunities for FES-related education for health care providers, providing families easier access to FES-assisted interventions, including adaptive cycles, equipment, and stimulation devices, promoting research related to efficacy and effectiveness of FES-assisted cycling would be instrumental in advancing the use of FES-assisted cycling in pediatric clinical care [130].

Multiple Sclerosis

Impact of Multiple Sclerosis on the Nervous System

Multiple sclerosis (MS) is an immune-mediate central nervous system (CNS) disorder that affects almost three million people living worldwide [131]. The hallmark neuropathological features of MS include demyelination, astrocytic gliosis, and axonal or neuronal loss, the latter of which is believed to be the main contributor to clinical disability in MS [132]. The clinical presentation of MS is heterogeneous across individuals depending on the location and extent of inflammation and damage within the CNS [132]. Common impairments and symptoms in MS include the loss of mobility, muscle weakness, spasticity, visual and cognitive impairments, bladder, bowel and sexual dysfunction, mood changes, and symptoms of fatigue and pain [133]. Comorbid health conditions are also common in MS, such as cardiovascular and psychiatric conditions, with important implications for management throughout the disease course [134, 135].

Significant advancements have been made in the development of disease-modifying therapies that target the neuroinflammatory component of MS; however, there has been less success in preventing or halting neurodegeneration, ultimately leading to disability progression and accumulation long-term [132, 136]. Consequently, looking to comprehensive approaches for managing disability and improving function in MS are critical [135]. This may be particularly relevant in the later stages of the disease where accumulated clinical disability has substantial impacts on daily functioning [137–139].

Rehabilitation, including exercise-based strategies, is an approach for managing disability impacts and improving function for people living with MS. Functional electrical stimulation (FES) cycling is one such approach. Two prior reviews published in 2019 [140] and 2020 [141] summarized the available literature on FES-cycling in MS considering acute responses, training interventions, and overall safety. To provide clinical guidance on the use and potential benefits of FES-cycling for people with MS, we conducted an updated review of the literature with a focus on prospective studies of FES-cycling training (i.e., FES-cycling protocols applied for at least 2 weeks in duration). All outcome types were considered.

Herein we summarize the research to date on FES-cycling interventions for people living with MS with respect to training protocols and training effects, and potential for clinical benefits. We review specific considerations for FES-cycling in MS and highlight next steps for addressing current gaps in the evidence base.

Application of Functional Electrical Stimulation Cycling in MS—Training Protocols and Effects

In total, 11 reports [142–152] from 9 studies involving FES-cycling training (n = 6 pre-post studies; n = 3 randomized controlled trials [RCT]) were reviewed and summarized (Tables 6.9 and 6.10). The nine studies reviewed included 83 people with MS. Most studies involved participants who were middle age (mean age range 48–57 years), with moderate-to-severe MS disability, and had a mean disease duration between 13 and 21.5 years (Table 6.10). In general, participants in the reviewed studies were older, had more severe disability, and had been living with MS longer compared to samples in other MS exercise interventions [153]. This participant profile is not surprising given the application of an adapted exercise intervention but remains important to keep in mind when considering training protocols and interpreting potential benefits.

Table 6.9 Summary of FES-cycling intervention parameters and training effects in people with multiple sclerosis

Reference	Training parameters	Cycling and stimulation parameters	Adherence and training effects reported
Pre-post trials			
[142]	Duration: 2 weeks Session frequency: 3×/week Session duration: 12–18 min (active training time)	Cadence: NR Pulse width: 300 µsec Frequency: 20 Hz Intensity: Up to 127 mA Muscle groups: Quadriceps and hamstrings	No change in cycling PO No change in cycling smoothness (roughness index)
[143]	Duration: 24 weeks Session frequency: 3×/week Session duration: 60 min	Cadence: NR Pulse width: 250 µsec Frequency: 33–45 Hz Intensity: NR Muscle groups: Quadriceps, hamstrings and gluteals	Mean sessions/week: 3.8 (range = 3.1–5.1) Increased cycling distance Increased cycling PO
[144]	Duration: 10 weeks Session frequency: 2–3×/week Session duration: 40 min	Cadence: 10 rpm Pulse width: 300 µsec Frequency: 35 Hz Intensity: 30 mA (initial) Muscle groups: Quadriceps, hamstrings and gluteals	Mean sessions/week: 1.8 Mean total training duration: 10 weeks Increased stimulation intensity: (max mean stimulation) - quadriceps = 91 ± 11 mA - hamstrings = 86 ± 18 mA - Gluteals = 69 ± 21 mA
[145]	Duration: 4 weeks Session frequency: 3×/week Session duration: 30 min	Cadence: 40–50 rpm Pulse width: NR Frequency: NR Intensity: NR Muscle groups: Quadriceps, hamstrings and gluteals	Increased cycling time (participants unable to cycle 30 min)[a] Increased cycling resistance (participants able to cycle 30 min)[a]

(continued)

Table 6.9 (continued)

Reference	Training parameters	Cycling and stimulation parameters	Adherence and training effects reported
[146]	Duration: 4 weeks Session frequency: 2–3×/week Session duration: 30 min	Cadence: 35–50 rpm Pulse width: 200 μsec Frequency: 50 Hz Intensity: Individualized Muscle groups: Quadriceps, hamstrings and gluteals	Increased active cycling time (participants unable to cycle 30 min; ES = 0.77)[a] Increased active cycling PO (participants unable to cycle 30 min; ES = 0.63) Increased cycling PO (participants able to cycle 30 min; ES = 5.25) Increased cycling resistance (participants able to cycle 30 min; ES = 2.53)[a]
[147]	Duration: 12 weeks Session frequency: 2×/week Session duration: 40 min Arm cycling: 20 min total; 30″ work (60% PO_{peak}/RPE = 14) /30″ rest intervals; cadence = 50 rpm (delivered concurrently with FES-cycling during last 20 min of the session)	Cadence: 10 rpm Pulse width: 300 μsec Frequency: 35 Hz Intensity: 30 mA (initial) Muscle groups: Quadriceps, hamstrings, gluteals and gastrocnemius	Mean session adherence: 80 ± 10.4% Mean stimulation intensity: 93.7 ± 14.4 mA Arm cycle ergometry: Intervals preformed at 30″ work/30″ rest intervals: 65% (summary of intervals below) Total time: 19.5 ± 4.0 min Mean number of intervals performed/session: 18.1 ± 4.2 Mean PO: 116 ± 44%PO_{peak} Mean RPE: 15.1 ± 2.1 Mean HR: 103 ± 15%HR_{peak}
RCTs			
[148]	Duration: 8 weeks Session frequency: 3×/week Session duration: 45 min Control: Active leg cycling	Cadence: 45 rpm Pulse width: 250 μsec (initial) Frequency: 43.5 Hz Intensity: Individualized Muscle groups: Quadriceps, hamstrings, gluteals, tibialis anterior and gastrocnemius	Increased cycling distance (FES-cycling [ES = 0.30]; active leg cycling [ES = 0.24]) Increased cycling PO (FES-cycling [ES = 0.66][a]; active leg cycling [ES = 0.72][a] groups)

(continued)

Table 6.9 (continued)

Reference	Training parameters	Cycling and stimulation parameters	Adherence and training effects reported
[149–151]	Duration: 24 weeks Session frequency: 3×/week Session duration: 10–30 min Control: Passive leg cycling	Cadence: 40–50 rpm Pulse width: 250 μsec Frequency: 50 Hz Intensity: Individualized Muscle groups: Quadriceps, hamstrings and gluteals	Mean session adherence: 84% (FES-cycling)/84% (passive leg cycling) Increased cycling distance (FES-cycling and passive leg cycling groups) Increased cycling PO (FES-cycling group only) Increased cycling resistance (FES-cycling group only)
[152]	Duration: 12 weeks Session frequency: 2–3×/week Session duration: 30 min Control: Wait period with usual activities and medications	Cadence: 35–50 rpm Pulse width: 200 μsec Frequency: 50 Hz Intensity: Individualized Muscle groups: Quadriceps, hamstrings and gluteals	Session adherence: 100% (5/6 participants); 103% (1/6 participants) Increased cycling resistance (participants who could cycle 30 min at beginning of study) Increased cycling time, resistance and distance (participants unable to cycle 30 min at start of training but could cycle 30 min by the end) No change in cycling distance and no resistance added (participants who could not cycle 30 min at beginning and did not increase cycling time)

Abbreviations: *ES* effect size, *FES* functional electrical stimulation, *HR* heart rate, *Hz* hertz, *mA* milliamps, *NR* not reported, *PO* power output, *RPE* rating of perceived exertion, *rpm* revolutions per minute, *μsec* microseconds

[a]Indicates statistically significant difference at $p < 0.05$ level

Training Protocols

Overall, considerable variability exists in the FES-cycling protocols applied in MS to date (Table 6.9). Relative to the six pre-post studies [142–147], intervention durations ranged between 2 and 24 weeks, with most sessions delivered for 30–60 min, 2–3 times per week. Similarly, training durations for the three RCTs [148–152] ranged between 8 and 24 weeks, with sessions delivered 2–3 times per week. One RCT incorporated a progressive increase in session duration, beginning with 10 min and extending up to 30 min [149–151], while the other two RCTs maintained constant training durations of 30 or 40 min [148, 152]. Only one pre-post study [143] was delivered in the home setting, while all other studies were delivered in supervised training settings.

Table 6.10 Summary of effects of FES-cycling interventions in people with multiple sclerosis

Reference	Participants	Study outcomes (non-cycling)	Main intervention effects
Pre-post trials			
[142]	n = 8 Age: 52.1 (7.5) years EDSS range: 4.0–7.5 Disease duration: 13.3 (8.0) years	Muscular strength (MMT: KE, KF) Walking speed (10-MWT) Spasticity (MAS)	↔: MMT; 10MWT; MAS
[143]	n = 5 Age: 50 (median) years EDSS range: 6.0–6.5 Disease duration: 13 years	Neurological disability/ neuroperformance (EDSS, MSFC) Muscular strength (MMT: HE, HF, KE, KF, DF) Walking speed (T25FWT) Walking endurance (2MWT) Agility (TUG) Spatiotemporal gait parameters (electronic walkway) Spasticity (LLSMS) Vibration sensation (2AFC) QOL (SF-36) Psychiatric functioning (SCL-90 global severity index) Cytokines, chemokines and growth factors	↔: EDSS; LLSMS; SCL-90; cytokines, chemokines and growth factors ↑: MSFC; MMT (HE, KE, KF); T25WT, 2 MW, TUG; some spatiotemporal gait parameters; 2AFC; SF-36 ↓: MMT (HF, DF)
[144]	n = 7 Age: 48.0 (9.0) years EDSS range: 6.5–8.5 Disease duration: NR	Thigh circumference Perceived therapeutic benefits	↑: Left and right thigh circumferences[a]; perceived improvements in transfer ability, circulation, strength, balance, pain and spasticity ↓: Perceived fatigue and leg stiffness
[145]	n = 8 Age: 54.5 (13.9) years EDSS: >6.0 Disease duration: 16.8 (6.9) years	m $\dot{V}O_2$ of right vastus lateralis	↑: m $\dot{V}O_2$ of right vastus lateralis[a]

(continued)

Table 6.10 (continued)

Reference	Participants	Study outcomes (non-cycling)	Main intervention effects
[146]	n = 14 Age: 55.3 (11.0) years EDSS range: NR Disease duration: 15.3 (7.4) years	Muscular strength (MMT: HF, KE, KF, DF) Spasticity (MAS) Fatigue (MFIS) Mental health inventory (MHI) Pain (MOS) QOL (MSQLI)	↔: MMT (ES = 0.04–0.11); MAS (ES = −0.07– −0.33); MHI; SF-36 (ES = 0.19 Total score) ↑: MFIS (ES = 0.41; Total score); MOS (ES = −0.55)
[147]	n = 7 Age: 57.1 (7.8) years EDSS range: 6.5–8.5 Disease duration: 18.4 (7.5) years	Cardiorespiratory fitness (PO_{peak} and $\dot{V}O_{2peak}$ predicted from PO_{peak}) Fatigue (MFIS)	↑: PO_{peak} (ES = 0.33); $\dot{V}O_{2peak}$ (ES = 0.30); MFIS (ES = −0.77; Total score)
RCTs			
[148]	n = 14 Age: 53.6 (10.2) years PDDS range: 3–6 Disease duration: 13.1 (12.1) years	Lower limb strength/ function (5XSST) Walking speed (T25FWT) Walking endurance (6MWT) Agility (TUG) Spatiotemporal gait parameters (waist-worn inertial sensor) Self-reported mobility (MSWS-12) Balance confidence (ABC) Fatigue (MFIS) QOL (MSQOL-54)	↔: T25FW (ES = 0.11–0.12); most spatiotemporal gait parameters; MSWS-12; ABC; MSQOL-54 physical ↑ (both groups): 5XSST (ES = 0.53–0.68; time effect[a]); 6MWT (ES = 0.19–0.30; time effect[a]); MFIS Total score (time effect[a]); MSQOL-54 mental (time effect[a]); MSQOL-54 overall (time effect[a]) ↑ (favours FES group): TUG (ES = −0.30 FES; ES = 0.15 active leg cycling)

(continued)

Table 6.10 (continued)

Reference	Participants	Study outcomes (non-cycling)	Main intervention effects
[149–151]	n = 8 Age: 52.9 (7.9) years EDSS range: 5.5–6.5 Disease duration: 21.5 (6.6) years	Cardiorespiratory fitness ($\dot{V}O_{2peak}$ and PO_{peak} from CPET) Muscular strength and asymmetry (seated dynamometer: KE, KF) Body composition (DXA) Walking speed (T25FWT) Walking endurance (2MWT) Agility (TUG) Self-reported mobility (MSWS-12) Cognition (SDMT) Fatigue (MFIS, FSS) Pain (MPQ) QOL (MSIS-29)	↔: KF strength (ES = −0.07); %BF (ES = −0.16); FFM (ES = 0.18); FM (ES = 0.00) ↑ (favours FES group): $\dot{V}O_{2peak}$ (ES = 0.34); PO_{peak} (ES = 0.65); KE strength (ES = 0.56); KE strength asymmetry (ES = −0.33); KF strength asymmetry (ES = −0.23); BMD (ES = 0.57); T25FWT (ES = 0.40), 2MWT (ES = 0.20), TUG (ES = −0.30), MSWS-12 (ES = −0.68); SDMT (ES = 0.53); MFIS (ES = −0.60; Total score); FSS (ES = −0.92); MPQ (ES = −0.67) ↓ (favours passive leg cycling group): MSIS-29 physical (ES = 0.33); MSIS-29 psychological (ES = 0.21)
[152]	n = 12 Age: 55.4 (10.3) years EDSS range: 7.0–8.5 Disease duration: NR	Muscular strength (MMT: HE, HF, HA, KE, KF, DF, PF) Spasticity (MAS) Fatigue (MFIS-5; FSMC) Depressive symptoms (PHQ-9) Pain (MOS) QOL (MSQOL-54) Exercise self-efficacy (ESES)	↔: MMT, MAS, MOS (ES = 0.10); MSQOL-54 mental health composite (ES = 0.06) ↑ (favours FES group): MFIS-5 (ES = 0.60); FSMC total (ES = 0.37; Total score); MSQOL-54 physical health composite (ES = 1.48); ESES (ES = 0.46) ↓ (favours control group): PHQ-9 (ES = 0.67; outlier removed: ES = 0.03)

Abbreviations: *2AFC* Two Alternative Forced Choice Procedure, *2MWT* 2-Minute Walk Test, *5XSST* 5-Times Sit-to-Stand, *6MWT* 6-Minute Walk Test, *10MWT* 10-Meter Walk Test (10MWT), *ABC* Activities-specific Balance Confidence scale, *DF* dorsiflexors, *DXA* dual-energy X-ray absorptiometry, *EDSS* Expanded Disability Status Scale, *ESSE* Exercise Self-Efficacy Scale, *FES* functional electrical stimulation; *FSMC* Fatigue Scale for Motor and Cognitive Functions, *FSS* Fatigue Severity Scale, *HA* hip adductors, *HE* hip extensors, *HF* hip flexors, *KE* knee flexors, *KF* knee extensors, *LLSMS* Lower Limb Spasticity Measurement System, *MAS* Modified Ashworth Scale, *MFIS/MFIS-5* (5-item) Modified Fatigue Impact Scale, *MHI* Mental Health Inventory, *MMT* manual muscle testing; *MOS* Medical Outcomes Study Pain Effects Scale, *MPQ* McGill Pain Questionnaire, *MSFC* Multiple Sclerosis Functional Composite, *MSIS-29* 29-item Multiple Sclerosis Impact Scale, *MSQLI* MS Quality of Life Inventory, *MSQOL-54* 54-item Multiple Sclerosis Quality of Life instrument, *MSWS-12* 12-item Multiple Sclerosis Walking Scale, *NR* not reported, *PDDS* Patient Determined Disease Steps, *PF* plantarflexors, *PHQ-9* Patient Health Questionnaire-9, PO_{peak} peak power output, *SCL-90* Symptom Checklist 90, *SDMT* Symbol Digit Modalities Test, *SF-36* Short Form 36, *T25FWT* Timed 25-Foot Walk Test, *TUG* Timed Up-and-Go, $\dot{V}O_{2peak}$ peak oxygen consumption

↔ Indicates no change; ↑ indicates improvement; ↓ Indicates worsening

[a]indicates statistically significant difference

Across all studies, cycling cadence ranged between 10 and 50 rpm, with stimulation parameters set at a pulse width of 200–300 μsec and frequency of 20–50 Hz. Protocols most consistently involved stimulation of the quadriceps, hamstrings, and gluteal muscle groups, while some also stimulated the tibialis anterior and/or the gastrocnemius muscles. Early studies used standardized FES stimulation parameters, but as the field evolved there was a shift toward personalized approaches. Researchers increasingly adopted individualized FES protocols, tailoring stimulation intensities to align with participants' capabilities and training goals. Training protocols have also varied depending on the goal of the intervention; some protocols have encouraged participants to actively cycle with FES, while others have instructed participants to voluntarily push during FES-cycling. Interestingly, one pre-post trial used a hybrid design combining FES leg cycling with upper body arm cycling exercise [147]. In that study, interval-based arm cycling exercise was performed concurrently with FES leg cycling during the last 20 min of the 40-min training sessions [147].

Training Effects

Few studies have reported on training adherence or compliance with FES-cycling interventions. Of the studies reporting on these outcomes, adherence with FES-cycling training has ranged between 80% and 103%, suggesting good adherence. Two studies reported on the change in stimulation intensity, where intensity was increase from 30 mA to a mean of 69–93.7 mA across the muscle groups stimulated over the 10–12 week interventions [144, 147].

Most studies have reported progression in cycling training parameters (e.g., increased cycling time, distance, power output (PO), and/or resistance) over the duration of FES-cycling interventions (Table 6.9). The one RCT that compared FES leg cycling to a passive leg cycling control condition reported an increase in cycling distance in both groups, whereas the FES leg cycling group also increased cycling PO and resistance over the course of the intervention [149–151]. Another RCT involving an active leg cycling control condition reported a small non-significant increase in cycling distance and a medium statistically significant increase in PO in both groups pre-post intervention [148].

Application of Functional Electrical Stimulation Cycling in MS—Clinical Benefits

Given the small sample sizes (range n = 5–14; Table 6.10) in the studies reviewed, many studies did not conduct statistical significance testing and/or presented findings based on effect size magnitudes. The outcomes collected and main intervention effects are summarized in Table 6.10. The most common outcomes of FES-cycling interventions in people with MS to date have included physiological fitness, primarily assessed as muscular strength, symptoms of fatigue and pain, spasticity, quality of life (QOL), and mobility (Table 6.10).

Regarding physiological fitness, the effects of FES-cycling on muscular strength, primarily based on manual muscle testing, suggest no change or mixed findings, with improvements reported for some muscle groups and not others [142, 143, 146, 149, 151, 152]. Two studies examined training effects on cardiorespiratory fitness; both studies reported small improvements in aerobic capacity ($\dot{V}O_{2peak}$; ES = 0.30–0.34) and small-moderate improvements in the peak PO achieved during cardiopulmonary exercise testing (ES = 0.33–0.65) [147, 149]. Other studies have reported improvement in some body composition metrics, including thigh circumference and bone mineral density [144, 149], and in measures of leg muscle metabolism (m$\dot{V}O_2$) using near-infrared spectroscopy [145].

One of the most consistently reported benefit of FES-cycling in MS has been for symptoms of fatigue, with studies reporting small-to-moderate reductions in overall fatigue scores (ES = 0.37–77) after FES-cycling training [146–148, 150, 152]. Interestingly, an overall effect of time but not group on fatigue symptoms was observed in the one RCT involving an active cycling control condition, suggesting FES and active leg cycling both improved fatigue symptoms [148]. Some studies have reported benefits of FES-cycling on pain symptoms (ES = 0.55–0.67) [146, 150], while others have not (ES = 0.10) [152]. There was consistently no change reported in spasticity in response to FES-cycling training; spasticity was most commonly measured using the Modified Ashworth Scale [142, 143, 146, 152].

The effects of FES-cycling on QOL have been inconsistent. Some studies have reported benefits of FES-cycling on QOL [143], while others have reported no change or a small decrease (i.e., worsening) in QOL in response to FES-cycling [146, 150]. Mixed findings within the same study have further been reported, such that some QOL subscales improved while others did not, without demonstrating a consistent pattern of change [148, 152]. Again, there were no group differences in training effects on QOL in the one RCT comparing FES-cycling to active leg cycling; an overall time effect was observed for overall and mental QOL, but not physical QOL [148].

A variety of outcomes have been used to examine the effect of FES-cycling on mobility in MS, such as short- and long-distance walking tests, walking agility, spatiotemporal gait parameters, and self-reported walking scales. Overall, mixed effects of FES-cycling on short-distance walking tests (e.g., Timed 25-Foot Walk Test), spatiotemporal gait parameters, and self-reported walking were noted, with some studies reporting improved mobility and others reporting no change [142, 143, 148, 149]. Small improvements (ES = 0.19–0.30) in long-distance walking performance (e.g., 2-Minute Walk Test) and agility (Timed-Up-Go [TUG] test) were reported in response to FES-cycling training [143, 148, 149]. Notably, changes in TUG performance favoured the FES-cycling group in the one RCT comparing FES to active leg cycling, suggesting potential additional benefits of FES [148]. Given the breadth of tests used to assess mobility and the heterogeneity in walking ability in the samples examined, it is unsurprising that effect of FES-cycling on mobility are inconclusive at this time.

Considerations for FES-Cycling in MS

When implementing FES-cycling for individuals with MS, it is crucial to consider prominent symptomatology of MS and adjust accordingly. Fatigue is a prevalent symptom in MS that is often cited as a barrier to initiating and maintaining exercise participation [154–156]. Consequently, a tailored and gradual approach to FES-cycling is essential to ensure that this form of exercise remains feasible, beneficial, and enjoyable for individuals who may experience fatigue symptoms. Importantly, the evidence to date suggests that symptoms of fatigue improve with FES-cycling training in MS.

To address fatigue during FES-cycling, incorporating rest periods into training sessions can prevent overexertion and may help to reduce fatigue symptoms. These intervals should be customized to the individual's needs, ensuring that exercise overload remains manageable. Another adjustment for individuals with MS who experience fatigue is starting with lower stimulation intensities and gradually increasing over time. This progression allows for manageable exercise demands, while reducing the risk of exacerbating fatigue. Gradual increases in stimulation can also promote neuromuscular adaptation, enabling the body to better tolerate exercise and improve physical function over time [157–159]. Individualized pacing is another strategy to account for fluctuations in fatigue levels. These tailored adjustments can be used to promote training adherence, as participants are more likely to feel motivated and empowered to continue training when it is customized to their specific needs and energy levels.

In addition to fatigue, potential motor impairments in MS must also be considered, and appropriate adjustments made to effectively engage in FES-cycling. Given the unpredictable progression of MS, disability accumulation can be substantial. It is estimated that over 30% of individuals with MS rely on wheelchairs for mobility [160], limiting their ability to use many conventional exercise modalities. A key advantage of FES-cycling is the capacity to accommodate individuals with varying levels of disability, including those with severe mobility impairment; FES-cycling can be delivered with the participant seated in a wheelchair or powered chair. Further, unlike traditional exercise modalities which require a baseline level of voluntary movement, FES-cycling bypasses voluntary muscle activation allowing for exercise engagement with even substantial motor impairment.

Furthermore, many modern FES-cycling systems include adaptive features, such as adjustable support for weakened limbs and customizable stimulation parameters, further enhancing the usability for individuals with severe motor impairment. For individuals with limited or no ability to transfer, home-based FES-cycling might also be a considered as it can provide a convenient option for remotely delivered exercise, provided the user receives appropriate training. The feasibility and potential benefits of home-based FES-cycling in MS have yet to be established and should be examined in future research.

Future Directions

Overall, the study of FES-cycling in individuals with MS is still in its infancy with generally low-quality evidence to date. Considering the limited evidence, optimal training prescriptions and stimulation parameters are unclear at this stage. Current evidence suggests the most consistent benefit of FES-cycling in MS is for reducing symptoms of fatigue. Other potential benefits may be related to improved aerobic capacity and walking endurance. This may have particular relevance with increasing disability status in MS, given the loss of aerobic capacity [161–163] and greater symptomatic burden [164, 165] with disability accumulation. Future studies should focus on determining optimal training prescriptions with consideration of individual participant needs and training goals. Further exploration of combined FES interventions, such as hybrid FES leg cycling and arm cycling, may be a promising avenue for optimizing training benefits in advanced MS. Additional outcomes of relevance should be included in future high-quality RCT designs to examine comprehensive benefits of FES-cycling in MS.

Neuromuscular Diseases

Neuromuscular diseases (NMDs) are a group of disorders that impair the communication between the nervous system and muscles, often leading to muscle weakness, fatigue, and loss of motor function (Fig. 6.5). These conditions can be inherited, autoimmune, or idiopathic, and they vary widely in their clinical presentation and progression. The underlying pathology may affect different components of the neuromuscular system, including motor neurons (e.g., *amyotrophic lateral sclerosis*), axons (e.g., *peripheral neuropathies*), Schwann cells (e.g., *chronic inflammatory demyelinating polyradiculoneuropathy*), the neuromuscular junction (e.g., *myasthenia gravis, Lambert-Eaton syndrome*), or the muscle tissue itself (e.g., *muscular dystrophies, inflammatory myopathies*). While most neuromuscular diseases affect the peripheral nervous system, some, such as ALS, also involve the central nervous system [166] (Fig. 6.5).

Rationale for FES-Cycling in NMDs

FES-cycling uses electrical stimulation to elicit patterned muscle contractions that produce a pedaling motion on a stationary cycle. This intervention offers several potential benefits for individuals with NMDs:

- Preservation of muscle mass and strength in partially denervated muscles
- Regulation of metabolism and myokine secretion
- Improved cardiovascular fitness through active aerobic training
- Prevention of secondary complications, such as venous stasis and pressure ulcers
- Enhancement of functional mobility and quality of life, especially in patients with residual voluntary movement

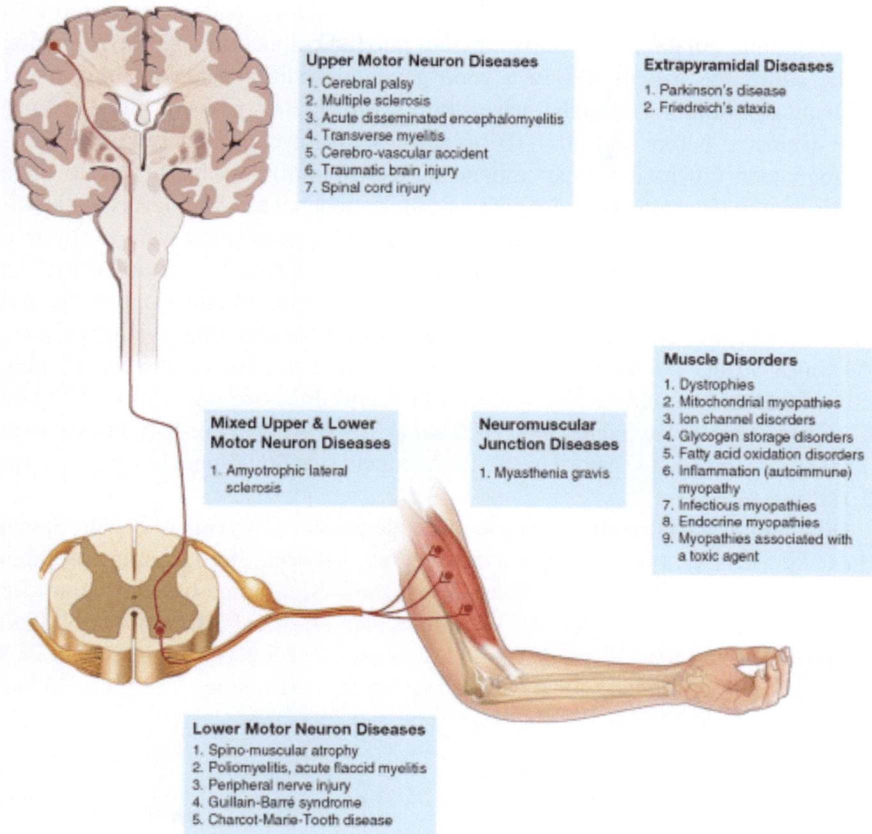

Fig. 6.5 Components of the neuromuscular system impairment according to pathology. (https://i0.wp.com/musculoskeletalkey.com/wp-content/uploads/2020/04/C29-FF1-1.gif?w=960)

FES-cycling is particularly relevant in early and intermediate stages of certain NMDs where sufficient motor units remain responsive to stimulation. It may also be used for maintaining muscle health and delaying deterioration in progressive conditions.

Evidence and Clinical Applications

Conventional electrical stimulation has been explored as a non-pharmacological intervention in individuals with muscular dystrophies [167] and other NMDs. Although the body of research is still developing, emerging evidence from case reports and small clinical trials supports the potential benefits of FES-cycling in this population, particularly for maintaining muscle volume, performance and metabolism, and delaying functional decline:

Frazão et al. [168] reported a case of a 49-year-old male patient diagnosed with severe chronic inflammatory demyelinating polyradiculoneuritis. At the beginning of the study, the patient was in a good general condition and breathing under mechanical ventilation through tracheostomy. Muscle ultrasound and blood glucose were evaluated before and after 10 sessions of FES-cycling. An isokinetic FES-cycling mode (20 rotations per minute during 10 min) was used. Due to huge impairment in the neuromuscular pathway, the patient needed high levels of electrical charge (high pulse width and intensity). The FES parameters were as follows: 75 Hz frequency, 800 μs to 900 μs pulse width and 170 mA to 210 mA intensity. The therapy was safe (no adverse events were reported during treatment), feasible and well tolerated. Rectus Femoris thickness increased 12% after FES-cycling (138 vs. 154 mm). Vastus Intermedius thickness was almost unchanged (96 vs. 98 mm, +2%). Mean blood glucose level reduced 21% after FES-cycling (162 vs. 128 mg/dL). There was a 27% reduction at 6:00 am (132 vs. 96 mg/dL), 15% reduction at 12:00 noon (166 vs. 142 mg/dL), and 21% reduction at 06:00 pm (187 vs. 147 mg/dL) (Fig. 6.6).

Gobbo et al. [169] reported a case of an adolescent (13 years old) with Spinal Muscular Atrophy type III that underwent an 18-week strengthening program divided into two stages. During Phase I (weeks: 1–8), a home-based program for quadriceps strengthening through neuromuscular electrical stimulation (NMES) was provided. In Phase II (weeks: 9–18), at-home NMES was combined with FES assisting volitional cycling for a broader, systemic conditioning. The protocol had

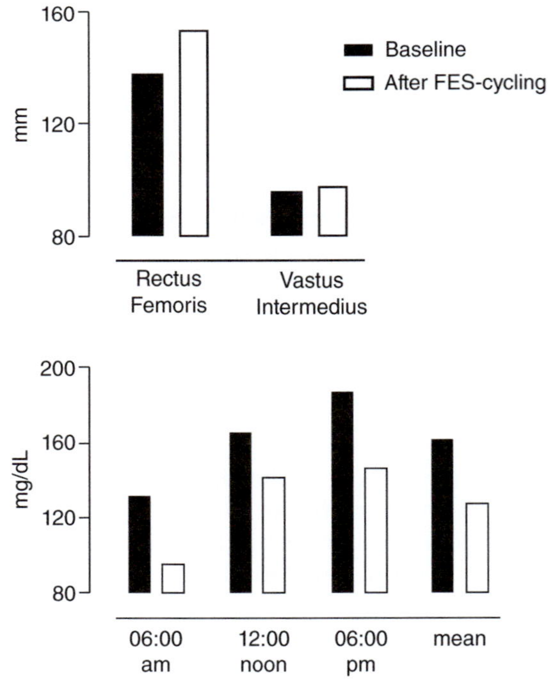

Fig. 6.6 Muscle thickness (top panel) and blood glucose level (bottom panel) (Frazão et al. [168])

duration of 25 min and was performed at the velocity of 30 rpm with pedal resistance gradually raised from 5 to 9 Nm. The stimulation amplitude was fixed at 45 mA for quadriceps, 30 mA for hamstring, and 25 mA for gluteal muscles. The treatment improved patient's structural and functional motor outcomes (quadriceps circumference and strength, Tinetti scale, and Hammersmith scale) as well as independence in stair climbing.

Cudia et al. [170] conducted a controlled pilot study with myotonic dystrophy type 1 patients. Eight patients (age, 39–67 years) fulfilled the inclusion criteria. Four participants performed FES-cycling training for 15 days (one daily session of 30 min for 5 days a week). The electrical stimulation was based on a rectangular waveform with the frequency of 30 Hz (pulse width, 200 ms) with an intensity modulated as the minimum to elicit muscle contraction. A control group, matched for clinical and genetic variables, who had contraindications to electrical stimulation, performed 6 weeks of conventional resistance and aerobic training. The modified Medical Research Council Scale and functional assessments were performed before and after treatment. Cohen d effect size was used for statistical analysis. FES-cycling was well tolerated and resulted in a greater improvement of tibialis anterior muscle strength (d = 1583), overall muscle strength (d = 1723), and endurance (d = 0,626) than conventional training.

Considerations and Limitations

- FES-cycling requires individualized protocols based on disease stage, degree of denervation, and residual muscle function.
- Monitoring for fatigue, muscle overuse, and skin integrity is essential.
- Not all NMD patients are candidates—severely denervated muscles may not respond adequately to stimulation or requires a high performance FES-cycling device.
- Clinical benefit often depends on early intervention, consistency of use, and integration with broader rehabilitation strategies.

Conclusions

FES-cycling has become a powerful tool in neurorehabilitation, offering benefits that extend beyond isolated muscle activation. By enabling patterned, repetitive, and task-oriented movement, FES-cycling addresses key challenges faced by individuals with neurological diseases such as spinal cord injury, stroke, cerebral palsy, and multiple sclerosis. Evidence demonstrates improvements in muscle strength, spasticity management, cardiovascular fitness, metabolic regulation, motor recovery, and quality of life. Importantly, these outcomes have been observed across different stages of recovery, confirming the broad applicability of this intervention.

Nonetheless, important gaps remain. The lack of standardized protocols, limited long-term follow-up, and variability in study populations hinder the ability to draw definitive conclusions about optimal implementation. In addition, practical barriers such as device availability, costs, and integration into health systems still restrict widespread adoption. Overcoming these challenges will require larger multicenter trials, better mechanistic studies linking physiological changes to functional outcomes, and the development of accessible, home-based, and hybrid solutions.

Looking ahead, FES-cycling holds the potential to become a cornerstone of neurological rehabilitation. With continued technological innovation, greater clinical integration, and stronger evidence, it may significantly enhance recovery, independence, and participation for people living with neurological conditions.

References

1. Geoffroy CG, Alilain W. Pathophysiology of spinal cord injury (SCI). Basel: MDPI; 2022.
2. Ditor DS, Hicks AL. Exercise therapy after spinal cord injury: the effects on heath and function. Biomed Eng. 2009;37(1–2):165–91.
3. Richardson A, Samaranayaka A, Sullivan M, Derrett S. Secondary health conditions and disability among people with spinal cord injury: a prospective cohort study. J Spinal Cord Med. 2021;44(1):19–28.
4. Margetis K, Das JM, Emmady PD. Spinal cord injuries. In: StatPearls [Internet]. Treasure Island (FL): StatPearls Publishing; 2025.
5. Xu X, Talifu Z, Zhang CJ, Gao F, Ke H, Pan YZ, Gong H, Du HY, Yu Y, Jing YL, Du LJ. Mechanism of skeletal muscle atrophy after spinal cord injury: a narrative review. Front Nutr. 2023;3(10):1099143.
6. Panisset MG, El-Ansary D, Dunlop SA, Marshall R, Clark J, Churilov L, Galea MP. Factors influencing thigh muscle volume change with cycling exercises in acute spinal cord injury–a secondary analysis of a randomized controlled trial. J Spinal Cord Med. 2022;45(4):510–21.
7. Popa C, Popa F, Grigorean VT, Onose G, Sandu AM, Popescu M, Burnei G, Strambu V, Sinescu C. Vascular dysfunctions following spinal cord injury. J Med Life. 2010;3(3):275–85.
8. Kirshblum SC, Burns SP, Biering-Sorensen F, Donovan W, Graves DE, Jha A, Johansen M, Jones L, Krassioukov A, Mulcahey MJ, Schmidt-Read M. International standards for neurological classification of spinal cord injury (revised 2011). J Spinal Cord Med. 2011;34(6):535–46.
9. Scale ASCIAAI. In: Physiopedia [Internet].
10. Yin L, Li N, Jia W, Wang N, Liang M, Yang X, Du G. Skeletal muscle atrophy: from mechanisms to treatments. Skeletal muscle atrophy: from mechanisms to treatments. Pharmacol Res. 2021;172:105807.
11. Björnholm M, Zierath JR. Insulin signal transduction in human skeletal muscle: identifying the defects in type II diabetes. Biochem Soc Trans. 2005;33(2):354–7.
12. Castro MJ, Apple DF Jr, Hillegass EA, Dudley GA. Influence of complete spinal cord injury on skeletal muscle cross-sectional area within the first 6 months of injury. Eur J Appl Physiol Occup Physiol. 1999;80:373–8.
13. Abrigo J, Simon F, Cabrera D, Vilos C, Cabello-Verrugio C. Mitochondrial dysfunction in skeletal muscle pathologies. Curr Protein Pept Sci. 2019;20(6):536–46.

14. Zhang S, Chen N. Regulatory role of MicroRNAs in muscle atrophy during exercise intervention. Int J Mol Sci. 2018;19(2):405.
15. Otzel DM, Lee J, Ye F, Borst SE, Yarrow JF. Activity-based physical rehabilitation with adjuvant testosterone to promote neuromuscular recovery after spinal cord injury. Int J Mol Sci. 2018;19(6):1701.
16. Moore CD, Craven BC, Thabane L, Laing AC, Frank-Wilson AW, Kontulainen SA, Papaioannou A, Adachi JD, Giangregorio LM. Lower-extremity muscle atrophy and fat infiltration after chronic spinal cord injury. J Musculoskelet Neuronal Interact. 2015;15(1):32.
17. Shah PK, Stevens JE, Gregory CM, Pathare NC, Jayaraman A, Bickel SC, Bowden M, Behrman AL, Walter GA, Dudley GA, Vandenborne K. Lower-extremity muscle cross-sectional area after incomplete spinal cord injury. Arch Phys Med Rehabil. 2006;87(6):772–8.
18. Kraft & Associates PC. Illustrations of complete vs. incomplete spinal cord injury – paraplegia and tetraplegia [Internet]. Dallas: KraftLaw.
19. Waters RL, Adkins RH, Yakura JS. Definition of complete spinal cord injury. Spinal Cord. 1991;29(9):573–81.
20. Kretzer RM. A clinical perspective and definition of spinal cord injury. Spine (Phila Pa 1976). 2016;41:S27.
21. Rupp R, Biering-Sørensen F, Burns SP, Graves DE, Guest J, Jones L, Read MS, Rodriguez GM, Schuld C, Tansey-Md KE, Walden K, Kirshblum S. International standards for neurological classification of spinal cord injury: revised 2019. Top Spinal Cord Inj Rehabil. 2021;27(2):1–22.
22. Problem WiSCISot.
23. Mastropietro A, Peruzzo D, Taccogna MG, Sanna N, Casali N, Nossa R, Biffi E, Ambrosini E, Pedroc-chi A, Rizzo G. Multiparametric MRI assessment of morpho-functional muscle changes following a 6-month FES-cycling training program: pilot study in people with a complete spinal cord injury. JMIR Rehabil Assist Technol. 2025;12:e6482.
24. Yaşar E, Yılmaz B, Göktepe S, Kesikburun S. The effect of functional electrical stimulation cycling on late functional improvement in patients with chronic incomplete spinal cord injury. Spinal Cord. 2015;53(12):866–9.
25. Gurcay E, Karaahmet OZ, Cankurtaran D, Nazlı F, Umay E, Güzel Ş, Gurcay AG. Functional electrical stimulation cycling in patients with chronic spinal cord injury: a pilot study. Int J Neurosci. 2022;132(4):421–7.
26. Johnston TE, Modlesky CM, Betz RR, Lauer RT. Muscle changes following cycling and/or electrical stimulation in pediatric spinal cord injury. Arch Phys Med Rehabil. 2011;92(12):1937–43.
27. Rosley N, Hamzaid NA, Hasnan N, Davis GL, Manaf H. Muscle size and strength benefits of functional electrical stimulation-evoked cycling dosage in spinal cord injury: a narrative review. Sains Malaysiana. 2019;48(3):607–12.
28. Johnston TE, Marino RJ, Oleson CV, Schmidt-Read M, Leiby BE, Sendecki J, Singh H, Modlesky CM. Musculoskeletal effects of 2 functional electrical stimulation cycling paradigms conducted at different cadences for people with spinal cord injury: a pilot study. Arch Phys Med Rehabil. 2016;97(9):1413–22.
29. Fornusek C, Davis GM, Russold MF. Pilot study of the effect of low-cadence functional electrical stimulation cycling after spinal cord injury on thigh girth and strength. Arch Phys Med Rehabil. 2013;94(5):990–3.
30. Skold C, Lonn L, Harms-Ringdahl K, Hultling C, Levi R, Nash M, Seiger A. Effects of functional electrical stimulation training for six months on body composition and spasticity in motor complete tetraplegic spinal cord-injured individuals. J Rehabil Med. 2002;34(1):25–32.

31. Sadowsky CL, Hammond ER, Strohl AB, Commean PK, Eby SA, Damiano DL, Wingert JR, Bae KT, McDonald JW. Lower extremity functional electrical stimulation cycling promotes physical and functional recovery in chronic spinal cord injury. J Spinal Cord Med. 2013;36(6):623–31.
32. Kuhn D, Leichtfried V, Schobersberger W. Four weeks of functional electrical stimulated cycling after spinal cord injury: a clinical cohort study. Int J Rehabil Res. 2014;37(3):243–50.
33. Fornusek C, Davis GM. Maximizing muscle force via low-cadence functional electrical stimulation cycling. J Rehabil Med. 2004;36(5):232.
34. Demchak TJ, Linderman JK, Mysiw WJ, Jackson R, Suun J, Devor ST. Effects of functional electric stimulation cycle ergometry training on lower limb musculature in acute sci individuals. J Sports Sci Med. 2005;4(3):263.
35. Thrasher TA, Ward JS, Fisher S. Strength and endurance adaptations to functional electrical stimulation leg cycle ergometry in spinal cord injury. NeuroRehabilitation. 2013;33(1):133–8.
36. Duffell LD, Donaldson N d N, Perkins TA, Rushton DN, Hunt KJ, Kakebeeke TH, Newham DJ. Long-term intensive electrically stimulated cycling by spinal cord–injured people: effect on muscle properties and their relation to power output. Muscle Nerve. 2008;38(4):1304–11.
37. Liu CW, Chen SC, Chen CH, Chen TW, Chen JJ, Lin CS, Huang MH. Effects of functional electrical stimulation on peak torque and body composition in patients with in-complete spinal cord injury. Kaohsiung J Med Sci. 2007;23(5):232–40.
38. Baldi JC, Jackson RD, Moraille R, Mysiw WJ. Muscle atrophy is prevented in patients with acute spinal cord injury using functional electrical stimulation. Spinal Cord. 1998;36(7):463–9.
39. van der Scheer JW, Goosey-Tolfrey VL, Valentino SE, Davis GM, Ho CH. Functional electrical stimulation cycling exercise after spinal cord injury: a systematic review of health and fitness-related outcomes. J Neuroeng Rehabil. 2021;18(1):99.
40. Ibitoye MO, Hamzaid NA, Ahmed YK. Effectiveness of FES-supported leg exercise for promotion of paralysed lower limb muscle and bone health – a systematic review. Biomed Tech (Berl). 2023;68(4):329–50.
41. Karamian BA, Siegel N, Nourie B, Serruya MD, Heary RF, Harrop JS, Vaccaro AR. The role of electrical stimulation for rehabilitation and regeneration after spinal cord injury. J Orthop Traumatol. 2022;23(1):2.
42. Mervis JS, Phillips TJ. Pressure ulcers: pathophysiology, epidemiology, risk factors, and presentation. J Am Acad Dermatol. 2019;81(4):881–90.
43. Brienza D, Krishnan S, Karg P, Sowa G, Allegretti AL. Predictors of pressure ulcer incidence following traumatic spinal cord injury: a secondary analysis of a prospective longitudinal study. Spinal Cord. 2018;56(1):28–34.
44. Vecin NM, Gater DR. Pressure injuries and management after spinal cord injury. J Pers Med. 2022;12(7):1130.
45. Smit CA, de Groot S, Stolwijk-Swuste JM, Janssen TW. Effects of electrical stimulation on risk factors for developing pressure ulcers in people with a spinal cord injury: a focused review of literature. Am J Phys Med Rehabil. 2016;95(7):535–52.
46. Gerrits HL, de Haan A, Sargeant AJ, van Langen H, Hopman MT. Peripheral vascular changes after electrically stimulated cycle training in people with spinal cord injury. Arch Phys Med Rehabil. 2001;82(6):832–9.
47. Dolbow D, Gorgey AS, Dolbow J, Gater D. Seat pressure changes after eight weeks of functional electrical stimulation cycling: a pilot study. Topn Spinal Cord Inj Rehabil. 2013;19(3):222–8.
48. Frazão M, de Gomes Figueiredo T, Cipriano G. Should we use the functional electrical stimulation-cycling exercise in clinical practice? Physiological and clinical effects systematic review with meta-analysis. Arch Phys Med Rehabil. 2025;106(3):404–23.

49. Atkins KD, Bickel CS. Effects of functional electrical stimulation on muscle health after spinal cord injury. Curr Opin Pharmacol. 2021;60:226–31.
50. Warburton D0, Enj JJ, Krassioukov A, Sproule S. Cardiovascular health and exercise rehabilitation in spinal cord injury. Top Spinal Cord Inj Rehabil. 2021;13(1):98–122.
51. Johnston TE, Smith BT, Mulcahey MJ, Betz RR, Lauer RT. A randomized controlled trial on the effects of cycling with and without electrical stimulation on cardiorespiratory and vascular health in children with spinal cord injury. Arch Phys Med Rehabil. 2009;90(8):1379–88.
52. Figoni SF, Dolbow DR, Crawford EC, White ML, Pattanaik S. Does aerobic exercise benefit persons with tetraplegia from spinal cord injury? A systematic review. J Spinal Cord Med. 2021;44(5):690–703.
53. Stampas A, Hook M, Korupolu R, Jethani L, Kaner MT, Pemberton E, Li S, Francisco GE. Evidence of treating spasticity before it develops: a systematic review of spasticity outcomes in acute spinal cord injury interventional trials. Ther Adv Neurol Disord. 2022;15:17562864211070657.
54. Couper SK, Smith M. The effects of functional electrical stimulation cycling on muscle spasticity in individuals with spinal cord injury: a systematic review. Top Spinal Cord Inj Rehabil. 2025;31(1):77–99.
55. Gorgey AS, Dudley GA. Spasticity may defend skeletal muscle size and composition after incomplete spinal cord injury. Spinal Cord. 2008;46(2):96–102.
56. Billington ZJ, Henke AM, Gater DR Jr. Spasticity management after spinal cord injury: the here and now. J Pers Med. 2022;12(5):808.
57. Bhimani R, Anderson L. Clinical understanding of spasticity: implications for practice. Rehabil Res Pract. 2014;2014:279175.
58. Sköld C, Levi R, Seiger Å. Spasticity after traumatic spinal cord injury: nature, severity, and location. Arch Phys Med Rehabil. 1999;80(12):1548–57.
59. Nelson RM, Hayes KW, Currier DP, editors. Clinical electrotherapy. Stamford: Appleton & Lange; 1999.
60. Hon AJ. Spasticity management after spinal cord injury. Curr Phys Med Rehabil Rep. 2020;8:159–71.
61. Fernández-Tenorio E, Serrano-Muñoz D, Avendaño-Coy J, Gómez-Soriano J. Transcutaneous electrical nerve stimulation for spasticity: a systematic review. Neurología (Engl Ed). 2019;34(7):451–60.
62. Alashram AR, Annino G, Mercuri NB. Changes in spasticity following functional electrical stimulation cycling in patients with spinal cord injury: a systematic review. J Spinal Cord Med. 2022;45(1):10–23.
63. Fang CY, Lien ASY, Tsai JL, Yang HC, Chan HL, Chen RS, Chang YJ. The effect and dose-response of functional electrical stimulation cycling training on spasticity in individuals with spinal cord injury: a systematic review with meta-analysis. Front Physiol. 2021;12:756200.
64. Bekhet AH, Bochkezanian V, Saab IM, Gorgey AS. The effects of electrical stimulation parameters in managing spasticity after spinal cord injury: a systematic review. Am J Phys Med Rehabil. 2019;98(6):484–99.
65. Sivaramakrishnan A, Soloman JM, Manikandan N. Comparison of transcutaneous electrical nerve stimulation (TENS) and functional electrical stimulation (FES) for spasticity in spinal cord injury-a pilot randomized cross-over trial. J Spinal Cord Med. 2018;41(4):397–406.
66. Dolbow DR, Gorgey AS, Daniels JA, Adler RA, Moore JR, Gater DR Jr. The effects of spinal cord injury and exercise on bone mass: a literature review. NeuroRehabilitation. 2011;29(3):261–9.
67. Sutor TW, Kura J, Mattingly AJ, Otzel DM, Yarrow JF. The effects of exercise and activity-based physical therapy on bone after spinal cord injury. Int J Mol Sci. 2022;23(2):608.

68. Lai CH, Chang WH-S, Chan WP, Peng CW, Shen LK, Chen JJ, Chen SC. Effects of functional electrical stimulation cycling exercise on bone mineral density loss in the early stages of spinal cord injury. J Rehabil Med. 2010;42(4):150–4.
69. Hangartner TN, Rodgers MM, Glaser RM, Barre PS. Tibial bone density loss in spinal cord injured patients: effects of FES exercise. J Rehabil Res Dev. 1995;31:50–61.
70. Mohr T, Podenphant J, Biering–Sørensen F, Galbo H, Thamsborg G, Kjaer M. Increased bone mineral density after prolonged electrically induced cycle training of paralyzed limbs in spinal cord injured man. Calcif Tissue Int. 1997;61(1):22–5.
71. Eser P, de Bruin ED, Telley I, Lechner HE, Knecht H, Stüssi E. Effect of electrical stimulation-induced cycling on bone mineral density in spinal cord-injured patients. Eur J Clin Investig. 2003;33(5):412–9.
72. Chen SC, Lai CH, Chan WP, Huang MH, Tsai HW, Chen JJ. Increases in bone mineral density after functional electrical stimulation cycling exercises in spinal cord injured patients. Disabil Rehabil. 2005;27(2):1337–41.
73. Kakebeeke TH, Hofer PJ, Frotzler A, Lechner HE, Hunt KJ, Perret C. Training and detraining of a tetraplegic subject: high-volume FES cycle training. Am J Phys Med Rehabil. 2008;87(1):56–64.
74. Frotzler A, Coupaud S, Perret C, Kakebeeke TH, Hunt KJ, Donaldson ND, Eser P. High-volume FES-cycling partially reverses bone loss in people with chronic spinal cord injury. Bone. 2008;43(1):169–76.
75. Lauer RT, Smith BT, Mulcahey MJ, Betz RR, Johnston TE. Effects of cycling and/or electrical stimulation on bone mineral density in children with spinal cord injury. Spinal Cord. 2011;49(8):917–23.
76. Calabrò RS, Portaro S, Tomasello P, Porcari B, Balletta T, Naro A. Paving the way for a better management of pain in patients with spinal cord injury: an exploratory study on the use of functional electric stimulation (FES)-cycling. J Spinal Cord Med. 2023;46(1):107–17.
77. Campbell BC, De Silva DA, Macleod MR, et al. Ischaemic stroke. Nat Rev Dis Primers. 2019;5(1):70.
78. Krishnamurthi RV, Ikeda T, Feigin VL. Global, regional and country-specific burden of ischaemic stroke, intracerebral haemorrhage and subarachnoid haemorrhage: a systematic analysis of the global burden of disease study 2017. Neuroepidemiology. 2020;54(2):171–9.
79. Brouns R, De Deyn PP. The complexity of neurobiological processes in acute ischemic stroke. Clin Neurol Neurosurg. 2009;111(6):483–95.
80. Stinear C. Prediction of recovery of motor function after stroke. Lancet Neurol. 2010;9(12):1228–32.
81. Grefkes C, Ward NS. Cortical reorganization after stroke: how much and how functional? Neuroscientist. 2014;20(1):56–70.
82. Sommerfeld DK, EUB E, Svensson AK, Holmqvist LW, von Arbin MH. Spasticity after stroke: its occurrence and association with motor impairments and activity limitations. Stroke. 2004;65(1):134–9.
83. Hilkens NA, et al. Stroke. Lancet. 2017;389(10069):641–54.
84. Langhorne P, Bernhardt J, Kwakkel G. Stroke rehabilitation. Lancet. 2011;377(9778):1693–702.
85. Ada L, O'Dwyer N, O'Neill E. Relation between spasticity, weakness and contracture of the elbow flexors and upper limb activity after stroke: an observational study. Disabil Rehabil. 2006;28(13–14):891–7.
86. Lance JW. The control of muscle tone, reflexes, and movement: Robert Wartenberg lecture. Neurology. 1980;30(12):1303–13.
87. Watkins CL, Leathley MJ, Gregson JM, Moore AP, Smith TL, Sharma AK. Prevalence of spasticity post stroke. Clin Rehabil. 2002;16(5):515–22.
88. Saunders DH, Sanderson M, Hayes S, Kilrane M, Greig CA, Brazzelli M, Mead GE. Physical fitness training for stroke patients. Cochrane Database Syst Rev. 2016;24(3):CD003316.
89. Billinger SA, Arena R, Bernhardt J, Eng JJ, Franklin BA, Johnson CM, MacKay-Lyons M, Macko RF, Mead GE, Roth EJ, Shaughnessy M, Tang A. Physical activity

and exercise recommendations for stroke survivors: a statement for healthcare professionals from the American Heart Association/American Stroke Association. Stroke. 2014;45(8):2532–53.
90. Kleim JAJT. Principles of experience-dependent neural plasticity: implications for rehabilitation after brain damage. J Speech Lang Hear Res. 2008;51(1):S225–39.
91. Howlett OA, Lannin NA, Ada L, McKinstry C. Functional electrical stimulation improves activity after stroke: a systematic review with meta-analysis. Arch Phys Med Rehabil. 2015;96(5):934–43.
92. Ambrosini E, Ferrante S, Pedrocchi A, Ferrigno G, Molteni F. Cycling induced by electrical stimulation improves motor recovery in postacute hemiparetic patients: a randomized controlled trial. Stroke. 2011;42(4):1068–73.
93. Daly JJ, Wolpaw JR. Brain-computer interfaces in neurological rehabilitation. Lancet Neurol. 2008;7(11):1032–43.
94. Sheffler LR, Chae J. Neuromuscular electrical stimulation in neurorehabilitation. Muscle Nerve. 2007;35(5):562–90.
95. Lo HC, Hsu Y-C, Hsueh YH, Yeh CY. Cycling exercise with functional electrical stimulation improves postural control in stroke patients. Gait Posture. 2012;35(3):506–10.
96. Ferrante S, Pedrocchi A, Ferrigno G, Molteni F. Cycling induced by functional electrical stimulation improves the muscular strength and the motor control of individuals with post-acute stroke. Europa Medicophysica-SIMFER 2007 award winner. Eur J Phys Rehabil Med. 2008;44(2):159–67.
97. Galvão WR, Silva LKC, Formiga MF, Thé GAP, Faria CDCM, Viana RT, Lima LAO. Cycling using functional electrical stimulation therapy to improve motor function and activity in post-stroke individuals in early subacute phase: a systematic review with meta-analysis. Biomed Eng Online. 2024;23(1):1.
98. Yeh CY, Tsai K-H, Su FC, Lo HC. Effect of a bout of leg cycling with electrical stimulation on reduction of hypertonia in patients with stroke. Arch Phys Med Rehabil. 2010;91(11):1731–6.
99. Sommerfeld DK, Eek EU-B, Svensson AK, Holmqvist LW, von Arbin MH. Spasticity after stroke: its occurrence and association with motor impairments and activity limitations. Stroke. 2004;35(1):134–9.
100. Ambrosini E, Ferrante S, Ferrigno G, Molteni F, Pedrocchi A. Cycling induced by electrical stimulation improves muscle activation and symmetry during pedaling in hemiparetic patients. IEEE Trans Neural Syst Rehabil Eng. 2012;20(3):320–30.
101. Bauer P, Krewer C, Golaszewski S, Koenig E, Müller F. Functional electrical stimulation-assisted active cycling–therapeutic effects in patients with hemiparesis from 7 days to 6 months after stroke: a randomized controlled pilot study. Arch Phys Med Rehabil. 2015;96(2):188–96.
102. Janssen TW, Beltman JM, Elich P, Koppe PA, Konijnenbelt H, de Haan A, Gerrits KH. Effects of electric stimulation-assisted cycling training in people with chronic stroke. Arch Phys Med Rehabil. 2008;89(3):463–9.
103. Dobkin BH. Training and exercise to drive poststroke recovery. Nat Clin Pract Neurol. 2008;4(2):76–85.
104. Sanger TD. Movement disorders in cerebral palsy. J Pediatr Neurol. 2015;13(4):198–207.
105. Data and Statistics for Cerebral Palsy | CDC Archive.
106. Zwier JN, van Schie PEM, Becher JG, Smits DW, Gorter JW, Dallmeijer AJ. Physical activity in young children with cerebral palsy. Disabil Rehabil. 2010;32(18):1501–8.
107. Carlon SL, Taylor NF, Dodd KJ, Shields N. Differences in habitual physical activity levels of young people with cerebral palsy and their typically developing peers: a systematic review. Disabil Rehabil. 2013;35(8):647–55.
108. Giuliani CA. Dorsal rhizotomy for children with cerebral palsy: support for concepts of motor control. Phys Ther. 1991;71(3):248–59.
109. Hof AL. Changes in muscles and tendons due to neural motor disorders: implications for therapeutic intervention. Neural Plast. 2001;8(1–2):71–81.

110. McLaughlin JF, Bjornson KF, Astley SJ, Hays RM, Heffinger SA, Armantrout EA, et al. The role of selective dorsal rhizotomy in cérébral palsy: critical evaluation of a prospective clinical series. Dev Med Child Neurol. 1994;36(9):755–69.
111. Hoffer MM. Management of the hip in cerebral palsy. JBJS. 1986;68(4)
112. Senghas MD. The diplegic child: evaluation and management. Rosemont: American Academy of Orthopaedic Surgeons; 1992. p. 259–70.
113. Johnston TE, Barr AE, Lee SCK. Biomechanics of submaximal recumbent cycling in adolescents with and without cerebral palsy. Phys Ther. 2024;87(5):572–85.
114. Kaplan SL. Cycling patterns in children with and without cerebral palsy. Dev Med Child Neurol. 1995;37(7):620–30.
115. Johnston TE, Prosser LA, Lee SCK. Differences in pedal forces during recumbent cycling in adolescents with and without cerebral palsy. Clin Biomech (Bristol, Avon). 2007;23(2):248.
116. Sansare A, Behboodi A, Johnston TE, Bodt B, Lee SCK. Characterizing cycling smoothness and rhythm in children with and without cerebral palsy. Front Rehabil Sci. 2021;2:690046.
117. Griffin L, Decker MJ, Hwang JY, Wang B, Kitchen K, Ding Z, et al. Functional electrical stimulation cycling improves body composition, metabolic and neural factors in persons with spinal cord injury. J Electromyogr Kinesiol. 2009;19:4.
118. Duffell LD, Donaldson N d N, Perkins TA, Rushton DN, Hunt KJ, Kakebeeke TH, et al. Long-term intensive electrically stimulated cycling by spinal cord-injured people: effect on muscle properties and their relation to power output. Muscle Nerve. 2008;38(4):1304–11.
119. Krause P, Szecsi J, Straube A. Changes in spastic muscle tone increase in patients with spinal cord injury using functional electrical stimulation and passive leg movements. Clin Rehabil. 2008;22(7):627–34.
120. Mohr T, Andersen JL, Biering-Sørensen F, Galbo H, Bangsbo J, Wagner A, et al. Long term adaptation to electrically induced cycle training in severe spinal cord injured individuals. Spinal Cord. 1997;35(1):1–16.
121. Johnston TE, Wainwright SF. Cycling with functional electrical stimulation in an adult with spastic diplegic cerebral palsy. Phys Ther. 2011;91(6):970–82.
122. Sansare A, Harrington AT, Wright H, Alesi J, Behboodi A, Verma K, et al. Aerobic responses to FES-assisted and volitional cycling in children with cerebral palsy. Sensors. 2021;21(22):7590.
123. Armstrong EL, Boyd RN, Horan SA, Kentish MJ, Ware RS, Carty CP. Functional electrical stimulation cycling, goal-directed training, and adapted cycling for children with cerebral palsy: a randomized controlled trial. Dev Med Child Neurol. 2020;62(12):1406–13.
124. Özen N, Unlu E, Karaahmet OZ, Gurcay E, Gundogdu I, Umay E. Effectiveness of functional electrical stimulation-cycling treatment in children with cerebral palsy. Malawi Med J. 2021;33(3):144–52.
125. Bryant E, Pountney T, Williams H, Edelman N. Can a six-week exercise intervention improve gross motor function for non-ambulant children with cerebral palsy? A pilot randomized controlled trial. Clin Rehabil. 2013;27(2):150–9.
126. Armstrong EL, Spencer S, Kentish MJ, Horan SA, Carty CP, Boyd RN. Efficacy of cycling interventions to improve function in children and adolescents with cerebral palsy: a systematic review and meta-analysis. Clin Rehabil. 2019;33(7):1113–29.
127. Fowler EG, Knutson LM, DeMuth SK, Siebert KL, Simms VD, Sugi MH, et al. Pediatric endurance and limb strengthening (PEDALS) for children with cerebral palsy using stationary cycling: a randomized controlled trial. Phys Ther. 2010;90(3):367–81.
128. Auchstaetter N, Luc J, Lukye S, Lynd K, Schemenauer S, Whittaker M, et al. Physical therapists' use of functional electrical stimulation for clients with stroke: frequency, barriers, and facilitators. Phys Ther. 2016;96(7):995–1005.

129. Swaffield E, Yang JF, Manns P, Chan K, Musselman KE. Parents' perceptions of functional electrical stimulation as an upper limb intervention for young children with hemiparesis: qualitative interviews with mothers. BMC Pediatr. 2022;22(1):1–12.
130. Musselman KE, Provad E, Djuric A, Bercovitch D, Yuen I, Kane KJ. Exploring the experiences and perceptions of pediatric therapists who use functional electrical stimulation in their clinical practice. Phys Occup Ther Pediatr. 2023;43(6):759–79.
131. Walton C, King R, Rechtman L, Kaye W, Leray E, Marrie RA, et al. Rising prevalence of multiple sclerosis worldwide: insights from the atlas of MS, third edition. Mult Scler. 2020;26(14):1816–21.
132. Thompson AJBS, Geurts J, Hemmer B, Ciccarelli O. Multiple sclerosis. Lancet. 2018;391(10130):1622–36.
133. Lakin L, Davis BE, Binns CC, Currie KM, Rensel MR. Comprehensive approach to management of multiple sclerosis: addressing invisible symptoms – a narrative review. Neurol Ther. 2021;10(1):75–98.
134. Marrie RA, Fisk JD, Fitzgerald K, Kowalec K, Maxwell C, Rotstein D, et al. Etiology, effects and management of comorbidities in multiple sclerosis: recent advances. Front Immunol. 2023;14:1197195.
135. Giovannoni G, Ford HL, Schmierer K, Middleton R, Stennett AM, Pomeroy I, et al. MS care: integrating advanced therapies and holistic management. Front Neurol. 2023;14:1286122.
136. Bebo BF, Banwell BL, Whitacre CC, Coetzee T, Dalgas U, De Jager PL, et al. The refined pathways to cures research roadmap for multiple sclerosis cures. Mult Scler. 2024;30(10):1242–51.
137. Conradsson D, Ytterberg C, von Koch L, Johansson S. Changes in disability in people with multiple sclerosis: a 10-year prospective study. J Neurol. 2018;265(1):119–26.
138. Salter AR, Cutter GR, Tyry T, Marrie RA, Vollmer T. Impact of loss of mobility on instrumental activities of daily living and socioeconomic status in patients with MS. Curr Med Res Opin. 2010;26(2):493–500.
139. van der Feen FE, de Haan GA, van der Lijn I, Heersema DJ, Meilof JF, Heutink J. Independent outdoor mobility of persons with multiple sclerosis – a systematic review. Mult Scler Relat Disord. 2020;37:101463.
140. Pilutti LAMR. Functional electrical stimulation cycling exercise for people with multiple sclerosis. Curr Treat Options Neurol. 2019;21(11):54.
141. Scally JBBJ, Baker JS, Rankin J, Renfrew L, Sculthorpe N. Evaluating functional electrical stimulation (FES) cycling on cardiovascular, musculoskeletal and functional outcomes in adults with multiple sclerosis and mobility impairment: a systematic review. Mult Scler Relat Disord. 2020;37:101485.
142. Szecsi J, Schlick C, Schiller M, Pöllmann W, Koenig N, Straube A. Functional electrical stimulation-assisted cycling of patients with multiple sclerosis: biomechanical and functional outcome–a pilot study. J Rehabil Med. 2009;41(8):674–80.
143. Ratchford JN, Shore W, Hammond ER, Rose JG, Rifkin R, Nie P, et al. A pilot study of functional electrical stimulation cycling in progressive multiple sclerosis. NeuroRehabilitation. 2010;27(2):121–8.
144. Fornusek C, Hoang P. Neuromuscular electrical stimulation cycling exercise for persons with advanced multiple sclerosis. J Rehabil Med. 2014;46(7):689–702.
145. Reynolds MA, McCully K, Burdett B, Manella C, Hawkins L. Backus D pilot study: evaluation of the effect of functional electrical stimulation cycling on muscle metabolism in nonambulatory people with multiple sclerosis. Arch Phys Med Rehabil. 2015;96(4):627–32.
146. Backus DBB, Hawkins L, Manella C, McCully KK. Sweatman M outcomes after functional electrical stimulation cycle training in individuals with multiple sclerosis who are nonambulatory. Int J MS Care. 2017;19(3):113–21.
147. Máté S, Soutter M, Liaros J, Hackett D, Barnett M, Singh MF, et al. The effects of hybrid functional electrical stimulation interval training on aerobic fitness and fatigue in people with

advanced multiple sclerosis: an exploratory pilot training study. Mult Scler Relat Disord. 2024;83:105458.
148. Hochman L. Effects of functional electrical stimulation cycling versus cycling only on walking performance and quality of life in individuals with multiple sclerosis: a randomized, clinical pilot study. Department of Physical Therapy Student Theses, Dissertations and Capstones.
149. Edwards T, Motl RW, Sebastião E, Pilutti LA. Pilot randomized controlled trial of functional electrical stimulation cycling exercise in people with multiple sclerosis with mobility disability. Mult Scler Relat Disord. 2018;26:103–11.
150. Pilutti LA, Edwards T, Motl RW, Sebastião E. Functional electrical stimulation cycling exercise in people with multiple sclerosis: secondary effects on cognition, symptoms, and quality of life. Int J MS Care. 2019;21(6):258–64.
151. Farrell JW, Edwards T, Motl RW, Pilutti LA. Effect of functional electrical stimulation cycling exercise on lower limb strength asymmetry in persons with multiple sclerosis. Int J MS Care. 2022;24(1):25–8.
152. Backus D, Moldavskiy M, Sweatman WM. Effects of functional electrical stimulation cycling on fatigue and quality of life in people with multiple sclerosis who are nonambulatory. Int J MS Care. 2020;22(4):193–200.
153. Gaemelke T, Frandsen JJ, Hvid LG, Dalgas U. Participant characteristics of existing exercise studies in persons with multiple sclerosis – a systematic review identifying literature gaps. Mult Scler Relat Disord. 2022;68:104198.
154. Stroud N, Minahan C, Sabapathy S. The perceived benefits and barriers to exercise participation in persons with multiple sclerosis. Disabil Rehabil. 2009;31(26):2216–22.
155. Asano M, Duquette P, Andersen R, Lapierre Y, Mayo NE. Exercise barriers and preferences among women and men with multiple sclerosis. Disabil Rehabil. 2013;35(5):353–61.
156. Moffat F, Paul L. Barriers and solutions to participation in exercise for moderately disabled people with multiple sclerosis not currently exercising: a consensus development study using nominal group technique. Disabil Rehabil. 2019;41(23):2775–83.
157. Guo Y, Phillips BE, Atherton PJ, Piasecki M. Molecular and neural adaptations to neuromuscular electrical stimulation; implications for ageing muscle. Mech Ageing Dev. 2021;193:111402.
158. Girsch W, Bijak M, Heger G, Koller R, Lanmüller H, Mayr W, et al. Monitoring of FES-induced muscle activity by continuous EMG-recording. Int J Artif Organs. 1995;18(6):340–4.
159. Everaert DG, Okuma Y, Abdollah V, Ho C. Timing and dosage of FES cycling early after acute spinal cord injury: a case series report. J Spinal Cord Med. 2021;44:S250–5.
160. Bishop M, Dennis KL, Bishop LA, Sheppard-Jones K, Bishop F, Frain M. The prevalence and nature of modified housing and assistive devices use among Americans with multiple sclerosis. J Vocat Rehabil. 2015;42(2):153–65.
161. Langeskov-Christensen M, Heine M, Kwakkel G, Dalgas U. Aerobic capacity in persons with multiple sclerosis: a systematic review and meta-analysis. Sports Med. 2015;45(6):905–23.
162. Madsen LT, Dalgas U, Hvid LG, Bansi J. A cross-sectional study on the relationship between cardiorespiratory fitness, disease severity and walking speed in persons with multiple sclerosis. Mult Scler Relat Disord. 2019;29:35–40.
163. Schlagheck ML, Bansi J, Langeskov-Christensen M, Zimmer P, Hvid LG. Cardiorespiratory fitness (VO2peak) across the adult lifespan in persons with multiple sclerosis and matched healthy controls. J Sci Med Sport. 2024;7(1):10–5.
164. Bakshi R, Shaikh ZA, Miletich RS, Czarnecki D, Dmochowski J, Henschel K, et al. Fatigue in multiple sclerosis and its relationship to depression and neurologic disability. Mult Scler. 2000;6(3):181–5.
165. Schmidt S, Jöstingmeyer P. Depression, fatigue and disability are independently associated with quality of life in patients with multiple sclerosis: results of a cross-sectional study. Mult Scler Relat Disord. 2019;35:262–9.

166. Morrison BM. Neuromuscular diseases. Semin Neurol. 2016;36(5):409–18.
167. Enza Leone AP, Rogers A, Kulshrestha R, Hill J, Philp F. Effectiveness of conservative non-pharmacological interventions in people with muscular dystrophies: a systematic review and meta-analysis. J Neurol Neurosurg Psychiatry. 2023;95(5):442–53.
168. Frazão M, de Lima DT, Nogueira AP, Leandro Guedes TDS, Pinto Dias AL, da Silva Lima MVD, Mota Fernandes IA. Effects of functional electrical stimulation-cycling on muscle thickness and blood glucose level in neuromuscular disease mechanically ventilated patient: case report. Clin Case Rep Int. 2024;8:1648.
169. Massimiliano Gobbo SL, Vacchi L, Gaffurini P, Bissolotti L, Padovani A, Filosto M. Exercise combined with electrotherapy enhances motor function in an adolescent with spinal muscular atrophy type III. Case Rep Neurol Med. 2019;2019(22):4839793.
170. Paola Cudia LW, Baba A, Kiper P, Marcante A, Rossi S, Angelini C, Piccione F. Effects of functional electrical stimulation lower extremity training in myotonic dystrophy type I: a pilot controlled study. Am J Phys Med Rehabil. 2016;95(11):809–17.

Clinical Applicability of FES-Cycling in Non-neurological Diseases

7

Murillo Frazão

Introduction

Rehabilitation strategies are essential for mitigating the systemic consequences of acute and chronic diseases. In non-neurological populations, prolonged immobility, muscle wasting, ventilatory inefficiency, cardiovascular deconditioning, and metabolic alterations are frequent barriers to recovery. Functional Electrical Stimulation (FES)-cycling has emerged as an innovative approach capable of overcoming many of these challenges. By combining neuromuscular electrical stimulation with rhythmic cycling, it allows for the activation of large muscle groups and the achievement of physiological exercise responses, even in individuals with severely reduced voluntary capacity. Although initially developed for neurological disorders, the scope of FES-cycling has expanded significantly. Clinical evidence now supports its applicability in diverse non-neurological conditions. FES-cycling not only attenuates muscle atrophy but also promotes cardiovascular, respiratory, and metabolic adaptations that are critical for recovery and long-term health.

This chapter reviews the mechanisms, clinical benefits, and practical considerations for implementing FES-cycling in non-neurological diseases. It highlights how the modality addresses the multisystem consequences of disease and ageing, while offering a feasible and safe therapeutic option that can be integrated into hospital, rehabilitation, and home settings.

Hospitalized Patients

Acquired muscle weakness is a common comorbidity during hospitalization. It mainly affects critically ill [1], but is not exclusive to this type of patients. Such dysfunction is related to the inflammatory level, but can appear independently of the

M. Frazão (✉)
Lauro Wanderley University Hospital – EBSERH/UFPB, João Pessoa, PB, Brazil
e-mail: murillo.frazao@gmail.com

M. Frazão (ed.), *Functional Electrical Stimulation Cycling in Clinical Practice*,
https://doi.org/10.1007/978-3-032-23937-2_7

underlying pathology that led to hospital admission. During hospitalization, bed rest induces alterations in neuromuscular control and muscle protein synthesis [2]. Physical activity and neuromuscular electrical stimulation help prevent significant muscle mass reduction and enhance muscle strength in individuals with acquired weakness. Furthermore, cycling exercise improves not only muscle strength but also overall functionality [3]. To promote the best clinical results, high electrical charge is needed in hospitalized patients [4]. The safety of high-intensity FES-cycling settings has already been demonstrated in this patient population [5].

FES-Cycling Effects on Muscle Mass and Performance

A systematic review with meta-analysis [6] showed favorable results for FES-cycling in terms of leg and total body muscle mass. A plausible physiological explanation is that high-intensity FES-cycling generates significant intramuscular tissue pressure. On one hand, the muscle tension is caused by the electrical stimulation, while on the other, additional muscle tension is created by the resistance generated during cycling. Muscle fiber splitting is a physiological response to extreme muscle loading that can occur during hypertrophy [7]. It's the branching or splitting of skeletal muscle fibers (Fig. 7.1). This increased intramuscular pressure also leads to ischemia [8], which in turn enhances metabolic stress [9] and promotes muscle adaptations. These high mechanical tension and high metabolic stress also leads autocrine/paracrine actions, releasing growth hormones [10].

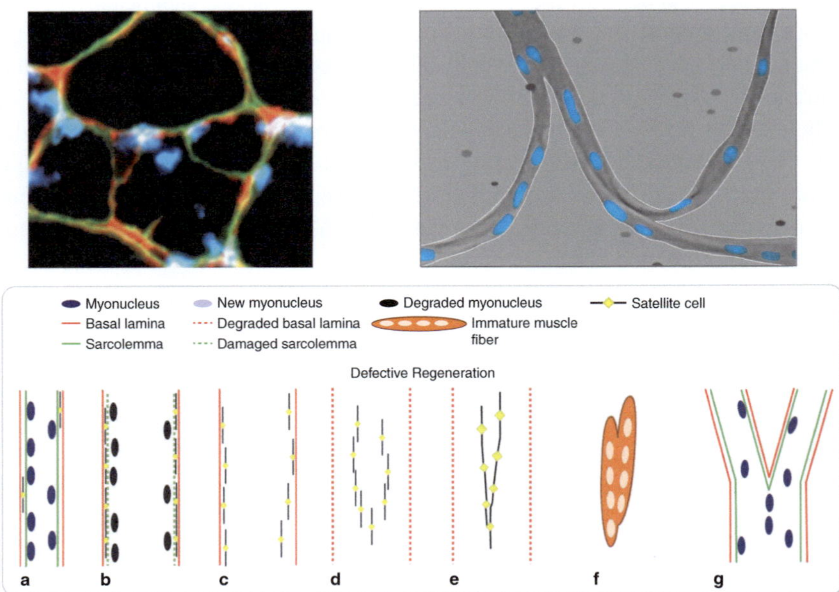

Fig. 7.1 Muscle fiber splitting secondary to muscle loading. (Adapted from Murach et al. [7])

FES-cycling also reduces the negative nitrogen balance [11] (when the patient consumes more than excrete) that is related to a catabolic state and muscle protein breakdown. However, it is important to emphasize that the muscle hypotrophy reduction effect is strictly related to the FES-cycling exercise intensity. Low [12] or very low [11] intensities have limited results in muscle cross-section area maintenance in hospitalized patients.

The previously mentioned systematic review with meta-analysis [6] also showed favorable results for FES-cycling in terms of torque and power. The increase in torque and power induced by FES-cycling strongly affect the motor recovery [13]. Electrical stimulation is an effective method for enhancing the rate of force development through neural activity [14]. The additional muscle tension generated by cycling may further amplify these effects. Moreover, neural adaptations typically occur before structural changes. The increased capacity for muscle force generation is primarily attributed to neuromuscular adaptations, rather than muscle hypertrophy [15].

In hospitalized patients, those benefits are strongly related to exercise intensity. Few sessions of high-intensity low-volume FES-cycling exercise can promote a mean 117% increase in torque and 61% in power [16] (Fig. 7.2). It also improves the neuromuscular efficiency. High-intensity low-volume FES-cycling reduces 33% of the stimulation cost [16] (Fig. 7.2). This means that fewer motor units are required to produce the same power output, or alternatively, greater power output is achieved with the same number of motor units.

FES-Cycling Effects on Physical Function and Ambulation Capacity

The physical function improvement depends on the FES-cycling exercise protocol. In hospitalized patients, the results will follow the intensity of the exercise. Waldauf et al. [11] used a very low-intensity, high-volume FES-cycling protocol, with pulse intensities ranging from 0 to 60 mA, frequency set at 40 Hz, and pulse width at 250 μs. The exercise protocol averaged 31 min per day, and patients received an average of 6.5 FES-cycling sessions. However, no improvements in muscle strength or physical function were observed compared to the control group. Berney et al. [12] implemented a low-intensity, high-volume protocol, with pulse intensity between 20 and 30 mA, frequency between 43.5 and 50 Hz, and pulse width of 250 to 300 μs. The median exercise duration was 51 min per day, with a median of 5 FES-cycling sessions. While muscle strength showed no significant improvements, physical function was 25% better than in the control group. Parry et al. [17] used a moderate-intensity, high-volume FES-cycling protocol, with pulse intensities up to 140 mA, frequencies between 30 and 50 Hz, and pulse widths ranging from 300 to 400 μs. The exercise duration ranged from 20 to 60 min per day, and patients received an average of 8.6 FES-cycling sessions. In this study, physical function improved by 83% compared to the control group. Frazão et al. [16] used a high-intensity, low-volume FES-cycling protocol, with pulse intensities up to 180 mA, 75 Hz frequency, and pulse widths ranging from 500 to 800 μs (Fig. 7.3). The

Fig. 7.2 Effects of high-intensity low-volume FES-cycling exercise on muscle performance in hospitalized patients. (Frazão et al. [16])

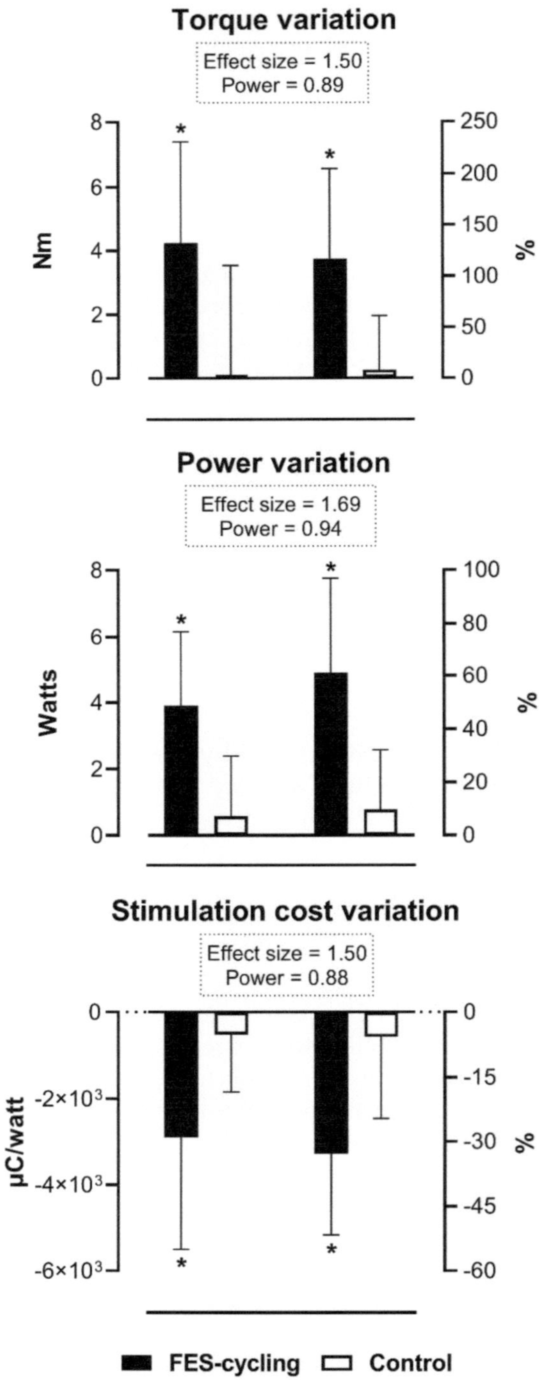

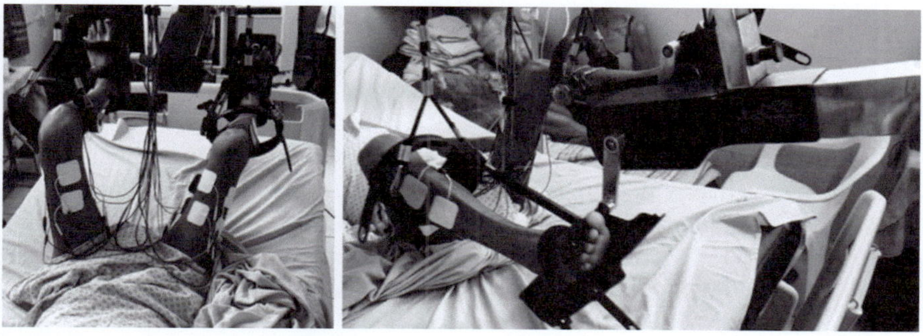

Fig. 7.3 High-intensity and low-volume FES-cycling exercise during hospitalization. (Frazão et al. [16])

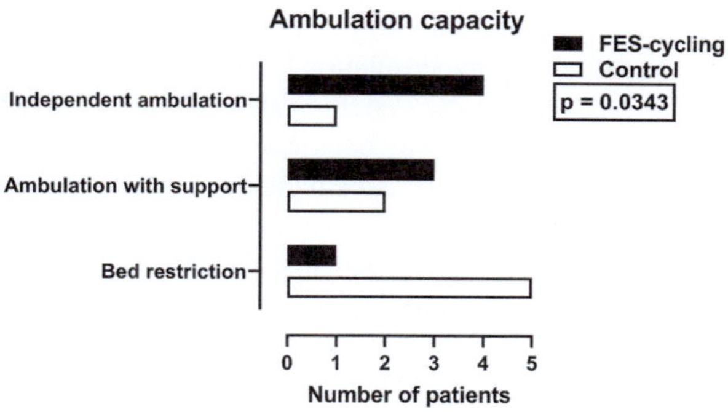

Fig. 7.4 Ambulation capacity after high-intensity and low-volume FES-cycling exercise treatment. (Frazão et al. [16])

exercise duration was 10 min per day, and patients received an average of 5 FES-cycling sessions. While muscle strength improved 117%, physical function was 200% better than in the control group.

The ambulation capacity shows improvement after a FES-cycling exercise program, likely as a result of the enhanced muscle performance. A strong link exists between torque variations and gait speed [18], and early ambulation has been shown to boost strength [19], creating a mutually beneficial relationship between these two outcomes.

It's important to highlight that ambulation capacity is closely connected to hospital length of stay and survival rates [20], making it a critical therapeutic goal. In this context, high-intensity, low-volume FES-cycling exercise may be the most appropriate modality for hospitalized patients (Fig. 7.4). During hospitalization, the focus should be on achieving short, impactful exercises (like a 100-m sprint competition) rather than long-duration activities (like a marathon). Patients typically cover only short distances, moving from their bed to the bathroom or walking through the ward/ICU halls. On the other hand, low-intensity, high-volume exercises may be more suitable for long-term programs aimed at improving cardiorespiratory fitness.

Chronic Obstructive Pulmonary Disease (COPD)

Impact of COPD on the Body

Chronic obstructive pulmonary disease leads to structural changes in the lung parenchyma, such as remodeling and airway obstruction, which reduce lung elastic recoil. These alterations disrupt the structures responsible for maintaining open airways during expiration, resulting in dynamic hyperinflation [21, 22]. The dynamic hyperinflation promotes lower respiratory neuromuscular efficiency at moderate exercise intensity [23] (Fig. 7.5).

Dynamic hyperinflation has a direct impact on the cardiovascular system [24]. It impairs ventricular filling, leading to smaller end-diastolic volumes and a reduction in the intrathoracic blood volume index, as well as the end-diastolic volumes of both the left and right ventricles and systolic volume [25, 26]. The performance of both ventricles is compromised by low preload, which is caused by thoracic hypovolemia due to pulmonary hyperinflation [27].

The skeletal muscle system is also affected by COPD. Eliason et al. [28] found that the severity of airway obstruction influences lower muscle capillarization, particularly in type I fibers. This reduced muscle perfusion also impacts muscle morphology. Gosker et al. [29] observed a decrease in mitochondrial density in the vastus lateralis of COPD patients, contributing to a reduction in muscle oxidative capacity, which leads to decreased performance and early fatigue. COPD patients also presents lower peripheral neuromuscular efficiency at light exercise intensity [23] (Fig. 7.6). Less efficient muscles require greater ventilatory effort, creating a harmful cycle.

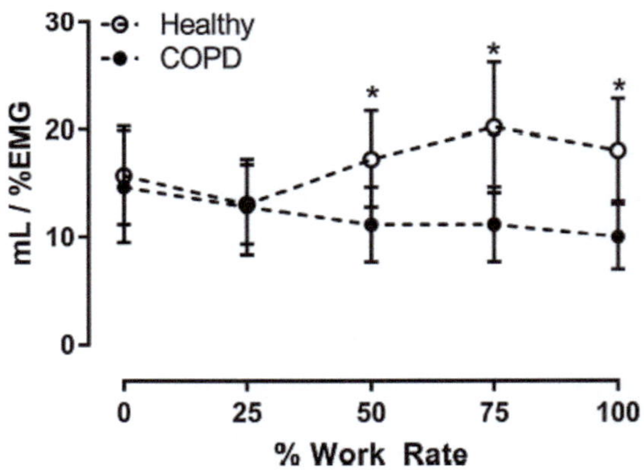

Fig. 7.5 Respiratory neuromuscular efficiency (amount of tidal volume per percentage of respiratory muscle activity). EMG: electromyographic activity. *$p < 0.05$ compared to COPD. (Frazão et al. [23])

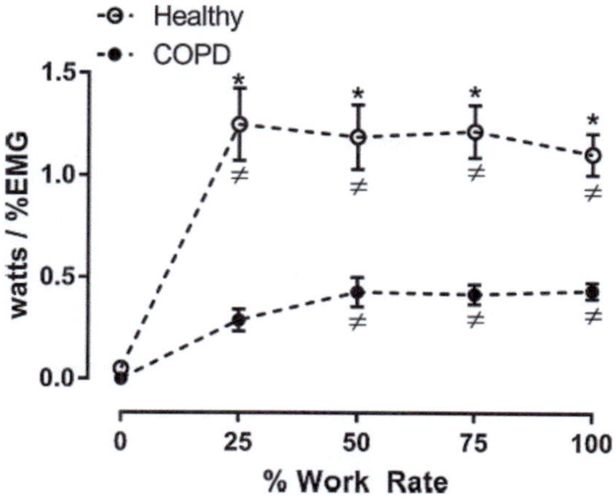

Fig. 7.6 Peripheral neuromuscular efficiency (amount of power output per percentage of quadriceps muscle activity). EMG: electromyographic activity. $*p < 0.05$ compared to COPD, $^{\neq}p < 0.05$ compared to 0% work rate. (Frazão et al. [23])

The Rationale for FES-Cycling Exercise in COPD

FES-cycling can enhance the metabolism during exercise. Medrinal et al. [30] analyzed 23 consecutive patients with COPD GOLD stage 2, 3 or 4 (mean FEV1 = 50.3% pred) who had recently begun a respiratory rehabilitation program. The patients performed two consecutive 30-minute sessions at a constant load with active and placebo FES-cycling. FES-cycling increased the physiological response more than the placebo, with a greater VO2 achieved of 36.6 mL/min ($p = 0.01$) (Fig. 7.7). There was also a greater increase in lactate after FES-cycling (+1.5 mmol/L; $p = 0.01$).

Despite been a more intense exercise, FES-cycling did not change dyspnea or muscle fatigue compared with the placebo condition [30, 31]. This finding has a major clinical impact on the management of a pulmonary rehabilitation program. This type of patient often cannot tolerate a more intense exercise due to dyspnea and muscle fatigue.

There is a high certainty of evidence that FES-cycling induces higher cardiorespiratory fitness in rehabilitation programs longer than 8 weeks, with a clinically important difference compared to other therapeutic modalities [6]. There is also a moderate certainty of evidence that FES-cycling induces higher peripheral muscle oxygen extraction with a clinically important difference compared to other therapeutic modalities [6]. These effects may improve the metabolic efficiency reducing the ventilatory demand, respiratory rate and, consequently, dynamic hyperinflation [32].

The dynamic hyperinflation reduction is a corner stone not only in ventilatory, but also in cardiac performances improvement in COPD patients [33] (Fig. 7.8). Reducing dynamic hyperinflation improves oxygen pulse and alleviates dynamic cardiac constraints. Cardiac mechanics are enhanced by lowering left ventricular afterload, which is typically elevated due to the high intrathoracic pressure swings required to overcome the increased elastic and resistive loads in COPD during

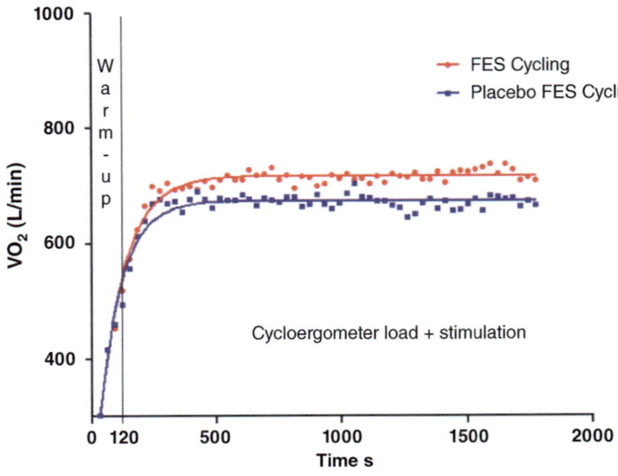

Fig. 7.7 Increased oxygen consumption during FES-cycling in COPD patients. (Medrinal et al. [30])

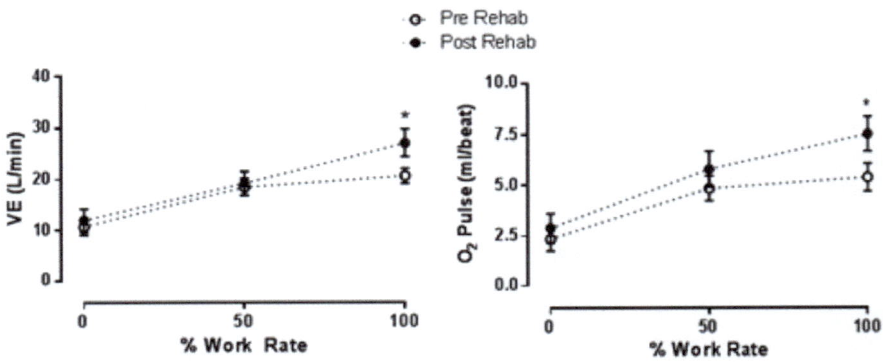

Fig. 7.8 Effects of pulmonary rehabilitation on ventilatory and cardiac performances of COPD patients. *$p < 0.05$

exercise [34]. The reduction in dynamic hyperinflation enhances blood return and preload, thereby optimizing cardiac performance.

Additionally, FES-cycling exercise improves muscle mass and performance [6], being an important tool for treating sarcopenia in this population. Sarcopenia is prevalent in a significant proportion of patients with COPD and negatively impacts upon important clinical outcomes.

Sepúlveda-Loyola et al. [35] showed that overall sarcopenia prevalence varies from 15.5% (combined muscle mass, strength, and/or physical performance criteria) to 34% (muscle mass criteria alone) and is greater in patients with more severe (37.6%) than in less severe (19.1%) lung disease. Patients with sarcopenia have poorer exercise tolerance and quality of life compared with those without sarcopenia.

Heart Failure

Impact of Heart Failure on the Body

Heart failure is a chronic, multi-etiological syndrome (commonly caused by cardiomyopathy, valvular disease, or other structural and functional cardiac abnormalities) that results in progressive multi-organ dysfunction. Its primary impact occurs within the heart, where the inability to sustain adequate stroke volume [36] triggers ventricular remodeling, typically characterized by cardiomegaly and altered chamber geometry. This remodeling process is not driven by a single mechanism but by a complex interplay of factors, including hemodynamic overload, neurohormonal activation, inflammatory pathways, and metabolic disturbances [37]. Beyond the heart, heart failure exerts profound secondary effects on pulmonary and skeletal muscle systems, further contributing to exercise intolerance and poor prognosis.

Left ventricular dysfunction increases end-diastolic pressure, which elevates left atrial pressure and subsequently raises pulmonary capillary pressure. The resulting hydrostatic imbalance promotes the movement of fluid from pulmonary capillaries into the interstitial and alveolar spaces, leading to pulmonary congestion [36]. The accumulation of fluid compromises the integrity and function of the alveolar-capillary membrane, reducing its diffusing capacity. This impaired gas exchange is a key determinant of limited pulmonary function in chronic heart failure and is strongly correlated with both maximal exercise capacity and overall functional status [38].

Additionally, the competition for intrathoracic space reduces lung capacity in advanced stages chronic heart failure patients. The change in cardiac size within a closed thoracic cavity may pose significant constraints on the lungs, resulting in reductions in lung volumes that likely play a major role in the restrictive breathing patterns often reported in patients with chronic heart failure [39]. During exercise, the close relationship between cardiac size and pulmonary mechanics becomes even more evident, as the enlarged heart further limits lung expansion, promoting tachypneic breathing [40].

In heart failure patients, the skeletal muscle dysfunction develops as a consequence of chronic inactivity, impaired perfusion, and neuromuscular and metabolic alterations. These alterations together lead to decreased exercise tolerance and overall physical capacity.

The reduction in maximal exercise capacity observed is largely attributed to impaired nutritive blood flow to skeletal muscle, leading to early onset of muscular fatigue. In the early 1980s, Wilson et al. [41] demonstrated that with increasing severity of exercise intolerance, there is a progressive decline in cardiac output and limb blood flow at any given workload. This hemodynamic limitation is further compounded by a reduction in leg oxygen extraction, highlighting a combined impairment in both oxygen delivery and utilization during exercise. Wilson et al. [41].

Sullivan et al. [42] demonstrated that patients with chronic heart failure exhibit significant histological and biochemical alterations in skeletal muscle, including a marked reduction in oxidative enzyme activity. These adaptations are accompanied by a shift in muscle fiber composition, characterized by a decreased proportion of type I fibers (which are highly oxidative and fatigue-resistant) and an increased proportion of fast-twitch type IIb fibers, which rely predominantly on glycolytic metabolism. Additionally, these patients show a reduced capillary-to-fiber ratio, indicating impaired muscle perfusion compared to healthy individuals. Collectively, these structural and metabolic changes contribute to early fatigue and reduced exercise tolerance in heart failure. Sullivan et al. [42]

Reduced aerobic enzyme activity in skeletal muscle is a key factor contributing to the early onset of anaerobic metabolism during exercise in patients with chronic heart failure. This metabolic limitation is evidenced by premature blood lactate accumulation, indicating a shift toward glycolytic pathways even at low workloads [43]. Such impairment not only constrains exercise tolerance but also influences the adaptive response to long-term interventions, including exercise training. Moreover, heart failure is associated with neuromuscular inefficiency, characterized by an accelerated onset of muscle fatigue, further compounding functional limitations during physical activity [44]. At the contractile level, heart failure induces alterations in myosin-actin cross-bridge dynamics, impairing muscle mechanics and further compromising skeletal muscle performance [45]. Sullivan et al. [43].

The Rationale for FES-Cycling Exercise in Heat Failure

FES-cycling has been shown to enhance stroke volume, heart rate, and cardiac output [6], all of which are critical for improving cardiac performance during the rehabilitation of patients with heart failure. These hemodynamic responses contribute to increased oxygen delivery to working muscles and improved systemic perfusion. Additionally, during moderate to vigorous FES-cycling intensities, a rise in systolic blood pressure is typically observed [46]. This controlled increase in systolic pressure induces a physiological myocardial overload, which is an essential stimulus for promoting favorable cardiac antiremodeling and adaptive cardiovascular responses over the course of rehabilitation.

Long-term exercise training has a beneficial antiremodeling effect on cardiac structure and function. In a 6-month home-based program, Hambrecht et al. [47], demonstrated that 20 min of daily ergometer training at 70% of peak oxygen uptake significantly reduced cardiomegaly. The training group achieved a 10% reduction in end-diastolic volume and a 15% reduction in end-systolic volume, while the control group showed increases of 5% and 1%, respectively. These findings were later corroborated by Giannuzzi et al. [48] in a multicenter study. In addition to reducing cardiomegaly, exercise training improved ejection fraction in the intervention group, whereas no change occurred in controls. Moreover, significant improvements in work capacity, peak VO_2, walking distance, and quality of life were observed exclusively among trained patients.

During FES-cycling exercise, ventilatory efficiency improves significantly. Gorgey and Lawrence [49] demonstrated a reduction in the ventilatory equivalent (amount of ventilation to promote gas exchange) for carbon dioxide (VE/VCO_2) during FES-cycling (Fig. 7.9). This enhancement in ventilatory efficiency is a key mechanism underlying the reduction of dyspnea in patients with heart failure. Guazzi et al. [50] investigated whether enhanced pulmonary diffusion contributes to the improvement in aerobic efficiency induced by physical training in patients with chronic heart failure. After training, the intervention group exhibited a 25% increase in lung diffusing capacity, a 15% increase in alveolar-capillary conductance, a 10% increase in pulmonary capillary blood volume, and a 13% rise in peak VO_2 (Fig. 7.10), in addition to VE/VCO_2 slope reduction. Additionally, pulmonary arteriolar resistance at peak exercise decreased by 28%. However, these benefits were dependent on continued exercise. Following an eight-week detraining period, all improvements regressed to values comparable to baseline and control levels, which clearly demonstrates the need for chronic treatment.

FES-cycling exercise markedly enhances muscular blood perfusion, contributing to improved oxygen delivery and utilization in individuals with limited mobility or cardiovascular impairment. Gojda et al. [51] demonstrated a 165% increase in leg blood flow index during FES-cycling. This effect is primarily mediated by significant arteriolar vasodilation within the active muscles, which increases regional perfusion [19]. The vasodilatory response is largely driven by enhanced endothelial function, secondary to the combined effects of rhythmic muscle contractions and electrical stimulation. These stimuli increase shear stress on the vascular endothelium, promoting nitric oxide release and reducing peripheral vascular resistance. In addition to increased perfusion, peripheral oxygen extraction is augmented during FES-cycling [52], improving the arterio-venous oxygen difference and overall oxygen utilization by working muscles. This integrated adaptation (greater blood flow and enhanced oxygen extraction) optimizes muscle metabolism and contributes to improved exercise tolerance, reduced fatigue, and better functional capacity.

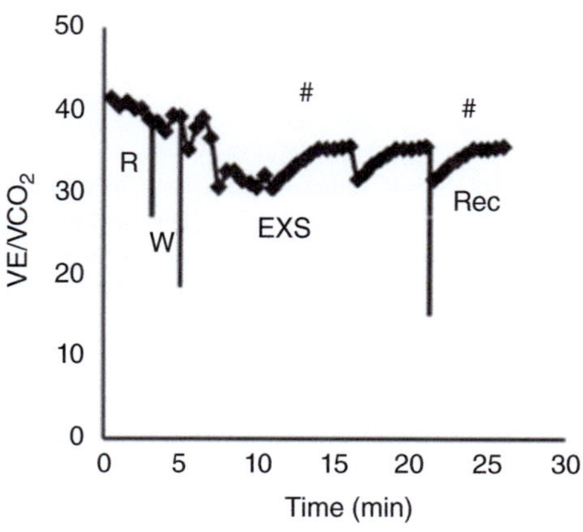

Fig. 7.9 Ventilatory equivalent of carbonic gas (ventilatory efficiency) during FES-cycling exercise. *R* rest, *W* warm-up, *EXS* exercise, *Rec* recovery. #Significant differences during EXS and recovery compared with rest and warm-up periods. (Gorgey and Lawrence [49])

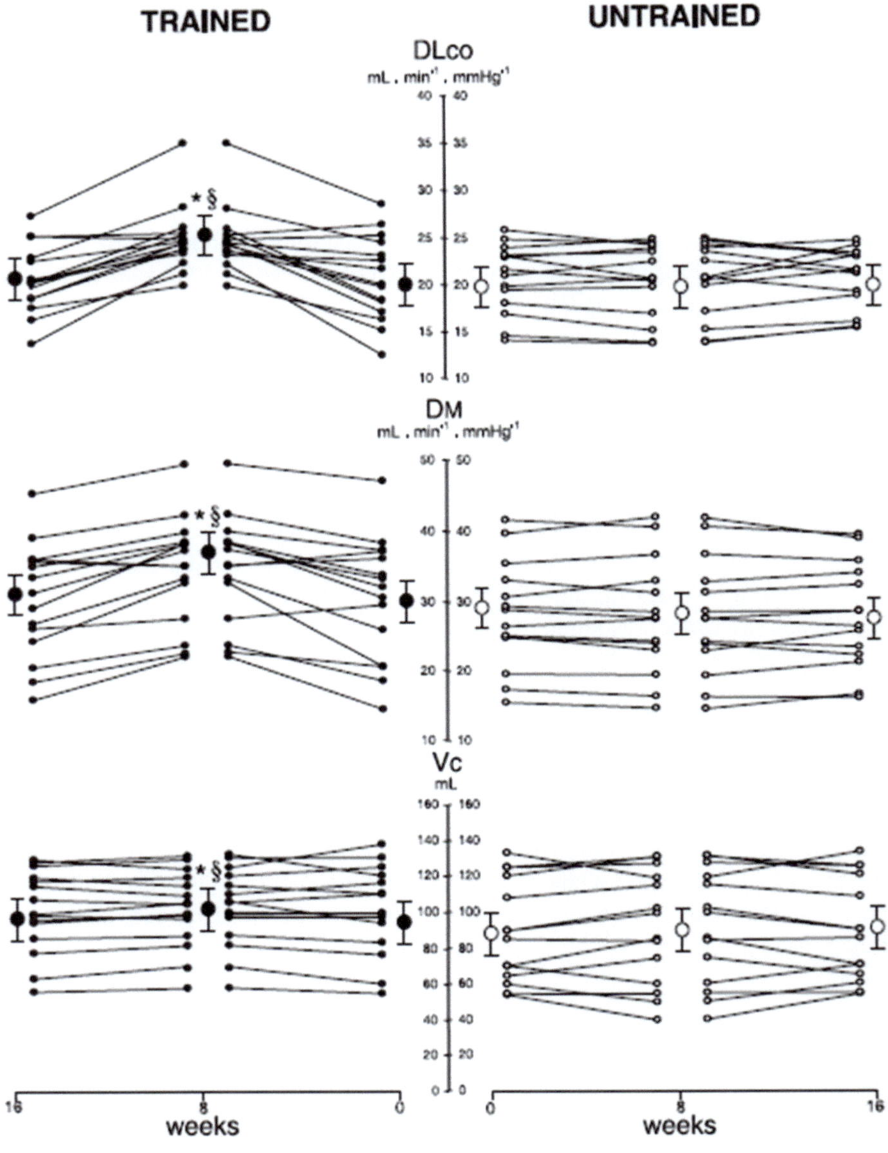

Fig. 7.10 Single values of diffusion capacity for CO (DLCO) and its subcomponents, alveolar-capillary membrane conductance (DM) and pulmonary capillary blood volume (Vc), in trained and untrained groups at baseline (*week 0*), at the end of training (8 week), and after detraining (16 week). *$P < 0.01$ vs. baseline. §$P < 0.01$ vs. corresponding untrained value. (Guazzi et al. [50])

Metabolic Disease

Obesity and Type 2 Diabetes

Metabolic disorders, including obesity, type 2 diabetes (T2DM), and metabolic syndrome, pose an escalating global health burden. Among these, obesity is the strongest risk factor for T2DM [53], primarily through its association with metabolic abnormalities that promote insulin resistance [54]. Although the exact mechanisms by which obesity drives T2DM and insulin resistance are not fully elucidated, evidence suggests a multifactorial process involving both cell-autonomous pathways and inter-organ crosstalk, including adipose tissue dysfunction, chronic low-grade inflammation, altered adipokine secretion, and ectopic lipid accumulation.

Skeletal muscle insulin resistance is widely regarded as the most critical extra-pancreatic contributor to the development of T2DM. Under physiological conditions, insulin promotes muscle glycogen synthesis by enhancing glucose uptake from the bloodstream. This process depends on three key rate-limiting components: glycogen synthase, hexokinase, and the glucose transporter GLUT4. When insulin binds to its receptor on the muscle cell surface, it activates a signaling cascade that triggers GLUT4 translocation from intracellular storage sites (such as the endosomal recycling compartment and the trans-Golgi network) to the plasma membrane. This translocation facilitates glucose entry into the cell, thereby promoting glycogen synthesis and reducing circulating glucose concentrations [55].

The Rationale for FES-Cycling Exercise in Obesity and Type 2 Diabetes

FES-cycling exercise increases energy expenditure [52] (Fig. 7.11), contributing to reductions in fat mass and improvements in body composition. To assess these effects, Dolbow et al. [56] conducted a study in which participants were divided into two groups: [1] FES-cycling combined with nutritional counseling (FES & Nutri), and [2] nutritional counseling alone (Nutri Only). The FES & Nutri group underwent high-intensity interval FES-cycling for 30 min, three times per week, over an

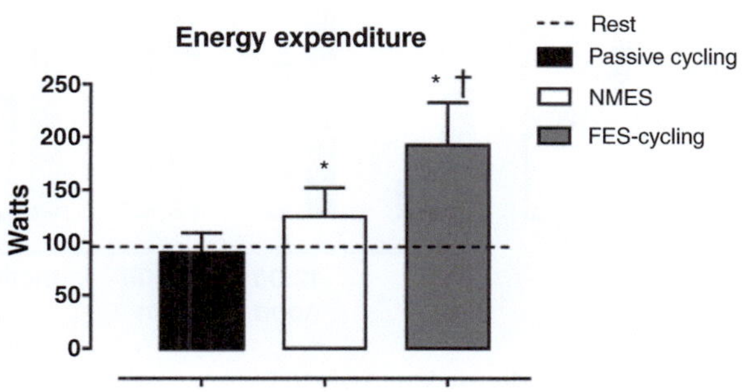

Fig. 7.11 Energy expenditure during FES-cycling (comparison to other rehabilitation modalities). (Frazão et al. [52])

eight-week period, in addition to receiving weekly 30-minute nutritional counseling sessions. The Nutri Only group received the same nutritional counseling without FES-cycling.

Results showed that participants in the FES & Nutri group experienced a significantly greater reduction in body fat percentage (mean change = −1.14%) compared to the Nutri Only group (mean change = +0.28%). Additionally, the FES & Nutri group gained more lean mass in the legs (mean = +0.66 kg), whereas the Nutri Only group showed a decrease (mean = −1.05 kg). These findings highlight the synergistic effect of FES-cycling and nutritional intervention on improving body composition.

Beyond body composition changes, FES-cycling can impact the glucose regulation. A recent case report showed a blood glucose level reduction after 10 FES-cycling exercise sessions (Fig. 7.12) [57]. Glucose uptake by contracting skeletal muscle occurs via facilitated diffusion, which requires both the presence of GLUT4 in the surface membrane and a favorable inward diffusion gradient for glucose. During exercise, skeletal muscle hyperemia, capillary recruitment, and GLUT4 translocation to the sarcolemma and T-tubules largely eliminate delivery and membrane transport as major limitations to glucose uptake. Under these conditions, glucose phosphorylation can become the rate-limiting step, particularly at high exercise intensities [58].

GLUT4 was identified in the late 1980s as the predominant isoform responsible for insulin- and contraction-stimulated glucose transport in skeletal muscle [59]. The contraction-induced increase in skeletal muscle glucose uptake is primarily driven by enhanced glucose transport across the sarcolemma and T-tubules. This reflects not only an increased abundance of GLUT4 in these membranes due to translocation but also, potentially, an increase in GLUT4 intrinsic activity.

During the early recovery period after exercise, skeletal muscle exhibits a sustained increase in glucose uptake even in the absence of insulin, followed by a secondary phase characterized by enhanced insulin sensitivity. This heightened insulin sensitivity reflects an increased capacity for insulin-stimulated GLUT4 translocation to the cell surface. However, whether this effect is mediated by alterations in

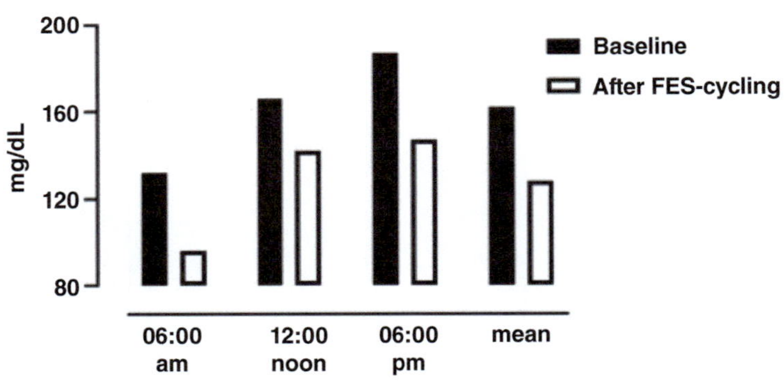

Fig. 7.12 Blood glucose level after 10 FES-cycling exercise sessions. (Frazão et al. [57])

insulin signaling pathways, GLUT4 trafficking dynamics, or both remains to be fully clarified. Importantly, the postexercise enhancement of skeletal muscle insulin sensitivity is strongly linked to glycogen depletion during exercise. Indeed, insulin-stimulated glucose transport has been shown to vary with muscle glycogen content, and it has been proposed that GLUT4-containing vesicles may directly associate with glycogen, providing a mechanistic link between glycogen status and glucose transport regulation [60].

Chronic Kidney Disease

Impact of Chronic Kidney Disease on the Body

Muscle loss is a frequent complication of chronic kidney disease, particularly in advanced stages and among patients undergoing hemodialysis. Beyond impairing physical function, muscle wasting in chronic kidney disease is strongly associated with poorer quality of life, depression, protein-energy wasting, increased risk of fractures, cardiovascular complications, transplant-related graft failure, postoperative complications, as well as higher rates of hospitalization and mortality [61].

The mechanisms driving muscle loss are multifactorial, involving both non-inflammatory and inflammatory pathways. Non-inflammatory contributors include metabolic acidosis, insulin resistance, vitamin D deficiency, hormonal imbalances (testosterone, IGF-1, GH resistance), amino acid losses during dialysis, and inadequate nutritional intake [62, 63]. Metabolic acidosis stimulates protein catabolism through caspase-3 and ubiquitin–proteasome activation, while vitamin D deficiency impairs insulin secretion and protein synthesis. Inflammatory factors are linked to the bioincompatibility of dialysis membranes [64] and, more recently, to gut dysbiosis and intestinal barrier dysfunction [65]. Dietary restrictions limiting fiber-rich foods exacerbate dysbiosis, leading to the accumulation of uremic toxins and endotoxins that trigger systemic low-grade inflammation, further contributing to muscle protein breakdown and negative energy balance in chronic kidney disease [65].

Such profound alterations in skeletal muscle structure and function, driven by mitochondrial dysfunction, inflammation, oxidative stress, metabolic acidosis, and other uremia-related factors, lead to significant declines in muscle strength, physical performance, and cardiorespiratory fitness. Fahal et al. [66] reported that dialytic patients show reduced quadriceps strength, particularly in those with malnutrition, and slower muscle relaxation compared to healthy controls. Muscle biopsies revealed abnormalities in 78% of patients, with atrophy in type I (45%) and type II fibers (40%), and a significantly smaller type II fiber area in malnourished individuals. Howden et al. [67] showed a 17% reduction in cardiorespiratory fitness (VO_2) and a high rate of physical inactivity in chronic kidney disease patients. In a large multiethnic study, Sui et al. [68] found an independent, inverse, and graded association between cardiorespiratory fitness and mortality.

The Rationale for FES-Cycling Exercise in Chronic Kidney Disease

In maintenance hemodialysis patients, habitual physical activity has been associated with a reduced risk of mortality over a median follow-up of 45 months [69]. Conversely, physical inactivity is a major contributor to chronic disease, and extensive evidence demonstrates that prolonged sedentary behavior increases the risk of all-cause and cardiovascular mortality. Data from the National Health and Nutrition Examination Survey III (NHANES III) revealed that 28% of individuals with chronic kidney disease reported being physically inactive, compared with 13.5% of non- chronic kidney disease individuals [70]. These findings highlight the critical role of physical activity in improving survival and overall health in patients with chronic kidney disease, particularly those receiving hemodialysis.

Physical exercise exerts well-documented benefits on cardiorespiratory fitness, muscular strength, and skeletal muscle integrity [71] in this type of patients. Beyond improvements in physical performance, Andrade et al. [72] demonstrated that supervised exercise in patients undergoing maintenance hemodiafiltration is associated with enhanced dialysis efficiency and treatment-related performance outcomes. These findings underscore the role of exercise as an effective adjunct therapy in this population, with clinical applicability both during the intradialytic period and in structured interdialytic exercise programs.

FES-cycling exercise fits like a glove in this scenario. It can promote significant physiological benefits for patients with chronic kidney disease, particularly those on maintenance hemodialysis who suffer from profound muscle wasting, reduced oxidative capacity, and impaired exercise tolerance. FES-cycling induces muscle contractions that enhance mitochondrial function, capillary density, and glucose uptake, thereby counteracting the metabolic and structural derangements typical of uremia. Furthermore, repeated FES-cycling sessions contribute to increased muscle cross-sectional area, improved contractile function, and attenuation of the progressive sarcopenia observed in advanced chronic kidney disease. From a metabolic standpoint, FES-cycling has been linked to improved insulin sensitivity, reduced markers of systemic inflammation, and better regulation of phosphate and potassium balance, which are critical in dialytic patients.

The intervention can also facilitate intradialytic exercise (Fig. 7.13) without excessive patient burden, as it is safe, well-tolerated, and feasible to implement during dialysis sessions. Roxo et al. [73] didn't observe any adverse event during or after sessions in a 30 min, three times per week, for 2 months conventional electrical stimulation intradialytic protocol. Additionally, by improving exercise tolerance and functional reserve, FES-cycling may decrease hospitalization risk, enhance transplant readiness, and ultimately lower all-cause mortality. These benefits position FES-cycling as a clinically relevant adjunct therapy to conventional chronic kidney disease management, with growing potential for integration into nephrology rehabilitation protocols.

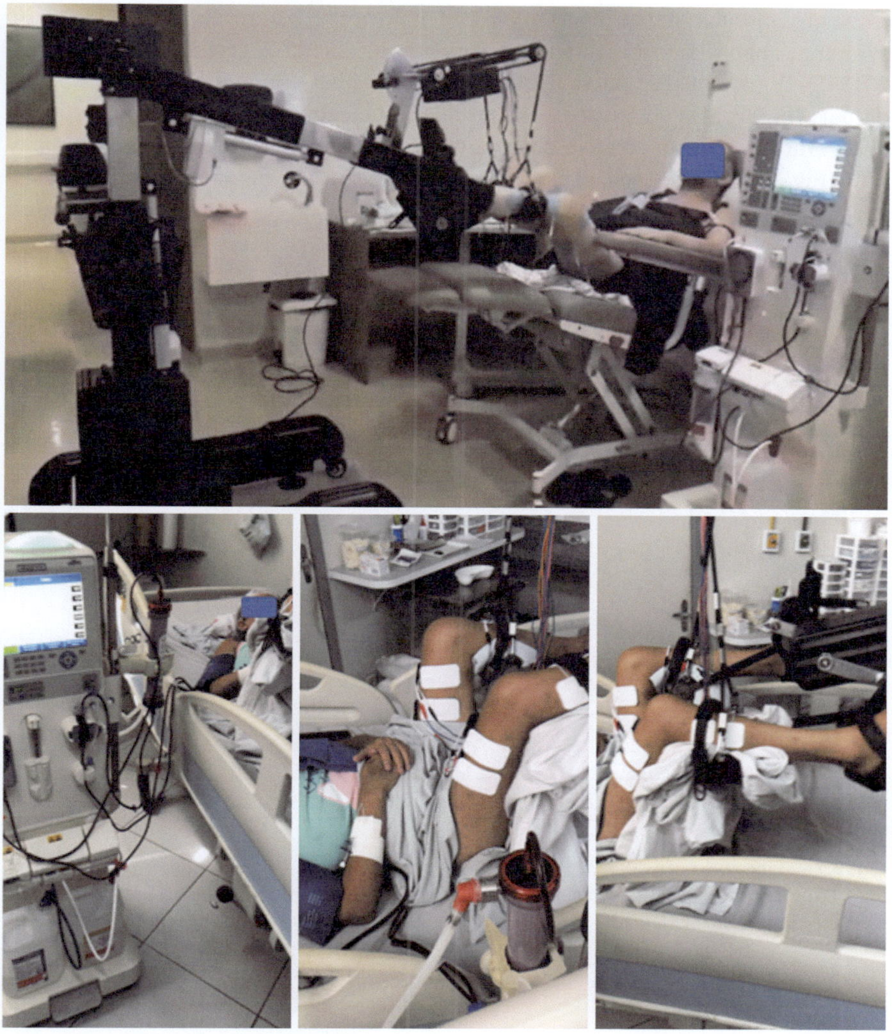

Fig. 7.13 Intradialytic FES-cycling exercise. (Source: The author)

Long COVID

Impact of COVID-19 on the Muscles

Muscle damage is quite common during the COVID-19 acute phase. SARS-CoV-2 activates inflammatory cytokines, causing inflammatory injury in muscle cells [74]. In a meta-analysis of prevalence based on each neurological manifestation, Pizon et al. [75] demonstrated that muscle injury or myalgia was the most common (19%) symptom in individuals with COVID-19.

Neuromuscular impairment associated with more severe acute disease phase symptoms appears to be implicated in limiting exercise capacity. Severe post-COVID-19 patients present activation of muscle fibers IIa and IIb at lower power outputs (Fig. 7.14) and lower neuromuscular efficiency (Fig. 7.15). The neuromuscular efficiency has a positive correlation with symptom-limited aerobic capacity [76] (Fig. 7.16). These changes are key elements in the fatigue and low physical capacity of long-COVID.

In patients hospitalized in the intensive care unit (ICU), these limitations are more pronounced. These individuals often experience intensive care-acquired muscle weakness and cardiopulmonary impairments. ICU survivors typically exhibit low ventilatory efficiency, requiring increased ventilation during exercise. As a result, persistent dyspnea is commonly linked to reduced physical fitness [77].

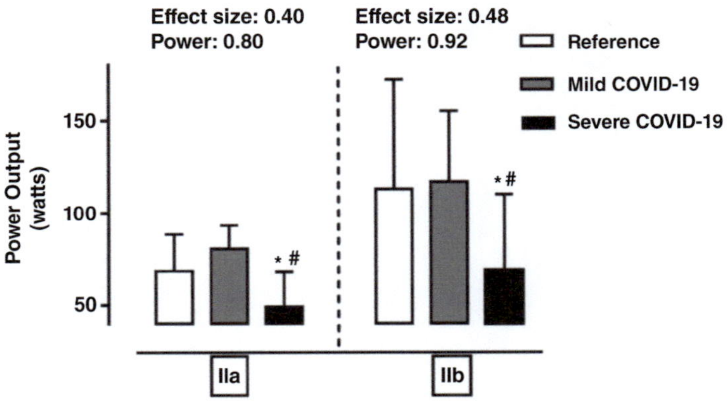

Fig. 7.14 Fiber type activation. *IIa* activation of type IIa fibers, *IIb* activation of type IIb fibers. $^*P \leq 0.05$ compared with the reference group. $^\#P \leq 0.05$ compared with the group that had mild COVID-19. (Frazão et al. [76])

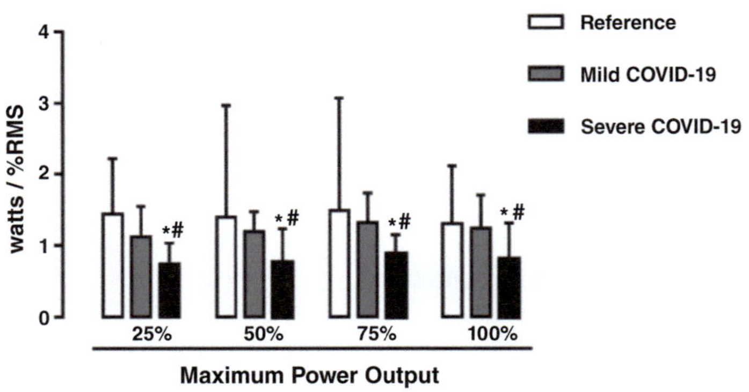

Fig. 7.15 Neuromuscular efficiency in each exercise intensity. *%RMS* percentage of root-mean-square obtained at the maximum effort. $^*P \leq 0.05$ compared with the reference group. $^\#P \leq 0.05$ compared with the group that had mild COVID-19. (Frazão et al. [76])

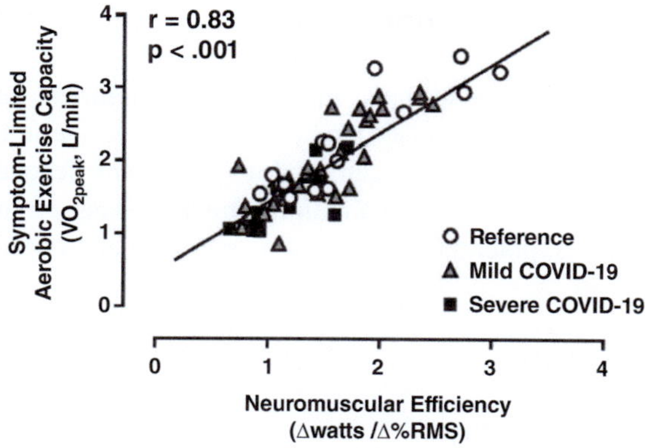

Fig. 7.16 Correlation between neuromuscular efficiency and symptom-limited aerobic capacity. *%RMS* percentage of root-mean-square obtained at the maximum effort. VO2peak = peak oxygen uptake. (Frazão et al. [76])

The Rationale for FES-Cycling Exercise in Long-COVID

As many long-COVID patients experience persistent muscle fatigue and neuromuscular inefficiency, improving muscle performance becomes a crucial aspect for rehabilitation. Strength and power are fundamental to a muscle's ability to perform work (muscle performance). To enhance this capacity, both strength and power must be considered. FES-cycling has been shown to significantly improve both strength and power [6], making this technology a valuable tool in long-COVID rehabilitation.

In a 4-week pragmatic proof-of-concept controlled study, Mateo et al. [78] demonstrated that FES-cycling could be safely used in combination with physiotherapy. The study included 14 patients who were admitted to the rehabilitation department following ICU hospitalization for a severe form of COVID-19. Cycling was incorporated into the rehabilitation program, with eight patients using FES (FES-cycling group) and six patients cycling without FES (cycling group). FES-cycling facilitated a faster restoration of an erect posture and a quicker resumption of spontaneous walking compared to rehabilitation without FES. Patients in the FES-cycling group reduced their sedentary time and increased their daily walking/running duration. Mateo et al. [78].

Another important finding in this study was the good tolerance of FES-cycling, both in terms of cardiovascular and pulmonary parameters, as well as the patients' subjective experience with FES administration. A notable example involved a patient who, initially out of breath while standing to set up the electrodes on the gluteus muscles, was able to cycle with FES for approximately 30 min with only a slight to moderate increase in dyspnea. Moreover, there was no need to modify, reschedule, or cancel physiotherapy sessions, suggesting that the fatigue induced by FES-cycling was minimal. These results indicate that FES-cycling could be effectively integrated with standard rehabilitation for patients recovering from critical COVID-19 [78].

Orthopedic Conditions

Orthopedic conditions, including joint injuries, post-surgical states, and chronic musculoskeletal disorders, often necessitate periods of reduced weight-bearing or immobilization that can lead to significant deconditioning. FES-cycling offers a potential means of maintaining muscle mass, strength, and function during these periods, potentially accelerating recovery and improving long-term outcomes.

The Rationale for FES-Cycling Exercise in Orthopedic Conditions

Joint Mobility

During FES-cycling exercise, the hip, knee, and ankle joints are mobilized repeatedly. The total number of movements depends on both cycling cadence and exercise duration. For example, at 10 RPM over 10 min, each joint is mobilized 100 times, whereas at 20 RPM over 20 min, mobilization increases to 400 repetitions. The effects on range of motion are determined by the biomechanical adjustments of the equipment. A closer positioning of the equipment to the patient increases range of motion. Moreover, unlike manual mobilization, FES-cycling provides consistent, rhythmic, and prolonged joint movement patterns, ensuring both repetition and uniformity throughout the exercise session.

The benefits of the continuous passive **motion** include reducing joint stiffness, minimizing swelling, and promoting cartilage health [79]. By gently moving the joint through a controlled range of motion, continuous passive motion facilitates edema clearance, helps maintain tissue compliance, and prevents the formation of adhesions. More than 30 years ago, Johnson [80] demonstrated in a prospective, randomized, controlled trial that continuous passive motion following knee arthroplasty significantly improved both early and late knee flexion, without impairing wound healing. More recently, Hong et al. [81] investigated the effects of continuous passive motion in patients with delayed rehabilitation progress (defined as failure to achieve 45° of active range of motion by postoperative day 3). Their findings showed that patients in the continuous passive motion group achieved a significantly greater mean active range of motion at discharge compared to controls (76.0° vs. 68.4°, $p = 0.02$).

Bone Density

Immobility and the absence of weight-bearing are well-recognized drivers of accelerated bone mineral density loss. A substantial body of literature has investigated the effects of FES-cycling on bone health in individuals with spinal cord injury, a population particularly vulnerable to disuse osteoporosis. Evidence suggests that early initiation and long-term application of FES-cycling may delay bone loss and, in some cases, even promote increases in bone mineral density.

Findings from multiple clinical trials demonstrate that FES-cycling exercise can produce significant improvements in bone mineral density, particularly in load-bearing regions such as the proximal tibia and distal femur. Interventions lasting 3–12 months consistently reported either bone mineral density gains or attenuation of bone loss, with increases of 6–13% in tibial and femoral sites [82, 83]. Longer training durations (≥12 months) were especially effective, as shown by a 10% increase in proximal tibia bone mineral density after 1 year [84] and a 32% improvement in hip bone mineral density among pediatric patients after 6 months of training [83]. Smaller cohorts and case studies further support these benefits, reporting modest yet clinically meaningful improvements in bone density [85, 86].

Nonetheless, outcomes were not uniform across all skeletal regions. Some trials reported no significant changes in lumbar spine or femoral neck bone mineral density [84], while others observed only a temporary attenuation of bone loss during early phases of training, with benefits diminishing after detraining [87]. The variability of response appears to be influenced by factors such as baseline bone status, age, and training frequency [88]. Overall, current evidence indicates that regular, intensive, and long-term FES-cycling can mitigate disuse-related bone loss and enhance bone health, although its effects are site-specific and require sustained application to be preserved.

Muscle Mass

During periods of immobilization, skeletal muscle undergoes profound physiological changes that accelerate atrophy. One of the central mechanisms underlying this process is the marked reduction in muscle blood flow, which compromises the delivery of oxygen and essential nutrients to myofibers. This impaired perfusion limits protein synthesis while simultaneously promoting protein degradation, thereby driving a rapid decline in muscle mass and strength. The resulting imbalance between anabolic and catabolic processes not only contributes to muscle wasting but also exacerbates metabolic dysfunction and reduces the capacity for functional recovery. FES-cycling has been shown to counteract these negative effects by markedly enhancing muscle perfusion. Gojda et al. [51] reported a increase in leg blood flow index during FES-cycling, underscoring its potent vascular effects. This improvement is primarily mediated by arteriolar vasodilation in the contracting musculature, which increases regional oxygen and nutrient delivery [19]. Enhanced blood flow may play a pivotal role in supporting muscle protein turnover, reducing atrophy.

FES-cycling exercise has been shown to substantially enhance lean mass, with consistent evidence emerging across clinical studies. A recent systematic review [6] confirmed that improvements were most pronounced under high-intensity stimulation protocols, often reaching current levels of up to 140 mA. These adaptations were not confined to the stimulated lower limbs, as increases in total body lean mass were also observed, raising the possibility that FES-cycling exerts systemic anabolic effects beyond localized muscle activation. Such findings are particularly relevant for individuals with long-term immobility, in whom lean mass preservation is critical for metabolic health, cardiovascular function, and overall rehabilitation outcomes.

At the molecular level, several mechanisms have been proposed to explain these muscle adaptations. High-intensity electrical stimulation has been associated with the up-regulation of IGF-1 and the modulation of MuRF-1, a muscle-specific ubiquitin ligase linked to protein degradation and atrophy. In parallel, FES-cycling can stimulate the expression of markers related to satellite cell differentiation and extracellular matrix remodeling, favoring muscle repair and adaptation. These changes contribute to enhanced muscle regeneration, reduced fibrosis, and an improved structural environment for contractile tissue maintenance [89]. Collectively, these findings highlight FES-cycling as a promising intervention not only to preserve but also to restore muscle mass.

Muscle Performance

Strength and power are fundamental components of muscle performance, as they determine the capacity of muscle to generate force and sustain work over time. In the context of orthopedic rehabilitation, optimizing these components is essential for restoring functional independence, improving mobility, and preventing secondary complications such as muscle atrophy and joint instability. For optimal rehabilitation outcomes, both aspects must be addressed through targeted interventions, since strength contributes to maximal force production, while power reflects the ability to rapidly generate force, which is critical for functional tasks such as rising from a chair, climbing stairs, or maintaining balance during locomotion.

FES-cycling has emerged as a potent modality to enhance both torque (strength) and power, demonstrating consistent improvements in neuromuscular performance across multiple studies [6]. High-intensity FES protocols promote increased motor unit recruitment. Such level of recruitment elevate intramuscular tissue pressure, and induce transient localized ischemia [90]. These physiological stimuli likely activate a cascade of adaptive responses within skeletal muscle, including enhanced excitation-contraction coupling, improved oxidative capacity, and increased resistance to fatigue. Moreover, these adaptations contribute to greater efficiency in repeated tension generation, enabling patients to perform functional tasks with reduced effort and higher endurance.

The observed gains in torque and power extend beyond isolated muscle performance, exerting a direct influence on overall motor recovery [91]. Improvements in muscle strength and power facilitate more coordinated and effective movement patterns, accelerate rehabilitation progress, and reduce dependency on compensatory strategies. Consequently, FES-cycling represents not only a tool for augmenting muscle performance but also a critical intervention for restoring autonomy and quality of life in individuals with orthopedic impairments. By integrating FES-cycling into rehabilitation programs, professionals can exploit both the neuromuscular and metabolic adaptations it elicits, thereby optimizing functional outcomes in patients with compromised musculoskeletal systems.

Pain

Pain is a common limiting factor in orthopedic rehabilitation, often reducing patient adherence, impairing functional recovery, and contributing to secondary muscle atrophy and joint stiffness. Effective interventions that reduce pain while promoting active participation are therefore essential to optimize rehabilitation outcomes. FES-cycling may have promising effects in modulating pain perception in patients with musculoskeletal disorders.

The analgesic effects of FES-cycling are thought to result from multiple physiological mechanisms. Repeated muscle contractions induced by FES enhance local circulation [51] and tissue oxygenation [52], promoting the clearance of inflammatory mediators and metabolic byproducts that can exacerbate pain. These effects contribute to reduced discomfort during and after exercise sessions, allowing patients to tolerate higher training intensities and longer sessions.

The muscle contractions may also help to modulate pain signals in the nervous system. Repeated activation of motor units, especially in the context of exercise and rehabilitation, can lead to pain relief. This is often achieved through a phenomenon called the repeated bout effect, where repeated muscle contractions, even if initially painful, can reduce pain sensitivity and improve muscle function. The repeated bout effect might involve a diminished inflammatory response after the second bout due to an attenuation of muscle damage markers concurrent with reductions in soreness and force losses [92]. Additionally, these contractions promote the release of endogenous opioids and other neurochemicals involved in pain inhibition, contributing to a natural analgesic effect.

Advanced Age

Effects of Advanced Age on the Body

Ageing is defined as the progressive physiological decline that typically begins after the age of 30. For a process to be considered part of ageing, it must meet four key criteria: it is universal, progressive, intrinsic, and deleterious. This decline affects all organ systems, leading to a reduced ability to maintain homeostasis when the body encounters stressors. Consequently, it can be difficult to distinguish between changes that are part of "normal" ageing and those resulting from pathology [93]. The physiological changes induce low cardiorespiratory fitness, low muscle performance, fatigue, and dyspnea in advanced age people.

With ageing, the lung parenchyma undergoes several structural changes, including loss of elastic recoil, alveolar dilatation, and reduced supporting tissue for peripheral airways [94]. Changes in the connective tissue increase chest stiffness and reduce the elastic component of the lungs, directly influencing respiratory mechanics. These alterations contribute to an increase in residual volume and declines in both forced vital capacity (FVC) and forced expiratory volume in 1 s (FEV1), resulting in reduced tidal volume. There is also an increase in physiological dead space, which promotes an increase in "ventilatory waste." The ventilatory inefficiency is related to poor cardiorespiratory fitness in the elderly [95].

Age itself is a strong independent risk factor for cardiovascular disease. Arterial walls thicken and stiffen over time, raising peripheral resistance and afterload. To adapt, the left ventricle undergoes hypertrophy but also becomes stiffer, reducing compliance and left ventricular reserve. It increases left atrial pressure and promotes atrial dilatation, contributing to the elevated risk of atrial fibrillation in older adults. Ageing is also associated with a higher incidence of valvular disease, particularly aortic stenosis. In addition, maximum heart rate, myocardial contractility, and adrenergic receptor sensitivity all decline with age. These structural and functional changes predispose older adults to heart failure [93].

Ageing is also associated with progressive skeletal muscle atrophy and loss of function, driven by both structural and metabolic alterations. Muscle mass declines at ~0.4–0.5% per year in midlife, accelerating after 75 years, and is markedly worsened during disuse. At the myocellular level, type II (fast-twitch) fibers undergo selective atrophy (10–40% smaller), while type I fibers are relatively preserved. This shift, compounded by reduced satellite cell content, impairs strength and limits performance in demanding tasks. Muscle quality also declines due to excitation–contraction coupling deficits. Structural remodeling, such as fat infiltration and fibrosis, and bioenergetic dysfunction with reduced mitochondrial content and ATP production further compromise performance. Collectively, these changes, exacerbated by anabolic resistance and impaired protein turnover, explain the progressive decline in muscle strength, endurance, and functional independence in older adults [96].

The Rationale for FES-Cycling Exercise in Advanced Age

Traditional exercise interventions are often limited by fatigue, pain, reduced mobility, or comorbidities that restrict voluntary participation. FES-cycling provides a unique rehabilitation strategy even in individuals with very low baseline performance [97]. This allows older adults to engage in exercise at intensities sufficient to induce beneficial neuromuscular, cardiovascular, and metabolic adaptations, while overcoming many of the barriers to conventional training.

From a cardiorespiratory perspective, FES-cycling enhances venous return, stroke volume, and cardiac output, thereby improving oxygen delivery to working tissues [6]. These adaptations help counteract the age-related reduction in maximal heart rate, myocardial contractility, and ventilatory efficiency. In addition, the rhythmic contraction of large muscle groups during cycling improves peripheral circulation and vascular endothelial function, reducing afterload and arterial stiffness (two hallmarks of cardiovascular ageing). Enhanced pulmonary ventilation and improved ventilation/perfusion matching may further mitigate ventilatory inefficiency, a critical contributor to exercise intolerance in advanced age.

At the musculoskeletal level, FES-cycling directly addresses sarcopenia and muscle weakness. By inducing repeated muscle contractions at controlled intensities, FES recruits both type I and type II fibers, including those prone to selective atrophy with ageing. This recruitment pattern promotes increases in torque, power, and muscle mass [6], while stimulating protein synthesis and mitochondrial biogenesis. Furthermore, electrical stimulation helps reduce intramuscular fat infiltration and fibrosis, thereby improving muscle quality [98]. These adaptations collectively translate into improved strength, endurance, and functional performance, enabling older adults to better perform activities of daily living and reducing the risk of falls and dependence.

Another key rationale is the metabolic and systemic impact of FES-cycling. Regular sessions might improve insulin sensitivity, glucose uptake [57], and lipid metabolism, thereby addressing common metabolic comorbidities in ageing such as type 2 diabetes and dyslipidemia. Additionally, the improved peripheral circulation and enhanced oxidative metabolism contribute to fatigue resistance, lowering the perception of effort and promoting adherence to long-term exercise programs. These systemic effects highlight FES-cycling as not only a rehabilitative tool but also a preventive intervention against chronic disease progression in the elderly.

Additionally, FES-cycling has a positive impact on symptoms such as fatigue [99] and pain [100], which often limit rehabilitation adherence in older populations. By improving muscle perfusion, stimulating afferent pathways that modulate nociception, and enhancing functional capacity, FES-cycling can reduce musculoskeletal discomfort and improve exercise tolerance. Importantly, the ability to perform guided, home-based, or supervised sessions makes FES-cycling accessible for individuals with mobility impairments, ensuring continuity of training and reducing sedentary behavior. Together, these attributes position FES-cycling as a powerful intervention to counteract the multisystem declines of ageing and support healthy longevity.

Conclusions

FES-cycling represents a clinically relevant and versatile rehabilitation tool that extends well beyond its neurological origins. In non-neurological diseases, it counteracts muscle wasting, enhances cardiovascular and pulmonary performance, improves metabolic control, and facilitates functional independence. The rationale provided in this chapter underscores its feasibility and therapeutic applicability across a wide range of conditions, including hospitalization-induced weakness, COPD, heart failure, metabolic disease, chronic kidney disease, orthopedic disorders, long COVID, and ageing.

Importantly, FES-cycling addresses the dual challenges of limited mobility and exercise intolerance, enabling patients with profound impairments to engage in effective training. Its integrative effects on muscular, cardiovascular, and metabolic systems make it a powerful intervention for promoting recovery, reducing complications, and improving quality of life. Future research should focus on optimizing stimulation protocols, long-term outcomes, and implementation strategies across healthcare settings.

References

1. Vanhorebeek I, Latronico N, Van den Berghe G. ICU-acquired weakness. Intensive Care Med. 2020;46(4):637–53.
2. Coker RH, Wolfe RR. Bed rest and sarcopenia. Curr Opin Clin Nutr Metab Care. 2012;15:7–11.
3. García-Pérez-de-Sevilla G, Sánchez-Pinto Pinto B. Effectiveness of physical exercise and neuromuscular electrical stimulation interventions for preventing and treating intensive care unit-acquired weakness: a systematic review of randomized controlled trials. Intensive Crit Care Nurs. 2023;74:103333.
4. Frazão MCJG, Silva PE. Does inflammation and altered metabolism impede efficacy of functional electrical stimulation in critically ill patients? Unleashing the potential of individualized functional electrical stimulation-cycling in critical illness. Crit Care. 2024;28(1):8.
5. Figueiredo TG, Frazão M, Werlang LA, Kunz A, Peltz M, Furtado VC, Júnior EB, únior JM, Silva RM, Sobral Filho DC. Safety and feasibility of a functional electrical stimulation cycling-based muscular dysfunction diagnostic method in mechanically ventilated patients. Artif Organs. 2024;48(7):713–22.
6. Frazão M, Figueiredo T, Cipriano JG. Should we use the functional electrical stimulation-cycling exercise in clinical practice? Physiological and clinical effects systematic review with meta-analysis. Arch Phys Med Rehabil. 2024;22:S0003-9993(24)01057-8.
7. Murach KA, Dungan CM, Peterson CA, McCarthy JJ. Muscle fiber splitting is a physiological response to extreme loading in animals. Exerc Sport Sci Rev. 2019;47(2):108–15.
8. Sadamoto T, Bonde-Petersen F, Suzuki Y. Skeletal muscle tension, flow, pressure, and EMG during sustained isometric contractions in humans. Eur J Appl Physiol Occup Physiol. 1983;51(3):395–408.
9. Pearson SJ, Hussain SR. A review on the mechanisms of blood-flow restriction resistance training-induced muscle hypertrophy. Sports Med. 2015;45(2):187–200.
10. Stokes K. Growth hormone responses to sub-maximal and sprint exercise. Growth Hormon IGF Res. 2003;13(5):225–38.
11. Waldauf P, Hrušková N, Blahutova B, Gojda J, Urban T, Krajčová A, Fric M, Jiroutková K, Řasová K, Duška F. Functional electrical stimulation-assisted cycle ergometry-based progressive mobility programme for mechanically ventilated patients: randomised controlled trial with 6 months follow-up. Thorax. 2021;76:664–71.
12. Berney S, Hopkins RO, Rose JW, Koopman R, Puthucheary Z, Pastva A, Gordon I, Colantuoni E, Parry SM, Needham DM, Denehy L. Functional electrical stimulation in-bed cycle ergometry in mechanically ventilated patients: a multicentre randomised controlled trial. Thorax. 2021;76:656–63.
13. Ferrante S, Pedrocchi A, Ferrigno G, Molteni F. Cycling induced by functional electrical stimulation improves the muscular strength and the motor control of individuals with post-acute stroke. Europa Medicophysica-SIMFER 2007 award winner. Eur J Phys Rehabil Med. 2008;44(2):159–67.
14. Nakanishi R, Takeuchi K, Akizuki K, Nakagoshi R, Kakihana H. The effect of neuromuscular electrical stimulation on muscle EMG activity and the initial phase rate of force development during tetanic contractions in the knee extensor muscles of healthy adult males. Phys Ther Res. 2020;23(2):195–201.
15. Kraemer WJ, Fleck SJ, Evans WJ. Strength and power training: physiological mechanisms of adaptation. Exerc Sport Sci Rev. 1996;24:363–97.
16. Frazão M, Martins FL, Cipriano G Jr. Recumbent FES-cycling exercise improves muscle performance and ambulation capacity in hospitalized patients: a randomized controlled trial. Artif Organs. 2025;49:1756.

17. Parry SM, Berney S, Warrillow S, El-Ansary D, Bryant AL, Hart N, Puthucheary Z, Koopman R, Denehy L. Functional electrical stimulation with cycling in the critically ill: a pilot case-matched control study. J Crit Care. 2014;29(4):695.e1–7.
18. Osawa Y, Chiles Shaffer N, Shardell MD, Studenski SA, Ferrucci L. Changes in knee extension peak torque and body composition and their relationship with change in gait speed. J Cachexia Sarcopenia Muscle. 2019;10(5):1000–8.
19. Jacob T, Higgins SKF, Lennie T, Rayens MK, Avila J. Early ambulation after injury is associated with increased muscle size and strength. Biol Res Nurs. 2020;22(4):527–35.
20. ECGE S, ACB S, Godoy CG, et al. Ambulation capacity, age, immunosuppression, and mechanical ventilation are risk factors of in-hospital death in severe COVID-19: a cohort study. Clinics. 2022;77:100075.
21. Lindberg A, Jonsson AC, Ronmark E, Lundger R, Larsson L-G, Lundba¨ck B. Prevalence of chronic obstructive pulmonary disease according to BTS, ERS, GOLD and ATS criteria in relation to doctor's diagnosis, symptoms, age, gender, and smoking habits. Respiration. 2005;72(5):471–9.
22. Celli BR, W MN. Standards for the diagnosis and treatment of patients with COPD: a summary of the ATS/ERS position paper. Eur Respir J. 2004;23(6):932–46.
23. Frazão M, Santos A, Araújo AA, et al. Neuromuscular efficiency is impaired during exercise in COPD patients. Respir Physiol Neurobiol. 2021;290:103673.
24. Frazão M, Silva P, Frazão W, et al. Dynamic hyperinflation impairs cardiac performance during exercise in COPD. J Cardiopulm Rehabil Prev. 2019;39(3):187–92.
25. Jörgensen K, et al. Reduced intrathoracic blood volume and left and right ventricular dimensions in patients with severe emphysema: an MRI study. Chest. 2007;131:1050–7.
26. Jörgensen K, et al. Left ventricular performance and dimensions in patients with severe emphysema. Anesth Analg. 2007;104:887–92.
27. Barr RG, et al. Percent emphysema, airflow obstruction and impaired left ventricular filling. N Engl J Med. 2010;362:217–27.
28. Eliason G. Alterations in the muscle-to-capillary interface in patients with different degrees of chronic obstructive pulmonary disease. Respir Res. 2010;11:97.
29. Gosker HR, et al. Reduced mitochondrial density in the vastus lateralis muscle of patients with COPD. Eur Respir J. 2007;30:73–9.
30. Medrinal C, Prieur G, Combret Y, Quesada AR, Debeaumont D, Bonnevie T, Gravier FE, Dupuis Lozeron E, Quieffin J, Contal O e. Functional electrical stimulation-a new therapeutic approach to enhance exercise intensity in chronic obstructive pulmonary disease patients: a randomized, controlled crossover trial. Arch Phys Med Rehabil. 2018;99(8):454–1461.
31. Prieur G, Combret Y, Bonnevie T, Gravier FE, Robledo Quesada A, Quieffin J, Lamia B, Medrinal C. Functional electrical stimulation changes muscle oxygenation in patients with chronic obstructive pulmonary disease during moderate-intensity exercise: a secondary analysis. COPD. 2019;16(1):30–6.
32. Osterling K, K MF, Gilbert R, Dechman G. The effects of high intensity exercise during pulmonary rehabilitation on ventilatory parameters in people with moderate to severe stable COPD: a systematic review. Int J Chron Obstruct Pulmon Dis. 2014;1(9):1069–78.
33. Frazão M, Frazão W. Pulmonary rehabilitation alters Ventilatory and cardiac performances profile during exercise in moderate to severe Copd: 5 cases report. Pulm Respir Med. 2016;6:320.
34. Montes de Oca M, Rassulo J, Celli BR. Respiratory muscle and cardiopulmonary function during exercise in very severe COPD. Am J Respir Crit Care Med. 1996;154(5):1284–9.
35. Sepúlveda-Loyola W, Osadnik C, Phu S, Morita AA, Duque G, Probst VS. Diagnosis, prevalence, and clinical impact of sarcopenia in COPD: a systematic review and meta-analysis. J Cachexia Sarcopenia Muscle. 2020;11(5):1164–76.
36. Kemp CD, Conte J. The pathophysiology of heart failure. Cardiovasc Pathol. 2012;21(5):365–71.

37. Cohn JN, Ferrari R, Sharpe N. Cardiac remodeling: concepts and clinical implications: a consensus paper from an international forum on cardiac remodeling. Am Coll Cardiol. 2000;35:569–82.
38. Puri S, Baker B, Dutka DP, Oakley CM, Hughes JM, Cleland JG. Reduced alveolar-capillary membrane diffusing capacity in chronic heart failure. Its pathophysiological relevance and relationship to exercise performance. Circulation. 1995;91(11):2769–74.
39. Olson TP, Beck K, Johnson JB, Johnson BD. Competition for intrathoracic space reduces lung capacity in patients with chronic heart failure: a radiographic study. Chest. 2006;130(1):164–71.
40. Olson TP, Johnson B. Influence of cardiomegaly on disordered breathing during exercise in chronic heart failure. Eur J Heart Fail. 2011;13(3):311–8.
41. Wilson JR, Martin J, Schwartz D, Ferraro N. Exercise intolerance in patients with chronic heart failure: role of impaired nutritive flow to skeletal muscle. Circulation. 1984;69:1079–87.
42. Sullivan MJ, Green HJ, Cobb FR. Skeletal muscle biochemistry and histology in ambulatory patients with long-term heart failure. Circulation. 1990;81(2):518–27.
43. Sullivan MJ, Green H, Cobb FR. Altered skeletal muscle metabolic response to exercise in chronic heart failure. Relation to skeletal muscle aerobic enzyme activity. Circulation. 1991;84(4):1597–607.
44. Buonocore M, Opasich C, Casale R. Early development of EMG localized muscle fatigue in hand muscles of patients with chronic heart failure. Arch Phys Med Rehabil. 1998;79(1):41–5.
45. Miller MS, P VB, LeWinter MM, Braddock JM, Ades PA, Maughan DW, Palmer BM, Toth MJ. Chronic heart failure decreases cross-bridge kinetics in single skeletal muscle fibres from humans. J Physiol. 2010;588(Pt 20):4039–53.
46. Fornusek C, Davis G. Cardiovascular and metabolic responses during functional electric stimulation cycling at different cadences. Arch Phys Med Rehabil. 2008;89(4):719–25.
47. Hambrecht R, Gielen S, Linke A, Fiehn E, Yu J, Walther C, Schoene N, Schuler G. Effects of exercise training on left ventricular function and peripheral resistance in patients with chronic heart failure: a randomized trial. JAMA. 2000;283(23):3095–101.
48. Giannuzzi P, Temporelli P, Corrà U, Tavazzi L, ELVD-CHF Study Group. Antiremodeling effect of long-term exercise training in patients with stable chronic heart failure: results of the exercise in left ventricular dysfunction and chronic heart failure (ELVD-CHF) trial. Circulation. 2003;108(5):554–9.
49. Gorgey AS, Lawrence J. Acute responses of functional electrical stimulation cycling on the ventilation-to-CO2 production ratio and substrate utilization after spinal cord injury. PM R. 2016;8(3):225–34.
50. Guazzi M, Reina G, Tumminello G, Guazzi MD. Improvement of alveolar-capillary membrane diffusing capacity with exercise training in chronic heart failure. J Appl Physiol (1985). 2004;97(5):1866–73.
51. Gojda J, Waldauf P, Hrušková N, Blahutová B, Krajčová A, Urban T, Tůma PŘKD. Lactate production without hypoxia in skeletal muscle during electrical cycling: crossover study of femoral venous-arterial differences in healthy volunteers. PLoS One. 2019;14(3):e0200228.
52. Frazão M, Werlang L, Azevedo C, Kunz A, Peltz M. Metabolic, ventilatory and cardiovascular responses to FES-cycling: a comparison to NMES and passive cycling. Technol Health Care. 2022;30(4):909–18.
53. Bellou V, Belbasis L, Tzoulaki I, Evangelou E. Risk factors for type 2 diabetes mellitus: an exposure-wide umbrella review of meta-analyses. PLoS One. 2018;13:e0194127.
54. Sinha R, Dufour S, Petersen KF, LeBon V, Enoksson S, Ma YZ, Savoye M, Rothman DL, Shulman GI, Caprio S. Assessment of skeletal muscle triglyceride content by (1)H nuclear magnetic resonance spectroscopy in lean and obese adolescents: relationships to insulin sensitivity, total body fat, and central adiposity. Diabetes. 2002;51:1022–7.

55. Galicia-Garcia U, Benito-Vicente A, Jebari S, Larrea-Sebal A, Siddiqi H, Uribe KB, Ostolaza H, Martín C. Pathophysiology of type 2 diabetes mellitus. Int J Mol Sci. 2020;21(17):6275.
56. Dolbow DR, Credeur D, Lemacks JL, Stokic DS, Pattanaik S, Corbin GN, Courtner AS. Electrically induced cycling and nutritional counseling for counteracting obesity after spinal cord injury: a pilot study. J Spinal Cord Med. 2021;44(4):533–40.
57. Frazão M, de Lima DT, Nogueira AP, TDS LG, Pinto Dias AL, MVD d SL, IA MF. Effects of functional electrical stimulation-cycling on muscle thickness and blood glucose level in neuromuscular disease mechanically ventilated patient: case report. Clin Case Rep Int. 2024;8:1–3.
58. Richter EA, Hargreaves M. Exercise, GLUT4, and skeletal muscle glucose uptake. Physiol Rev. 2013;93(3):993–1017.
59. Birnbaum MJ. Identification of a novel gene encoding an insulin-responsive glucosetransporter protein. Cell. 1989;57:305–15.
60. Flores-Opazo M, Hargreaves M, Hargreaves M. Exercise and GLUT4. Exerc Sport Sci Rev. 2020;48(3):110–8.
61. Sabatino A, Cuppari L, Stenvinkel P, Lindholm B, Avesani CM. Sarcopenia in chronic kidney disease: what have we learned so far? J Nephrol. 2021;34(4):1347–72.
62. Workeneh BT, Mitch W. Review of muscle wasting associated with chronic kidney disease. Am J Clin Nutr. 2010;91(4):1128s–32s.
63. Molina P, Carrero J, Bover J, Chauveau P, Mazzaferro S, Torres P. Vitamin D, a modulator of musculoskeletal health in chronic kidney disease. J Cachexia Sarcopenia Muscle. 2017;8(5):686–701.
64. Stenvinkel P, Carrero J, von Walden F, Ikizler T, Nader G. Muscle wasting in end-stage renal disease promulgates premature death: established emerging and potential novel treatment strategies. Nephrol Dial Transplant. 2016;31(7):1070–7.
65. Sabatino A, Regolisti G, Brusasco I, Cabassi A, Morabito S, Fiaccadori E. Alterations of intestinal barrier and microbiota in chronic kidney disease. Nephrol Dial Transplant. 2015;30(6):924–33.
66. Fahal I, Bell G, Bone J, Edwards R. Physiological abnormalities of skeletal muscle in dialysis patients. Nephrol Dial Transplant. 1997;12(1):119–27.
67. Howden EJ, Weston K, Leano R, Sharman JE, Marwick TH, Isbel NM, Coombes JS. Cardiorespiratory fitness and cardiovascular burden in chronic kidney disease. J Sci Med Sport. 2015;18(4):492–7.
68. Sui X, Kokkinos P, Faselis C, Samuel IBH, Pittaras A, Gollie J, Patel S, Lavie CJ, Zhang J, Myers J. Cardiorespiratory fitness and mortality in patients with chronic kidney disease: a prospective cohort study. Mayo Clin Proc. 2025;100(6):962–9.
69. Matsuzawa R, Matsunaga A, Wang G, Kutsuna T, Ishii A, Abe Y, et al. Habitual physical activity measured by accelerometer and survival in maintenance hemodialysis patients. Clin J Am Soc Nephrol. 2012;7:2010–6.
70. Beddhu S, Baird B, Zitterkoph J, Neilson J, Greene T. Physical activity and mortality in chronic kidney disease (NHANES III). Clin J Am Soc Nephrol. 2009;4:1901–6.
71. Gollie JM, Cohen S, Patel SS. Physical activity and exercise for cardiorespiratory health and fitness in chronic kidney disease. Rev Cardiovasc Med. 2022;23(8):273.
72. Andrade JLF, Heitmann A, Rodrigues MK, Marchand DK, Rodrigues AM, Biluca BP, Freitas R, Reis T, Goes MA, Oliveira MF. Exercise as an adjunctive therapy for patients on maintenance hemodiafiltration. Kidney Res Clin Pract. 2025. https://doi.org/10.23876/j.krcp.24.243.
73. Roxo RS, Xavier V, Miorin LA, Magalhães AO, Sens YA, Alves VL. Impact of neuromuscular electrical stimulation on functional capacity of patients with chronic kidney disease on hemodialysis. J Bras Nefrol. 2016;38(3):344–50.
74. Fotuhi MMA, Meysami S, Raji CA. Neurobiology of COVID-19. J Alzheimer's Dis. 2020;76(1):3–19.

75. Pinzon RTWV, Buana RB. Neurologic characteristics in coronavirus disease 2019 (COVID-19): a systematic review and meta-analysis. Front Neurol. 2020;11:1–11.
76. Frazão MSA, Silva PE, et al. Impaired neuromuscular efficiency and symptom-limited aerobic exercise capacity 4 weeks after recovery from COVID-19 appear to be associated with disease severity at onset. Phys Ther. 2023;103(2):pzac167.
77. David Debeaumont FB, Ferrand-Devouge E, et al. Cardiopulmonary exercise testing to assess persistent symptoms at 6 months in people with COVID-19 who survived hospitalization: a pilot study. Phys Ther. 2021;101(6):pzab099.
78. BV MS, Cheminon M, et al. Functional electrical stimulation-cycling favours erectus position restoration and walking in patients with critical COVID-19. A proof-of-concept controlled study. Ann Phys Rehabil Med. 2021;64:101516.
79. Nugent-Derfus GE, Takara T, O'neill JK, Cahill SB, Görtz S, Pong T, Inoue H, Aneloski NM, Wang WW, Vega KI, Klein TJ, Hsieh-Bonassera ND, Bae WC, Burke JD, Bugbee WD, Sah RL. Continuous passive motion applied to whole joints stimulates chondrocyte biosynthesis of PRG4. Osteoarthr Cartil. 2007;15(5):566–74.
80. Johnson DP. The effect of continuous passive motion on wound-healing and joint mobility after knee arthroplasty. J Bone Joint Surg Am. 1990;72(3):421–6.
81. Hong CM, Lee J, Yee Esther CW. Effectiveness of continuous passive motion in total knee replacement patients with slow rehabilitation under ERAS pathway. J Orthop Trauma Rehabil. 2023;30(1). https://doi.org/10.1177/22104917221150532.
82. Chen SC, Lai C, Chan WP, Huang MH, Tsai HW, Chen JJ. Increases in bone mineral density after functional electrical stimulation cycling exercises in spinal cord injured patients. Disabil Rehabil. 2005;27(22):1337–41.
83. Lauer RT, Smith B, Mulcahey MJ, Betz RR, Johnston TE. Effects of cycling and/or electrical stimulation on bone mineral density in children with spinal cord injury. Spinal Cord. 2011;49(8):917–23.
84. Mohr T, Podenphant J, Biering–Sørensen F, Galbo H, Thamsborg G, Kjaer M. Increased bone mineral density after prolonged electrically induced cycle training of paralyzed limbs in spinal cord injured man. Calcif Tissue Int. 1997;61(1):22–5.
85. Kakebeeke TH, Hofer P, Frotzler A, Lechner HE, Hunt KJ, Perret C. Training and detraining of a tetraplegic subject: high-volume FES cycle training. Am J Phys Med Rehabil. 2008;87(1):56–64.
86. Frotzler A, Coupaud S, Perret C, Kakebeeke TH, Hunt KJ, Donaldson ND, Eser P. High-volume FES-cycling partially reverses bone loss in people with chronic spinal cord injury. Bone. 2008;43(1):169–76.
87. Lai CH, Chang WH, Chan WP, Peng CW, Shen LK, Chen JJ, Chen SC. Effects of functional electrical stimulation cycling exercise on bone mineral density loss in the early stages of spinal cord injury. J Rehabil Med. 2010;42(2):150–4.
88. Eser PDBE, Telley I, Lechner HE, Knecht H, Stüssi E. Effect of electrical stimulation-induced cycling on bone mineral density in spinal cord-injured pa-tients. Eur J Clin Investig. 2003;33(5):412–9.
89. Kern HBL, Löfler S, Sbardella S, Burggraf S, Fruhmann H, Carraro U, Mosole S, Sarabon N, Vogelauer M, Mayr W, Krenn M, Cvecka J, Romanello V, Pietrangelo L, Protasi F, Sandri M, Zampieri S, Musaro A. Electrical stimulation counteracts muscle decline in seniors. Front Aging Neurosci. 2014;24(6):189.
90. Sadamoto TB-PF, Suzuki Y. Skeletal muscle tension, flow, pressure, and EMG during sustained isometric contractions in humans. Eur J Appl Physiol Occup Physiol. 1983;51(3):395–408.
91. Ferrante SPA, Ferrigno G, Molteni F. Cycling induced by functional electrical stimulation improves the muscular strength and the motor control of individuals with post-acute stroke. Europa Medicophysica-SIMFER 2007 award winner. Eur J Phys Rehabil Med. 2007;44(2):159–67.

92. Calvo-Rubio MG-DE, Tamayo-Torres E, Soto-Rodríguez S, Olaso-Gonzalez G, Ferrucci L, de Cabo R, Gómez-Cabrera MC. The repeated bout effect evokes the training-induced skeletal muscle cellular memory. Free Radic Biol Med. 2024;225:247–54.
93. Preston JBB. The physiology of ageing and how these changes affect older people. Medicine. 2021;49(1):1–5.
94. Sicard DHA, Choi KM, Craig AR, Fredenburgh LE, Tschumperlin DJ. Aging and anatomical variations in lung tissue stiffness. Am J Physiol Lung Cell Mol Physiol. 2018;314(6):964–55.
95. Frazão MFL, Bezerra SCM, Silva PE. Relationship of ventilatory inefficiency and low cardiorespiratory fitness in the elderly: a retrospective observational study. Rev Bras Geriatr Gerontol. 2019;22(4):e190025.
96. Tieland MTI, Clark BC. Skeletal muscle performance and ageing. J Cachexia Sarcopenia Muscle. 2018;9(1):3–19.
97. Baldi JCJR, Moraille R, Mysiw WJ. Muscle atrophy is prevented in patients with acute spinal cord injury using functional electrical stimulation. Spinal Cord. 1998;36(7):463–9.
98. Gorgey AS, Venigalla S, Deitrich JN, Ballance WB, Carter W, Lavis T, Adler RA. Electrical stimulation paradigms on muscle quality and bone mineral density after spinal cord injury. Osteoporos Int. 2025;36(6):1039–51.
99. Backus DMM, Sweatman WM. Effects of functional electrical stimulation cycling on fatigue and quality of life in people with multiple sclerosis who are nonambulatory. Int J MS Care. 2020;22(4):193–200.
100. Calabrò RSPS, Tomasello P, Porcari B, Balletta T, Naro A. Paving the way for a better management of pain in patients with spinal cord injury: an exploratory study on the use of functional electric stimulation (FES)-cycling. J Spinal Cord Med. 2023;46(1):107–17.

FES-Cycling for Competition and Leisure

8

Efe Anil Aksöz and Kenneth J. Hunt

Introduction

Functional Electrical Stimulation (FES) cycling is an innovative technology that enables individuals with spinal cord injuries (SCI) to engage in physical activity by electrically stimulating paralyzed muscles to produce coordinated leg movements. This approach allows individuals with motor impairments to participate in both recreational and competitive cycling, promoting mobility, autonomy, and social inclusion [1]. Initially developed in the early 1980s, FES cycling has since evolved into a widely used modality in rehabilitation and assistive sports, offering a practical means to counteract the physiological decline associated with paralysis [2, 3].

FES cycling has been associated with a range of health benefits, including improved cardiovascular function [4, 5], increased muscle mass [6], enhanced blood circulation [7], and better metabolic regulation [8]. Regular use can help prevent muscle atrophy [9, 10], reduce the incidence of pressure ulcers and osteoporosis [11, 12], and support psychological well-being through increased participation and perceived independence [13]. Despite its promise, the technology still faces challenges related to muscle fatigue, variability in stimulation effectiveness [14, 15], and high costs of equipment and training, which can limit broader accessibility [1].

Most FES cycling systems use surface electrodes to deliver stimulation to key leg muscles involved in the pedalling motion. These include the quadriceps, hamstrings, gluteus, and some cases tibialis anterior, gastrocnemius, and peroneal nerve regions. Stimulation is typically timed to correspond with the crank cycle, often using continuous or asynchronous modes to optimize force output and avoid joint

E. A. Aksöz (✉) · K. J. Hunt
rehaLab—The Laboratory for Rehabilitation Engineering, Division of Mechatronics and Systems Engineering, School of Engineering and Computer Science, HuCE—Institute for Human Centred Engineering, Bern University of Applied Sciences, Biel, Switzerland
e-mail: efeanil.aksoez@bfh.ch; kenneth.hunt@bfh.ch

M. Frazão (ed.), *Functional Electrical Stimulation Cycling in Clinical Practice*,
https://doi.org/10.1007/978-3-032-23937-2_8

compression. Synchronous stimulation patterns are less common due to their potential to cause mechanical strain or inefficiency.

In recent years, FES cycling has extended beyond clinical and training settings into organized sports and leisure domains. Mobile FES tricycles have been developed to enable outdoor use and participation in community activities. These are often adapted from commercial cycles or custom-built to meet individual needs, sometimes incorporating auxiliary electric motors to compensate for the limited power output generated by muscle stimulation alone [16–18]. The proportion of power contributed by the user and the assisting actuator can be adjusted or pre-set, depending on the system design and user capability.

Despite the physiological challenges faced by individuals with SCI, such as rapid muscle atrophy and reduced aerobic capacity, many users of FES-cycling systems have shown measurable improvements in strength and cardiovascular performance. The growing popularity of FES cycling in national and international competitions highlights its role not only in rehabilitation, but also in fostering active, inclusive lifestyles through assistive technology. One major international event that showcases FES cycling at a competitive level is the Cybathlon,[1] an elite competition where athletes with physical disabilities compete using cutting-edge assistive technologies, including FES bikes. This event not only promotes innovation but also raises public awareness and inspires collaboration between engineers, clinicians, and users.

The aim of this book chapter is to explore how FES cycling has evolved from a rehabilitative intervention into a multifaceted platform for physical fitness, recreational activity, and elite competition. This chapter will provide an overview of the physiological principles, technological developments, and practical applications of FES cycling, with a particular focus on its use in structured training programs and competitive settings. Emphasis will be placed on evidence-based strategies for optimizing performance, the role of user-centered design in equipment development, and the impact of international events such as the Cybathlon in advancing the field. Through this lens, the chapter aims to inform clinicians, researchers, athletes, and technology developers about the current state and future directions of FES cycling as both a therapeutic tool and a vehicle for inclusion, empowerment, and excellence.

Training Routine

Development of a Training Routine with FES-Cycling

A well-structured training regimen is fundamental for optimizing performance, physical conditioning, and neuromuscular adaptation in Functional Electrical Stimulation (FES)-cycling. Training should be individualized based on the participant's baseline physical condition, neurological impairment level, and physiological response to electrical stimulation.

[1] www.cybathlon.com

An effective FES-cycling program should be focused on enhancing both strength and endurance through structured FES cycling exercises. A recent study with eight SCI participants completed a six-week training program [19]. The sessions took place three times per week and involved a structured exercise routine that lasted 45 minutes per session. Each session included a three-minute warm-up, followed by four intervals of 4 min at 85–90% of peak power output, alternating with 4 min of active recovery at 50% effort. The study found notable improvements in muscle strength and volume. Quadriceps peak torque increased by up to 25.6%, hamstring peak torque by up to 23.3%, and leg volume showed gains of up to 18.2%. These findings suggest that HIIT-FES cycling is a promising and safe approach to enhancing lower limb muscle function in individuals with incomplete SCI.

To optimize neuromuscular engagement, FES-cycling programs should integrate progressive overload principles. The training approach used by PULSE Racing for the Cybathlon Global Edition followed a structured progression, beginning with a base training phase, followed by a specific training phase, and ending with a tapering phase [20]. Progressive overload was applied by adjusting stimulation parameters (amplitude, pulse-width and stimulation frequency), resistance levels, and ride time. High-intensity training weeks (12 h of training, increased stimulation frequency, added resistance) were alternated with recovery weeks (6 h of training, reduced stimulation frequency, passive stretching [20]). Different modes of exercise were incorporated to maximize neuromuscular efficiency, including FES cycling, arm cranking, hybrid cycling, and separate electrical stimulation of specific muscle groups. Each method targeted different physiological adaptations while minimizing monotony for the athlete.

The team from Cleveland used implanted pulse generators (IPGs), offering more selective muscle activation compared to traditional surface stimulation. Their approach led to significant improvements in strength, endurance, and cycling power, allowing their pilot to win gold at the Cybathlon [21]. The training program was designed to address initial challenges, as pilots initially fatigued quickly, generating only 30 W of power for 15–20 s before dropping to 10–15 W. Adjustments were made to improve both endurance and power output. The program incorporated strength and endurance protocols, where strength training involved 60 s of electrical stimulation followed by 30 s of rest for up to an hour, while endurance training consisted of four 10-min cycling bouts with 5-min rest intervals. Pilots trained three to four times per week on a stationary trainer, using real trikes instead of stationary FES bikes to ensure independent power generation without motor assistance. To enhance race-specific performance, pilots trained on a regulation-size ramp to practice race starts and gear shifts, developed breathing strategies to compensate for delayed ventilatory responses, and refined gear-shifting techniques to maintain efficiency as they fatigued. This structured approach significantly improved their performance, ultimately leading to their success in the Cybathlon.

Training Frequency

The optimal training frequency for FES-cycling depends on the individual's fitness level, neurological condition, and rehabilitation or performance goals. Research suggests that three to five weekly sessions (each lasting half an hour to 1 h) yield significant muscular and cardiovascular adaptations [22].

For cardiovascular and muscular benefits, four to five sessions per week are recommended. For rehabilitation or maintenance, two to three sessions per week are sufficient to sustain muscle integrity and cardiovascular fitness [23]. A balance between high-intensity interval sessions (shorter, with higher resistance) and moderate-intensity continuous sessions (longer duration, lower resistance) optimizes both strength and endurance adaptations can prove effective in increasing lean muscle mass and improving systemic vascular endothelial health in individuals with chronic SCI [24].

To prevent fatigue-related complications, rest periods between sessions should be individualized. Studies indicate that it could be beneficial to imposing rest breaks at least double of active cycling time could be effective in reducing neuromuscular fatigue while maintaining training consistency [25].

Based on the experience of PULSE Racing, an effective training frequency consisted of five FES cycling sessions per week, each lasting at least 90 min [20]. Training frequency was structured according to the following principles:

- Cardiovascular and muscular improvements: four to five FES cycling sessions per week
- Maintenance or rehabilitation: two to three sessions per week
- Intensity variation: Alternation between high-intensity sessions (shorter, with higher resistance) and moderate-intensity continuous sessions (longer duration, lower resistance)

Training Phases

FES-cycling training typically follows structured *periodization phases*, which allow for systematic neuromuscular adaptation:

1. *Preparation Phase (Base Training)*
   - *Goal*: Develop endurance and muscle adaptation
   - *Duration*: ~8 months
   - *Intensity*: Low-to-moderate electrical stimulation
   - *Progression*: Gradual increase in session duration (starting at 20–30 min per session)
   - *Training Focus*: Establishing personalized stimulation parameters, improving aerobic capacity, and optimizing resistance settings
2. *Performance Phase (Specific Training)*
   - *Goal*: Enhance neuromuscular efficiency and power output

- *Duration*: ~10 weeks
- *Intensity*: Progressive increases in resistance and stimulation amplitude (e.g., frequency increase from 20 to 50 Hz)
- *Monitoring*: Weekly performance tests a smart trainer
- *Training Strategies:*
  - High-intensity interval training to maximize power generation
  - Endurance-focused sessions to improve capillarization and muscle fascicle length

3. *Recovery Phase (Tapering)*
   - *Goal*: Allow for neuromuscular recovery and optimize race-day readiness
   - *Duration*: ~2–3 weeks
   - *Intensity*: Reduced training volume (40–60% of peak) with light resistance and passive stretching
   - *Training Adjustments*: Focus on testing and fine-tuning bike setup, adjusting starting speeds, and optimizing cadence

Training Components

Effective FES-cycling training incorporates multiple components targeting different physiological adaptations. Resistance training enhances muscle endurance through sustained electrical stimulation, preventing atrophy and improving fatigue resistance. Muscular strength training involves higher-intensity bursts, aimed at maximizing force output and improving power generation capacity. Cardiovascular conditioning is developed through sustained cycling sessions, improving heart and lung function while enhancing overall metabolic efficiency. The integration of these components ensures a comprehensive approach to training, promoting balanced development and functional improvements.

FES-cycling training consists of multiple physiological components to maximize adaptation:

1. Resistance Training:
   - Goal: Prevent muscle atrophy and improve fatigue resistance
   - Strategy: Sustained electrical stimulation with increasing resistance (5–10% increments)
2. Muscular Strength Training:
   - Goal: Enhance force output
   - Strategy: Short bursts of high-intensity stimulation (above 60 Hz)
3. Cardiovascular Conditioning:
   - Goal: Improve heart and lung function
   - Strategy: Sustained cycling at 50–70% VO_2 max, monitored via heart rate sensors [23]

Progress Monitoring

Tracking progress in FES-cycling is crucial to adjusting training plans and optimizing results. Key metrics such as power output, heart rate, and muscle endurance (fatigue index) should be regularly monitored to evaluate performance and ensure appropriate stimulation levels [26]. Data collection through sensors and performance tracking software enables real-time analysis, allowing for adjustments in intensity, frequency, and duration [27]. Modifying stimulation parameters based on physiological feedback can prevent muscle overstimulation, mitigate fatigue, and enhance the overall effectiveness of the training regimen. Performance metrics include:

- Power output (W): Measured via cycling ergometers
- Heart rate (BPM): Maintained at 50–85% of maximum heart rate for endurance benefits
- Muscle endurance (time to fatigue): Extended over time to measure improvement [22]

Parameter Sets/Technology Specificities for Competition

Parameter Settings for FES-Cycling Competitions

The effectiveness of FES-cycling in competitive settings depends on precise adjustment of key parameters, including intensity, frequency, and pulse width. These parameters must be optimized based on the athlete's physiological response, muscle composition, and endurance capacity. Customization is essential to ensure that muscle contractions are strong and sustained without leading to premature fatigue. Adjustments in stimulation settings should align with the athlete's goals, whether focused on power output, endurance, or sprint performance.

Competitive FES-cycling requires precise stimulation parameter settings to optimize muscle recruitment while minimizing fatigue.

- Frequency: 30–50 Hz (higher frequencies increase power but cause fatigue)
- Pulse width: 200–500 μs (adjusted based on muscle response)
- Intensity: 0–120 mA (adjusted based on fatigue resistance and performance goals)

Some FES stimulators provide higher parameter ranges. For example, the P24 Science from Hasomed, Germany, delivers a maximum voltage output of 150 V, a current amplitude of up to 130 mA, and pulse widths ranging from 10 to 65,520 μs. This extended range allows for more precise customization of stimulation parameters, which can be beneficial for optimizing muscle contraction efficiency and endurance in FES cycling applications.

Advanced stimulation strategies have emerged to overcome key limitations of conventional surface stimulation, such as rapid fatigue and limited power output. One particularly promising method is Spatially Distributed Sequential Stimulation (SDSS), which involves replacing large single electrodes with multiple smaller electrodes placed over the same or synergistic muscles. These smaller electrodes deliver stimulation with staggered timing, reducing the frequency per electrode while maintaining the total effective frequency. SDSS has been shown to significantly enhance both power output and fatigue resistance in individuals with spinal cord injury (SCI). For example, in a dynamic knee extension study simulating recumbent cycling, SDSS produced up to 132% greater mean power output compared to single-electrode stimulation and improved fatigue indices in most participants [28]. By activating motor units in a more dispersed and temporally shifted fashion, SDSS minimizes metabolic stress and delays muscle fatigue, both crucial for competition-level performance.

In addition to SDSS, stochastic modulation of the inter-pulse interval (IPI) is another effective strategy. Rather than using a constant frequency, pulse intervals are varied randomly within a physiological range. This approach mimics natural motor unit firing patterns and has been shown to increase short-term power output during repetitive knee extensions, although its impact on fatigue remains inconsistent [29].

These stimulation strategies (SDSS, IPI modulation) demonstrate the potential of optimizing not only stimulation parameters but also *how* the stimulation is delivered. Future developments in FES-cycling equipment can also incorporate programmable multi-electrode arrays and adaptive stimulation algorithms to enable real-time strategy adjustment based on athlete feedback and performance data.

Technological Specificities

Advanced technology plays a crucial role in FES-cycling competitions by providing real-time performance monitoring and feedback. State-of-the-art stimulation units integrate sensors that track power output, cadence, and heart rate, allowing athletes and coaches to make dynamic adjustments. Live feedback systems enable fine-tuning of stimulation parameters during competition, ensuring optimal muscle activation and coordination. This technological integration enhances performance consistency and minimizes inefficiencies in muscle recruitment.

Advanced stimulation units in competitive FES-cycling incorporate real-time performance monitoring and biofeedback. Features include:

- Virtual reality racing feedback [30]
- EMG feedback to optimize stimulation parameters [31]
- AI-driven adjustments for individualized stimulation settings [32]

Differences Between Competition and Recreational FES-Cycling

FES-cycling for competition requires high-intensity stimulation with precise control over pulse parameters to maximize performance. In contrast, recreational FES-cycling prioritizes moderate intensity, allowing for greater flexibility in parameter settings to accommodate comfort and long-term engagement. Competitive FES-cycling demands rigorous monitoring and adjustments to enhance power and speed, whereas recreational cycling emphasizes sustainable exercise routines that support overall health and well-being.

Factors Influencing Performance

Several external and biomechanical factors influence performance in FES-cycling. Environmental conditions such as ambient temperature, road surface type, and competition duration can affect muscle endurance and stimulation efficacy. Biomechanical aspects, including body positioning on the bike and synchronization of muscle stimulation with pedalling cadence, play a significant role in optimizing efficiency and power output. Proper adaptation to these factors through training and technology can enhance an athlete's ability to perform at peak levels during competition [33].

- Environmental conditions (e.g., temperature, road surface)
- Biomechanical efficiency (e.g., proper pedal-stroke synchronization)
- Technology adaptation (customized stimulation parameters to individual physiology)

By integrating optimized training routines, individualized stimulation settings, and advanced technology, FES-cycling can maximize performance, rehabilitation outcomes, and long-term neuromuscular health.

Main Required Equipment

Essential Equipment for Competitive FES-Cycling

Electrodes

Electrodes play a crucial role in FES-cycling by delivering precise electrical stimulation to targeted muscle groups. High-quality electrodes are essential for optimizing muscle contraction and ensuring user comfort. These electrodes must be durable to withstand repeated use and flexible enough to conform to different body shapes and positions.

There are two primary types of electrodes used in FES-cycling:

- Surface Electrodes: These are non-invasive, placed on the skin over specific muscle groups. They are cost-effective and easy to apply but require precise positioning to ensure optimal stimulation. Recently some studies explore ultrasound-compatible [34], textile based [35], aerogel based [36] and screen printed [37] electrodes and their effectiveness.
- Implanted Electrodes: Surgically placed within the body, these electrodes provide more targeted stimulation and can improve efficiency. However, they are more expensive and require medical procedures for implantation [38].

For prolonged use, electrodes should have high conductivity to ensure effective transmission of electrical pulses. Skin-friendly materials to prevent irritation or burns. Secure adhesion while allowing breathability for extended use proper electrode placement and maintenance are essential to prevent skin irritation, enhance stimulation efficiency, and prolong the life of the equipment.

Controllers and Stimulation Units

The controller and stimulation unit form the core of an FES-cycling system. These components regulate the electrical impulses sent to the electrodes, dictating the intensity, frequency, and duration of muscle contractions [39].

Key Features of Controllers and Stimulation Units:

- Adjustable Stimulation Parameters: Allows fine-tuning of pulse width, amplitude, and frequency to match the user's muscle condition and training objectives.
- Real-time Monitoring: Some advanced units feature feedback systems that adjust stimulation intensity based on muscle fatigue, ensuring optimal training efficiency and reducing the risk of overuse.
- Battery Efficiency: Portable stimulation units are designed for prolonged battery life to accommodate extended training sessions without frequent recharging.
- Advanced stimulation units integrate sensors that measure power output, muscle response, and heart rate, providing real-time feedback that helps optimize training efficiency and prevent fatigue-related injuries.
- By combining high-quality electrodes with precise and adaptable stimulation units, FES-cycling provides a more controlled and effective means of muscle activation, making the experience safer and more beneficial for both competitive and recreational users.

Stationary FES Cycling Ergometers for Training

Functional Electrical Stimulation (FES) cycling ergometers are specialized rehabilitation devices designed to assist individuals with neuromuscular impairments in regaining movement, improving circulation, and maintaining muscle mass. Several leading companies manufacture FES cycling systems tailored for clinical and home use.

- MYOLYN[2] (USA)—The MyoCycle series offers FES-enabled cycling systems designed for home users and rehabilitation clinics, helping individuals with spinal cord injuries, stroke, or neuromuscular disorders engage in active cycling.
- Restorative Therapies[3] (USA)—Their RT300 series provides advanced FES cycling technology for lower and upper limbs, supporting individuals in neurological rehabilitation. The systems are widely used in hospitals and therapy centers.
- MOTOmed[4] (Germany)—Known for its MOTOmed Viva2, MOTOmed Muvi, and MOTOmed Loop+FES systems, the company integrates motor-assisted cycling with optional FES, catering to users with spinal cord injuries, multiple sclerosis, and stroke recovery needs.
- BerkelBike[5] (Netherlands)—Combining arm and leg cycling with FES technology, the BerkelBike Pro and Connect models allow individuals with neurological impairments to engage in full-body exercise. These bikes are designed for both rehabilitation and outdoor use, making them a versatile solution for users seeking mobility and strength improvements.

These companies play a vital role in advancing adapted cycling technology, helping individuals with limited or no voluntary movement maintain muscle function and improve overall health through electrical stimulation-assisted exercise.

Main Competitions

Major International Competitions

Cybathlon

The Cybathlon is a global competition organized by ETH Zürich, bringing together teams from around the world to develop and showcase assistive technology innovations. One of its key disciplines is Functional Electrical Stimulation (FES) Cycling, where pilots with spinal cord injuries use electrical stimulation to activate their leg muscles and power a recumbent tricycle.

The inaugural Cybathlon 2016[6] (Fig. 8.1) took place in Zürich, Switzerland, as the first international event of its kind, emphasizing real-world applications of assistive technologies. In the FES Cycling race, teams competed to complete a set distance using only FES-controlled muscle contractions. The competition highlighted the varying capabilities of different FES systems and the need for individualized stimulation protocols. The winning team in the FES Cycling category demonstrated

[2] https://myolyn.com/

[3] https://restorative-therapies.com/

[4] https://www.motomed.com/

[5] https://berkelbike.com/

[6] https://cybathlon.com/de/events/edition/cybathlon-2016

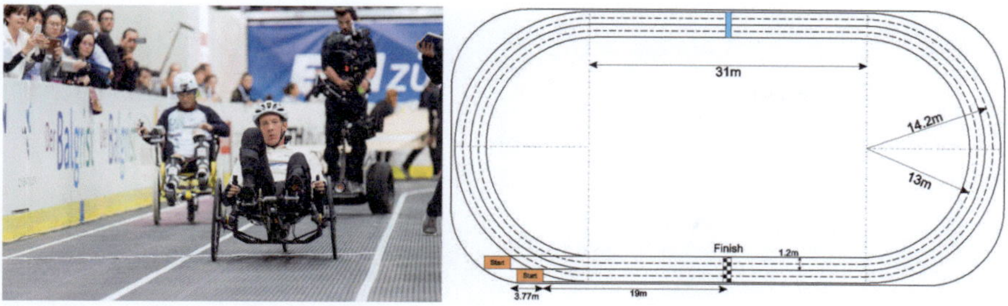

Fig. 8.1 Cybathlon 2016: First Edition of Cybathlon FES Race and Race Course

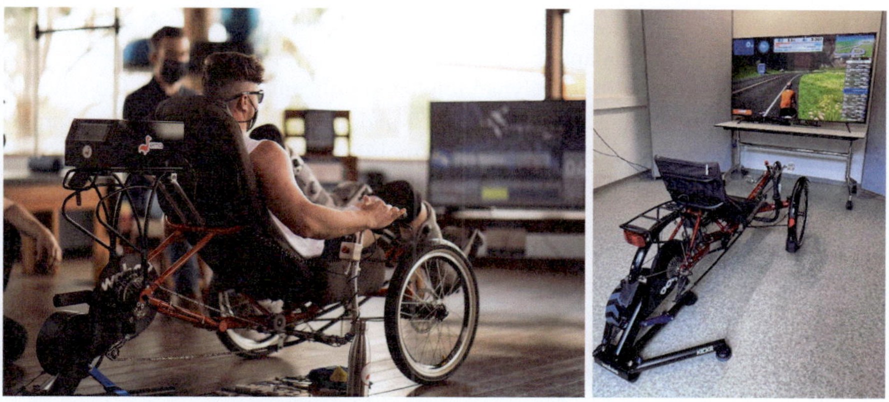

Fig. 8.2 Cybathlon 2020: Global Edition and task set-up

superior muscle endurance and control, showcasing the effectiveness of their training and stimulation strategies.

Due to the COVID-19 pandemic, the Cybathlon 2020 Global Edition[7] (Fig. 8.2) was held remotely, with teams competing in their home countries under standardized conditions. The event featured 51 teams from 20 countries, each performing in their own setup while adhering to strict competition rules. Despite the logistical challenges, the FES Cycling race showcased significant advancements in muscle stimulation technology, real-time feedback systems, and improved training methodologies. The competition results underscored the growing competitiveness of FES-assisted cycling, with several teams achieving remarkable power output and endurance improvements.

The Cybathlon 2024 edition[8] (Fig. 8.3) continues the evolution of assistive sports, integrating further technological advancements in FES and adaptive cycling. This edition is expected to introduce improved biomechanical analysis and refined stimulation protocols to enhance pilot performance. The event will again bring

[7] https://cybathlon.com/de/events/edition/cybathlon-2020

[8] https://cybathlon.com/de/events/edition/cybathlon-2024

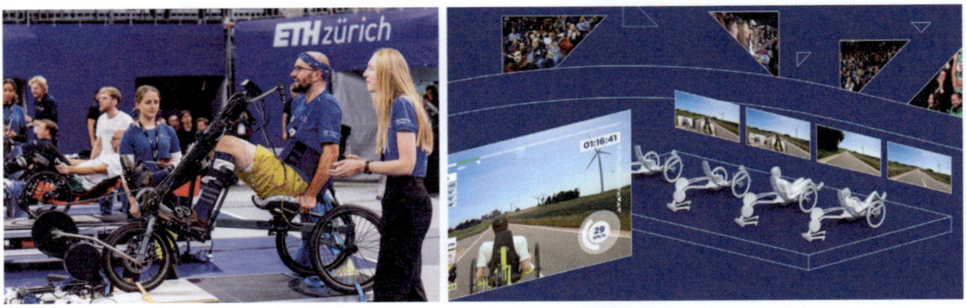

Fig. 8.3 Cybathlon 2024 and virtual scenario

together researchers, engineers, and athletes to push the boundaries of what is possible in FES cycling and adaptive technology.

Through its various editions, Cybathlon has significantly contributed to advancing FES cycling, providing a platform to test and improve neuromuscular stimulation strategies, ultimately leading to better mobility solutions for individuals with spinal cord injuries.

FES Bike Race as Part of Lyon Cyber Days

Lyon Cyber Days[9] (Fig. 8.4) is an annual event organized by ANTS (Advanced Neurorehabilitation Therapies & Sport, Lyon, France), dedicated to promoting technological advancements in motor rehabilitation and adapted physical activities for individuals with neuromotor disabilities. The event is held in collaboration with the Lyon Free Bike and consists of two main highlights over 2 days: a scientific conference and a Functional Electrical Stimulation (FES) bike race demonstration.

The second day of the event, held at Parc de Gerland in Lyon, France, is dedicated to FES cycling demonstrations and races. Participants, including FES cycling pilots and individuals with spinal cord injuries, engage in a competitive and friendly environment that showcases the capabilities of FES technology in sports. Over the years, the event has hosted thrilling races featuring top FES-pilots such as: Julien Jouffroy (Cybathlon 2016 bronze medallist, Swiss team), Mohammed Ackloufi (Pulse Racing, Netherlands).

These races not only demonstrate the athletic potential of FES cycling but also raise public awareness about the benefits of neurorehabilitation through sports. In addition to the races, Lyon Cyber Days offers workshops designed to engage the public in adapted physical activities and disability awareness. Attendees have the opportunity to experience: Wheelchair basketball and blind football, to understand the challenges and skills involved in adaptive sports, demonstrations of assistive technology, such as tricycles with electric assistance and adapted vehicle solutions, exhibitions by partners, including research institutions and accessibility-focused organizations. These activities emphasize the importance of inclusivity and

[9] https://ants-asso.com/en/lyon-cyber-days-en/

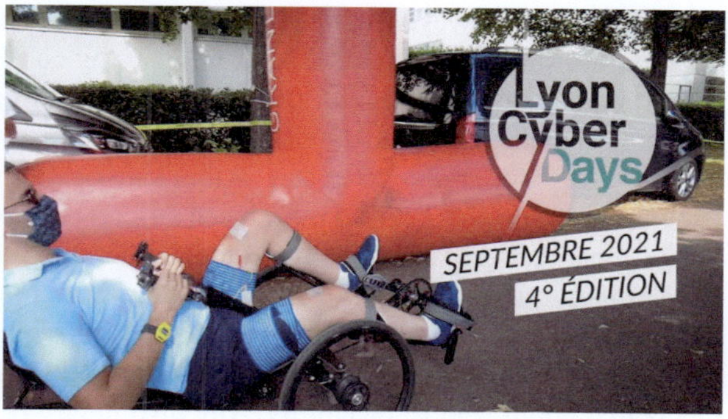

Fig. 8.4 Lyon Cyber Days 2021

accessibility in sports while encouraging broader participation in adaptive physical activities.

Since its first edition in 2018, Lyon Cyber Days has continued to expand, drawing more participants, researchers, and spectators each year. With ongoing advancements in FES technology, Lyon Cyber Days is set to play an even greater role in shaping the future of neurorehabilitation and adaptive sports.

Rules and Regulations

Cybathlon 2016: Rules and Regulations for FES Bike Race

The 2016 edition of Cybathlon introduced Functional Electrical Stimulation (FES) bike racing as a discipline where pilots with spinal cord injuries competed using electrical stimulation to activate their leg muscles and propel a recumbent tricycle. Each pilot-controlled muscle contractions through pre-programmed stimulation patterns, optimizing cadence and force for speed and endurance.

The race was conducted on a flat track, covering a predefined distance that required athletes to complete the circuit within a specified time. To ensure fair play, the competition prohibited external mechanical assistance, meaning only muscle power generated through stimulation was allowed. Competitors had to remain in their designated lane, avoiding interference with others.

Equipment used by teams had to adhere to technical guidelines, including stimulation parameters such as pulse width, frequency, and amplitude, which were restricted to safe limits. Referees closely monitored the race, enforcing penalties for rule violations, including early starts, unapproved modifications to the FES system, or unsportsmanlike conduct. The final ranking was determined by completion time, with the fastest pilot winning, and in cases where multiple racers failed to complete the course, partial distance covered was used for ranking.

Cybathlon 2019: Rules and Regulations for FES Bike Race

The 2019 Cybathlon edition refined race conditions and expanded the regulations governing FES bike competitions. The core objective remained the same, pilots used electrical stimulation to power their leg muscles, driving a recumbent cycle around a track. However, updated rules introduced new performance monitoring systems and standardized race distances, ensuring consistency across competitors.

Participants had to program their stimulation settings before the race, with no real-time manual adjustments allowed. Stimulation settings, including frequency and intensity, were required to stay within safe operating ranges to protect the athlete's health. The competition introduced stricter requirements for equipment compliance, mandating that teams submit their FES setup for approval before the race to prevent unfair advantages through custom hardware modifications.

The race format included multiple heats, with rankings based on time and distance completed. Pilots had to demonstrate controlled cycling without erratic movements that could lead to instability. Any involuntary or unsafe movements leading to loss of control resulted in disqualification. Additionally, more sophisticated tracking systems were introduced to ensure precise timing and performance evaluation. The final standings were based on both completion time and consistency, rewarding steady pedalling efficiency.

Cybathlon 2024: Rules and Regulations for FES Bike Race

By 2024, the Cybathlon further optimized the race structure, integrating real-time monitoring and improving safety measures. Competitors continued to use FES-controlled muscle activation to propel their bicycles, but the rules now emphasized even stricter control over electrical stimulation parameters, ensuring pilot safety and competitive fairness.

Pilots were required to pre-program their muscle stimulation patterns before the race, with no modifications allowed once the event began. The track layout was adjusted to provide a standardized challenge across all participants, eliminating potential advantages due to external factors. A time cap was introduced, requiring racers to complete the course within a specified duration to remain in contention.

Technology advancements enabled real-time feedback for referees, who closely monitored FES intensity levels, cadence, and power output. Any irregularities, such as excessive stimulation levels or unintended system modifications, resulted in penalties or disqualification. The competition also increased emphasis on biomechanical efficiency, rewarding pilots who demonstrated optimal synchronization between stimulation and cycling mechanics.

Discussion and Conclusions

This chapter sets out to examine how Functional Electrical Stimulation (FES) cycling has evolved from a therapeutic intervention into a multidimensional activity that supports physical fitness, recreational participation, and high-level competition among individuals with spinal cord injuries and other neuromuscular impairments. By reviewing the physiological foundations, training methodologies, and technological innovations of FES-cycling, the chapter highlights both the opportunities and challenges associated with its broader implementation.

FES-cycling represents a unique intersection of rehabilitation, engineering, and sport. While it was originally developed to maintain muscle mass and circulation in individuals with paralysis, it has since expanded to include structured exercise, competitive racing, and mobile outdoor applications. These developments reflect a growing recognition of the importance of long-term physical activity and autonomy in individuals with disabilities. In particular, the increasing participation in international competitions such as the Cybathlon illustrates the potential of FES-cycling not only as a rehabilitative modality but also as a means of fostering athletic identity, community engagement, and technological innovation.

A key theme in this chapter has been the importance of structured, evidence-based training approaches. Programs that incorporate periodized routines, including base training, specific performance phases, and tapering, have demonstrated measurable improvements in muscle strength, endurance, and cardiovascular capacity. High-intensity interval training (HIIT), when properly managed, has proven effective in promoting neuromuscular adaptation while avoiding overstimulation. These findings support the notion that individuals with SCI can benefit from training principles similar to those used in able-bodied athletic preparation, provided that stimulation parameters and recovery strategies are carefully tailored.

Technological developments have also played a critical role in advancing FES-cycling. New stimulation strategies, such as spatially distributed sequential stimulation and inter-pulse interval modulation, offer improved control over fatigue and muscle activation. In parallel, adaptive stimulation units and performance monitoring systems are enabling real-time adjustments based on physiological feedback. While these innovations are particularly relevant for competitive applications, they also hold promise for improving safety, efficiency, and user experience in recreational settings.

Despite the progress, several limitations remain. Muscle fatigue, high equipment costs, and the need for ongoing technical support continue to hinder widespread adoption. Additionally, the gap between recreational users and elite athletes is widening as advanced technologies become increasingly specialized. Addressing these challenges will require a focus on affordability, ease of use, and scalable training models that can be implemented outside of specialized research or clinical environments.

Looking ahead, the future of FES-cycling will likely depend on parallel advances in three areas. First, continued technological refinement is needed to improve stimulation efficiency and user comfort. Second, efforts to expand access through insurance coverage, open-source designs, or community-based programs. It will be essential to reach a broader population. Third, there is a need for longitudinal studies to better understand the long-term physiological and psychosocial impacts of FES-cycling in both competitive and recreational contexts.

In conclusion, FES-cycling offers a compelling model for how assistive technologies can promote physical activity, independence, and inclusion among individuals with significant motor impairments. By combining structured training, user-centered design, and interdisciplinary collaboration, the field can continue to evolve in ways that support both high-performance outcomes and everyday well-being. The growing interest in FES-cycling among clinicians, engineers, athletes, and end-users suggests a strong foundation for future innovation, provided that the field remains committed to both excellence and accessibility.

References

1. Ragnarsson KT. Functional electrical stimulation after spinal cord injury: current use, therapeutic effects and future directions. Spinal Cord. 2008;46(4):255–74.
2. Petrofsky JS, Heaton H, Phillips CA. Outdoor bicycle for exercise in paraplegics and quadriplegics. J Biomed Eng. 1983;5(4):292–6.
3. Petrofsky JS, Phillips CA, Heaton HH, Glaser RM. Bicycle ergometer for paralyzed muscle. J Clin Eng. 1984;9(1):13–20.
4. Berry HR, Kakebeeke TH, Donaldson N, Perret C, Hunt KJ. Energetics of paraplegic cycling: adaptations to 12 months of high volume training. Technol Health Care. 2012;20(2):73–84.
5. Hettinga DM, Andrews BJ. Oxygen consumption during functional electrical stimulation-assisted exercise in persons with spinal cord injury: implications for fitness and health. Sports Med. 2008;38(10):825–38.
6. Dolbow DR, Gorgey AS, Ketchum JM, Moore JR, Hackett LA, Gater DR. Exercise adherence during home-based functional electrical stimulation cycling by individuals with spinal cord injury. Am J Phys Med Rehabil. 2012;91(11):922–30.
7. Van Der Scheer JW, Goosey-Tolfrey VL, Valentino SE, Davis GM, Ho CH. Functional electrical stimulation cycling exercise after spinal cord injury: a systematic review of health and fitness-related outcomes. J Neuroeng Rehabil. 2021;18(1):99.
8. Dolbow D, Gorgey A, Ketchum J, Gater D. Home-based functional electrical stimulation cycling enhances quality of life in individuals with spinal cord injury. Top Spinal Cord Inj Rehabil. 2013;19(4):324–9.
9. Griffin L, Decker MJ, Hwang JY, Wang B, Kitchen K, Ding Z, et al. Functional electrical stimulation cycling improves body composition, metabolic and neural factors in persons with spinal cord injury. J Electromyogr Kinesiol. 2009;19(4):614–22.
10. Duffell LD, Donaldson NDN, Perkins TA, Rushton DN, Hunt KJ, Kakebeeke TH, et al. Long-term intensive electrically stimulated cycling by spinal cord–injured people: effect on muscle properties and their relation to power output. Muscle Nerve. 2008;38(4):1304–11.
11. Chen SC, Lai CH, Chan WP, Huang MH, Tsai HW, Chen JJJ. Increases in bone mineral density after functional electrical stimulation cycling exercises in spinal cord injured patients. Disabil Rehabil. 2005;27(22):1337–41.
12. Frotzler A, Coupaud S, Perret C, Kakebeeke TH, Hunt KJ, Donaldson NDN, et al. High-volume FES-cycling partially reverses bone loss in people with chronic spinal cord injury. Bone. 2008;43(1):169–76.
13. Alashram AR, Annino G, Mercuri NB. Changes in spasticity following functional electrical stimulation cycling in patients with spinal cord injury: a systematic review. J Spinal Cord Med. 2022;45(1):10–23.
14. Hunt KJ, Fang J, Saengsuwan J, Grob M, Laubacher M. On the efficiency of FES cycling: a framework and systematic review. Technol Health Care. 2012;20(5):395–422.
15. Hunt KJ, Saunders BA, Perret C, Berry H, Allan DB, Donaldson N, et al. Energetics of paraplegic cycling: a new theoretical framework and efficiency characterisation for untrained subjects. Eur J Appl Physiol. 2007;101(3):277–85.
16. Gföhler M, Loicht M, Lugner P. Exercise tricycle for paraplegics. Med Biol Eng Comput. 1998;36(1):118–21.

17. Chen JJ, Yu N-Y, Huang D-G, Ann B-T, Chang G-C. Applying fuzzy logic to control cycling movement induced by functional electrical stimulation. IEEE Trans Rehabil Eng. 1997;5(2):158–69.
18. Pons DJ, Vaughan CL, Jaros GG. Cycling device powered by the electrically stimulated muscles of paraplegics. Med Biol Eng Comput. 1989;27(1):1–7.
19. Manaf H, Hamzaid NA, Hasnan N, Yiwei C, Mohafez H, Hisham H, et al. High-intensity interval training with functional electrical stimulation cycling for incomplete spinal cord injury patients: a pilot feasibility study. Artif Organs. 2024;48(12):1449–57.
20. Docter H, Podvinšek K, Koomen S, PULSE Racing III, Kaman BE, Visser I, et al. Practical approaches of PULSE Racing in training their athlete for the cybathlon global edition functional electrical stimulation bike race: a case report. J NeuroEngineering Rehabil. 2023;20(1):30.
21. McDaniel J, Lombardo LM, Foglyano KM, Marasco PD, Triolo RJ. Cycle training using implanted neural prostheses: team Cleveland. Eur J Transl Myol. 2017;27(4):7087.
22. Sadowsky CL, Hammond ER, Strohl AB, Commean PK, Eby SA, Damiano DL, et al. Lower extremity functional electrical stimulation cycling promotes physical and functional recovery in chronic spinal cord injury. J Spinal Cord Med. 2013;36(6):623–31.
23. Johnston TE, Marino RJ, Oleson CV, Schmidt-Read M, Leiby BE, Sendecki J, et al. Musculoskeletal effects of 2 functional electrical stimulation cycling paradigms conducted at different cadences for people with spinal cord injury: a pilot study. Arch Phys Med Rehabil. 2016;97(9):1413–22.
24. Dolbow DR, Credeur DP. Effects of resistance-guided high intensity interval functional electrical stimulation cycling on an individual with paraplegia: a case report. J Spinal Cord Med. 2018;41(2):248–52.
25. Gelenitis K, Foglyano K, Lombardo L, Triolo R. Selective neural stimulation methods improve cycling exercise performance after spinal cord injury: a case series. J Neuroeng Rehabil. 2021;18(1):117.
26. Sanna N, Nossa R, Biffi E, Guanziroli E, Diella E, Ferrante S, et al. Evaluating the health and fitness benefits of a 6-month FES-cycling program on a recumbent trike for individuals with motor complete SCI: a pilot study. J Neuroeng Rehabil. 2025;22:55.
27. Nabi F, Malaty A, Shah DJ. Stress cardiac magnetic resonance. Curr Opin Cardiol. 2011;26(5):385–91.
28. Laubacher M, Aksoez EA, Brust AK, Baumberger M, Riener R, Binder-Macleod S, et al. Stimulation of paralysed quadriceps muscles with sequentially and spatially distributed electrodes during dynamic knee extension. J Neuroeng Rehabil. 2019;16(1):5.
29. Aksöz EA, Laubacher M, Binder-Macleod S, Hunt KJ. Effect of stochastic modulation of interpulse interval during stimulated isokinetic leg extension. Eur J Transl Myol. 2016;26(3):6160.
30. Duffell LD, Paddison S, Alahmary AF, Donaldson N, Burridge J. The effects of FES cycling combined with virtual reality racing biofeedback on voluntary function after incomplete SCI: a pilot study. J Neuroeng Rehabil. 2019;16(1):149.
31. Schauer T. Sensing motion and muscle activity for feedback control of functional electrical stimulation: ten years of experience in Berlin. Annu Rev Control. 2017;44:355–74.
32. Wannawas N, Faisal AA. Towards AI-controlled movement restoration: learning FES-cycling stimulation with reinforcement learning. In: 2023 international conference on rehabilitation robotics (ICORR). Singapore, Singapore. Piscataway: IEEE; 2023. p. 1–6.
33. Gfohler M, Lugner P. Dynamic simulation of FES-cycling: influence of individual parameters. IEEE Trans Neural Syst Rehabil Eng. 2004;12(4):398–405.
34. Moon S, Xue X, Ganesh V, Shukla D, Kreager BC, Cai Q, et al. Ultrasound-compatible electrode for functional electrical stimulation. Biomedicine. 2024;12(8):1741.
35. Dell'Eva F, Oliveri V, Sironi R, Perego P, Andreoni G, Ferrante S, et al. Ink-based textile electrodes for wearable functional electrical stimulation: a proof-of-concept study to evaluate comfort and efficacy. Artif Organs. 2024;48(10):1138–49.

36. Marquez-Chin M, Saadatnia Z, Naguib HE, Popovic MR. Development of an aerogel-based wet electrode for functional electrical stimulation. IEEE Trans Neural Syst Rehabil Eng. 2023;31:4085–95.
37. Yang K, Freeman C, Torah R, Beeby S, Tudor J. Screen printed fabric electrode array for wearable functional electrical stimulation. Sens Actuators Phys. 2014;213:108–15.
38. Pellot-Cestero JE, Herring EZ, Graczyk EL, Memberg WD, Kirsch RF, Ajiboye AB, et al. Implanted electrodes for functional electrical stimulation to restore upper and lower extremity function: history and future directions. Neurosurgery. 2023;93(5):965–70.
39. Popović-Maneski L, Mateo S. MotiMove: multi-purpose transcutaneous functional electrical stimulator. Artif Organs. 2022;46(10):1970–9.

Practical FES-Cycling Guideline Based on Functional Outcomes

9

Murillo Frazão

Introduction

Functional Electrical Stimulation (FES) cycling has emerged as a promising therapeutic modality for individuals with neurological impairments, offering substantial benefits in improving muscle strength, mobility, and cardiorespiratory fitness. By combining electrical stimulation with cycling movements, FES helps activate paralyzed or weakened muscles, allowing patients to engage in functional exercise, even when voluntary movement is limited. Despite its effectiveness, the lack of standardized protocols for FES-cycling (such as optimal intensity, frequency, duration, and cycling cadence) can make it challenging for clinicians to apply the therapy consistently and effectively. This practical guideline aims to address this gap by providing evidence-based recommendations on the best practices for FES-cycling, focusing on achieving functional outcomes in rehabilitation.

This guideline will focus on specific functional outcomes that FES-cycling can target, including improvements in muscle strength and power, spasticity reduction, cardiorespiratory fitness, and overall functional capacity. By synthesizing current research and clinical insights, the guideline will offer practical advice on setting the appropriate parameters to maximize the effectiveness of FES-cycling for different patient populations. This resource will serve as a comprehensive tool for clinicians, helping them tailor FES-cycling programs to improve patients' functional independence and quality of life.

M. Frazão (✉)
Lauro Wanderley University Hospital – EBSERH/UFPB, João Pessoa, PB, Brazil
e-mail: murillo.frazao@gmail.com

M. Frazão (ed.), *Functional Electrical Stimulation Cycling in Clinical Practice*,
https://doi.org/10.1007/978-3-032-23937-2_9

Parameters Sets and Training Routine for Strength and Power Improvement and Muscle Hypertrophy

Regular use of FES-cycling enhances blood circulation, increases muscle strength, and improves overall muscle performance, making it an essential component of physical rehabilitation programs. In addition to boosting muscle performance, FES-cycling plays a crucial role in muscle trophism. When muscles are not regularly used due to injury or disability, they can undergo atrophy, leading to a loss of strength and size. By engaging muscles through electrical stimulation, FES-cycling helps prevent muscle atrophy by maintaining muscle activity and stimulating protein synthesis.

Several studies have analyzed the positive effects of FES-cycling on muscle performance and trophism. However, despite the promising outcomes, the optimal parameters for FES-cycling, such as pulse intensity, frequency, pulse width, and duration, have not yet been standardized. Below, the results of some key studies are presented, highlighting the respective protocols used and the improvements observed.

Strength

There is an improvement in strength favors to FES-cycling compared to others therapies, with a clinically significant difference [1]. For this improvement to be reached, many studies used high FES intensity levels. Higher intensities induce higher motor unit recruitment, higher intramuscular tissue pressure, and, consequently, ischemia [2].

The studies mentioned highlight the significant benefits of FES-cycling in improving muscle strength and performance across a range of protocols. Ferrante et al. [3] reported a remarkable improvement, with a mean increase of 84 Newtons, using FES-cycling at 40 rotations per minute (RPM) for 35 min, seven times a week over 4 weeks. However, specific details on pulse intensity, width, and frequency were not disclosed. Johnston et al. [4] found a 142% strength increase after 6 months of FES-cycling at 50 RPM, 33 Hz, and a pulse width of 150–300 μs, with up to 140 mA intensity. The sessions lasted 60 min, three times per week. Backus et al. [5] showed a mean 59% improvement in resistance after 6 months of training at 60 min per session, three times a week, using pulse widths of 250 μs and frequencies between 33 and 45 Hz, but pulse intensity was not reported.

Further studies, such as Sadowsky et al. [6], demonstrated a 35% improvement in muscle strength after 3 months of FES-cycling at 50 RPM, 100 Hz, and pulse widths of 500 μs, with a maximum intensity of 140 mA. Sessions lasted between 45 and 60 min, performed three times a week. Ratchford et al. [7] also reported a mean 19% improvement in strength, with a large effect size, after 4 weeks of FES-cycling at 30-minute sessions, three times per week, using pulse widths of 250 μs and 35–40 Hz frequency. These studies emphasize the positive impact of FES cycling on muscle strength, although variation in protocols (intensity, pulse width, frequency, and duration) suggests that further research could clarify the optimal parameters for muscle rehabilitation.

Power

FES-cycling shows a significant improvement in power compared to other therapies, with a clinically meaningful difference and high certainty of evidence. To achieve this improvement, many studies have utilized high FES intensity levels. The adaptation mechanisms for the repeated muscle tension generation may be involved in muscle performance improvement [1].

The studies mentioned provide a range of insights into the effects of FES-cycling on muscle power, with varying protocols and outcomes. Brurok et al. [8] demonstrated an impressive 420% increase in power after 8 weeks of FES-cycling, with sessions held three times per week at 35–50 RPM and up to 140 mA. This protocol highlights the potential for significant power gains with appropriate stimulation parameters. Ferrante et al. [3] also reported a substantial improvement, with a mean 250% increase in power after 4 weeks of cycling at 40 RPM, seven times per week, for 35 min per session. However, details regarding pulse intensity, width, and frequency were not provided, suggesting the need for further investigation into these parameters.

Other studies further support the efficacy of FES-cycling in enhancing muscle power. Armstrong et al. [9] observed an 84% increase in power after 8 weeks of training at 40–50 Hz, using pulse widths of 200–250 μs and intensities ranging from 10 to 50 mA, with sessions lasting 30 min, three times per week. Janssen et al. [10] found a 33% power increase with a different protocol, using 450 μs, 60 Hz, and sessions lasting 25–30 min, twice a week for 6 weeks. In contrast, Bakkun et al. [11] showed a more modest 15% increase in power over 16 weeks, using up to 150 mA and sessions lasting 18–32 min, twice a week. These studies indicate that while FES-cycling can lead to significant improvements in muscle power, the extent of the improvement may depend on factors such as stimulation parameters, frequency of training, and duration of the program.

Muscle Hypertrophy

FES-cycling demonstrates an improvement in muscle trophism compared to other therapies, with a clinically significant difference [1]. The studies report high FES intensity levels. Beyond leg lean mass, total body mass also improves, suggesting that a systemic growth effect may be involved. High-intensity current stimulation induces up-regulation of IGF-1 and modulation of MuRF-1 (a muscle-specific atrophy-related gene). It also induces upregulation of relevant markers of differentiating satellite cells and extracellular matrix remodeling, reducing fibrosis [12].

The studies presented highlight the effectiveness of FES-cycling in improving muscle mass, with varying results depending on the stimulation parameters and duration of the programs. Demchak et al. [13] demonstrated a significant 63% improvement in the vastus lateralis cross-sectional area after 13 weeks of FES-cycling at 35–50 RPM, 60 Hz, with pulse widths of 375 μs and up to 140 mA intensity, three times per week for 30 min. This study showcases the potential of FES-cycling in significantly enhancing muscle size, particularly in the quadriceps region. Similarly, Sadowsky et al. [6] observed a 36% improvement in quadriceps muscle mass after 3 months of cycling at 50 RPM, 100 Hz, and pulse widths of 500 μs, with a maximum intensity of 140 mA. Sessions were conducted for 45–60 min, three times per week, indicating that a slightly longer protocol can yield substantial increases in muscle mass.

Other studies, such as those by Baldi et al. [14] and Dolbow et al. [15], show more modest improvements in muscle mass. Baldi et al. found a 9.3% increase in lower limb muscle mass after 6 months of FES cycling using 375 μs pulse width, 60 Hz frequency, and up to 140 mA intensity at 35–50 RPM, with 30-min sessions, three times per week. Dolbow et al. observed a 7% improvement in quadriceps muscle mass after 8 weeks of FES cycling at 350 μs pulse width, 40 Hz frequency, and up to 140 mA intensity at 35 RPM, with sessions lasting 30 min, three times per week. These studies suggest that while longer-term FES-cycling protocols can lead to notable gains in muscle mass, more modest improvements can still be achieved with shorter durations or less frequent stimulation, indicating that muscle adaptation depends on a range of factors, including the intensity and frequency of the electrical stimulation.

Recommendation

Based on FES-cycling parameters of these several studies, it is recommended a 300–500 μs pulse width, the highest tolerated pulse intensity (usually >100 mA), a 33–60 Hz pulse frequency, a 35–50 RPM cycling cadence and a 30–60 min exercise duration (Fig. 9.1; Table 9.1).

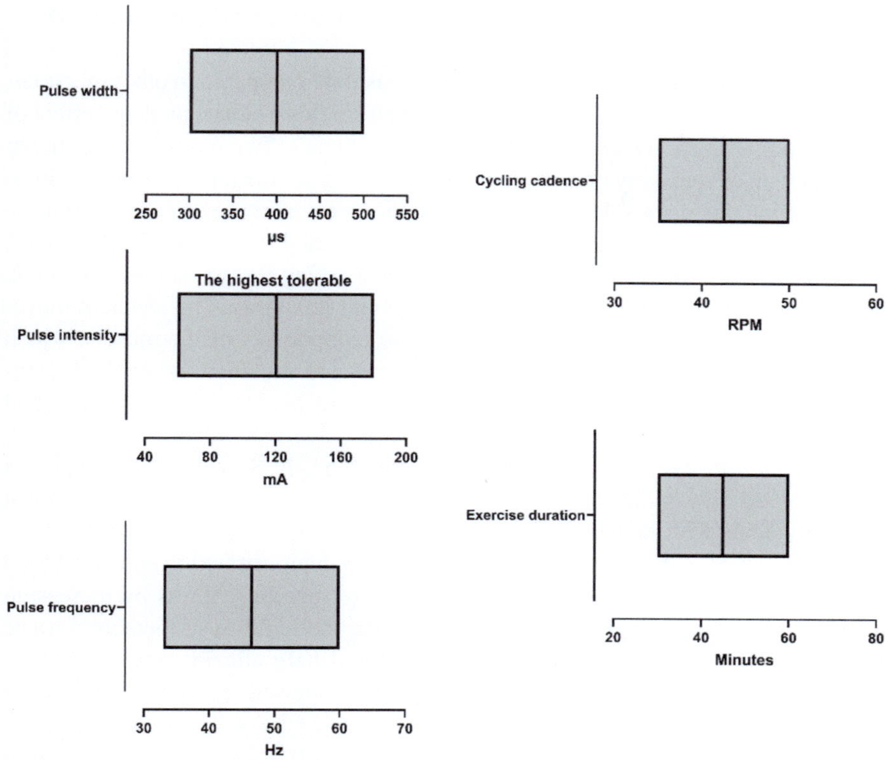

Fig. 9.1 Parameters sets and training routine for strength and power improvement and muscle hypertrophy

Table 9.1 Practical guideline for parameters set

	Pulse width (µs)	Intensity (mA)	Frequency (Hz)	Cycling cadence (RPM)	Exercise duration (min)
Strength, power and muscle hypertrophy	300–500	Highest tolerated (usually >100)	33–60	35–50	30–60
Spasticity	300–500	Comfortable intensity (usually <100)	20–33	Comfortable cycling cadence	20–60
Cardiorespiratory fitness	150–300	Highest tolerated (usually >100)	33–50	35–50	30–60
Muscle performance and physical function in hospitalized patients	400–800	Highest tolerated (usually >100)	50–75	10–20	10–20

Parameters Sets and Training Routine for Spasticity Reduction

FES-cycling shows a significant reduction in spasticity compared to other therapies, with a clinically meaningful difference [1]. Most studies evaluate an acute effect of FES-cycling using a low electrical stimulation frequency. Two plausible reasons for the reduction of spasticity observed with FES-cycling are the repetitive and reciprocal stretching that occurs during cycling, and the direct effects of electrical stimulation on muscle tone. The act of cycling involves repeated stretching of the muscles, particularly the agonist and antagonist muscles working in opposition, which can help reduce spasticity by promoting relaxation and flexibility. This cyclical movement may affect the elastic and parallel elastic components of the muscle, which influence the resistance encountered when muscles are stretched. When these components are altered through repeated stretching, it may lead to reduced stiffness and tone, contributing to a decrease in spasticity [16].

In addition to the mechanical effects of stretching, FES-cycling also improves muscle blood flow, which is crucial in reducing muscle tone. Studies have shown that individuals with higher levels of spasticity tend to experience reduced whole-leg blood flow [17]. Electrical stimulation has been demonstrated to enhance blood circulation to the muscles, which may help reduce muscle stiffness by increasing oxygen and nutrient supply, while also facilitating the removal of metabolic waste products [18, 19]. The improved circulation could help alleviate the heightened muscle tone associated with spasticity, supporting muscle relaxation and better overall function.

Several studies have demonstrated the positive effects of FES-cycling on spasticity, particularly through improvements in the relaxation index and reductions in spasticity-related measurements such as the Ashworth Scale and the Hoffman reflex (H/M ratio). Krause et al. [20] reported a significant 168% improvement in the relaxation index during the pendulum test. This was achieved using a 500 μs pulse width, up to 99 mA of pulse intensity, and a frequency of 20 Hz for 60 min. However, the cycling cadence during the protocol was not specified. Similarly, Lo et al. [21] showed an 18% improvement in the relaxation index during the pendulum test, as well as a 20% reduction in the Hoffman reflex (H/M ratio), using a 300 μs pulse width, 40–64 mA intensity, and a frequency of 20 Hz. The study mentioned a "comfortable cycling cadence," but did not provide specifics regarding the duration of the exercise.

Further research by Yeh et al. [16] showed a 15% improvement in the relaxation index during the pendulum test, along with a 50% reduction in the Ashworth Scale, after using a 300 μs pulse width, up to 100 mA of intensity, and 20 Hz frequency for 20 min. The cycling cadence was also described as comfortable but not quantified. Ralston et al. [22] demonstrated a 50% reduction in the Ashworth Scale, employing a 350 μs pulse width, up to 140 mA intensity, and a frequency of 33 Hz, with sessions lasting between 30 and 45 min at a comfortable cycling cadence. These studies underline the effectiveness of FES-cycling in reducing spasticity, with variations in pulse width, intensity, frequency, and duration, but no clear consensus on the ideal parameters for optimal results.

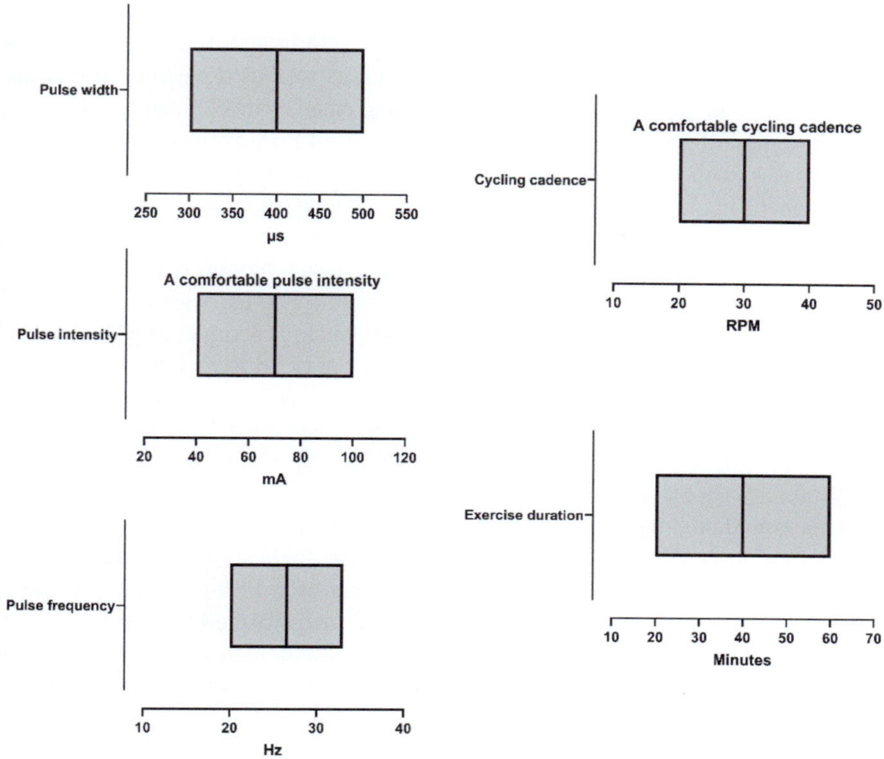

Fig. 9.2 Parameters sets and training routine for spasticity reduction

Recommendation

Based on FES-cycling parameters of these several studies, it is recommended a 300–500 μs pulse width, a comfortable pulse intensity (usually <100 mA), a 20–33 Hz pulse frequency, a comfortable cycling cadence and a 20–60 min exercise duration (Fig. 9.2; Table 9.1).

Parameters Sets and Training Routine for Cardiorespiratory Fitness Improvement

Interventions with more than 8 weeks show a cardiorespiratory fitness improvement favors FES-cycling compared to other therapies, with a clinically meaningful difference and high certainty of evidence. Interventions up to 8 weeks show limited effects on cardiorespiratory fitness compared to other therapies [1]. The relation between cardiorespiratory fitness improvement and exercise program duration is well established. Nonoyama et al. [23] previously reported an improvement in VO_2 during rehabilitation programs in individuals with respiratory, cardiac, or no comorbidities. Ward et al. [24] highlighted the importance of total training volume, demonstrating greater improvements in VO_2 peak with programs lasting more than 12 weeks compared to those lasting 6–12 weeks, as well as a positive correlation between the total number of training sessions and changes in VO_2 peak.

The studies offer valuable insights into the effects of FES-cycling on cardiorespiratory fitness, with varying protocols and outcomes. Brurok et al. [8] reported a 24% improvement in cardiorespiratory fitness after 8 weeks of FES-cycling, with sessions held three times per week at 35–50 RPM and up to 140 mA intensity. Johnston et al. [25] found a more modest 16% improvement after 6 months of FES-cycling at 50 RPM, 33 Hz frequency, and a pulse width of 150–300 μs, with up to 140 mA intensity. Sessions lasted 60 min, three times per week. Bakkun et al. [11] demonstrated a 12% increase in cardiorespiratory fitness after 16 weeks of FES-cycling, with sessions lasting 18–32 min, twice a week, and using up to 150 mA intensity.

In contrast, Sansare et al. [26] observed a non-significant 5% increase in cardiorespiratory fitness. Participants performed FES-cycling for 30 min, three times a week, over 8 weeks, targeting cycling power corresponding to 50–80% of their Karvonen-predicted target heart rate from a baseline incremental test. They maintained a mean cycling cadence of 45 RPM. These studies highlight the varying degrees of improvement in cardiorespiratory fitness from FES-cycling, suggesting that factors such as program and session duration, intensity, and frequency, as well as individual baseline fitness levels, may influence the outcomes. Further research is needed to determine the most effective parameters for optimizing cardiovascular benefits through FES cycling.

Recommendation

Based on FES-cycling parameters of these several studies, it is recommended a 150–300 μs pulse width, the highest tolerated pulse intensity (usually >100 mA), a 33–50 Hz pulse frequency, a 35–50 RPM cycling cadence and a 30–60 min exercise duration (Fig. 9.3; Table 9.1).

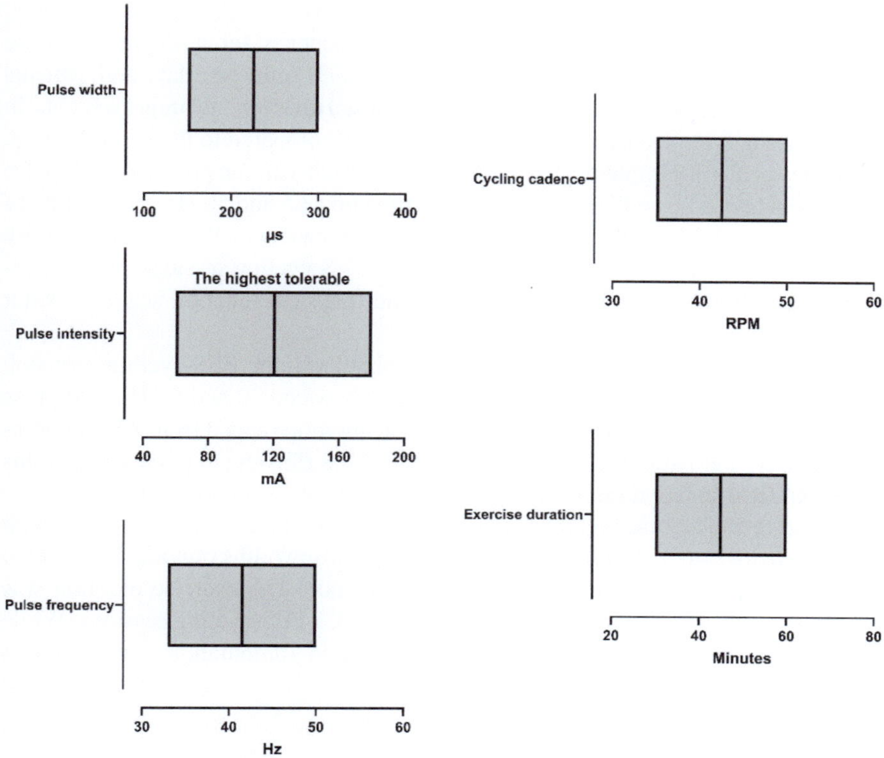

Fig. 9.3 Parameters sets and training routine for cardiorespiratory fitness improvement

Parameters Sets and Training Routine for Muscle Performance and Physical Function Improvement in Hospitalized Patients

Acquired muscle weakness is a common comorbidity during hospitalization. It mainly affects critically ill patients [27], but is not exclusive to this type of patient. Neuromuscular efficiency can be worsened in only 5 days of bed rest, reducing the strength produced for the same neural activation [28].

FES-cycling shows a significant improvement in physical function in hospitalized patients compared to other therapies, with a clinically meaningful difference and high certainty of evidence [1]. This physical function and muscle performance improvement depend on the FES-cycling exercise intensity and volume.

Waldauf et al. [29] used a very low-intensity, high-volume FES-cycling protocol, with pulse intensities ranging from 0 to 60 mA, frequency set at 40 Hz, and pulse width at 250 μs. The exercise protocol averaged 31 min per day, and patients received an average of 6.5 FES-cycling sessions. However, no improvements in muscle strength or physical function were observed compared to the control group.

Berney et al. [30] implemented a low-intensity, high-volume protocol, with pulse intensity between 20 and 30 mA, frequency between 43.5 and 50 Hz, pulse width of 250–300 μs and 35 rotations per minute of cycling cadence. The median exercise duration was 51 min per day, with a median of 5 FES-cycling sessions. While muscle strength showed no significant improvements, physical function was 25% better than in the control group.

Parry et al. [31] used a moderate-intensity, high-volume FES-cycling protocol, with pulse intensities up to 140 mA, frequencies between 30 and 50 Hz, and pulse widths ranging from 300 to 400 μs. The exercise duration ranged from 20 to 60 minutes per day, and patients received an average of 8.6 FES-cycling sessions. In this study, physical function improved by 83% compared to the control group.

Frazão et al. [32] used a high-intensity, low-volume FES-cycling protocol, with pulse intensities up to 180 mA, 75 Hz frequency, pulse widths ranging from 500 to 800 μs and 15 rotations per minute cycling cadence. The exercise duration was 10 min per day, and patients received an average of 5 FES-cycling sessions. While muscle strength improved 117%, physical function (ambulation capacity) was 200% better than in the control group.

Recommendation

Based on these main studies in hospitalized patients, it is recommended a 400–800 μs pulse width, the highest tolerated pulse intensity (usually >100 mA), a 50–75 Hz pulse frequency, a 10–20 rotation per minute cycling cadence and a 10–20 min exercise duration (usually 10 min) (Fig. 9.4; Table 9.1).

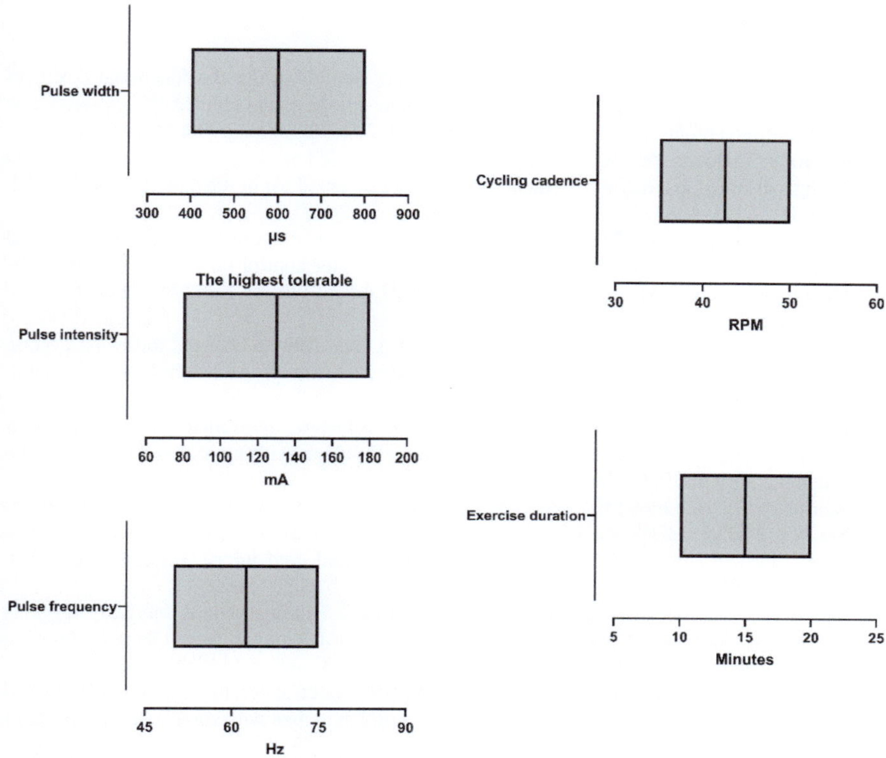

Fig. 9.4 Parameters sets and training routine for muscle performance and physical function improvement in hospitalized patients

The Following Table Brings a Pocket Guideline for FES-Cycling Parameters Set Based on Functional Outcomes

Although this table provides practical values to be used in the clinical practice, it is important to emphasize that the magnitude of electrically evoked force is the only valid indicator of electrical stimulation dose and the main determinant of treatment effectiveness [33]. The parameters recommended in this table for pulse width, intensity, and frequency will be sufficient to achieve the desired clinical outcome in the vast majority of cases. However, in specific conditions (e.g., limb edema, neuropathy, etc.), the parameters required for successful therapy may exceed those recommended in this table.

References

1. Frazão M, de Gomes Figueiredo T, Cipriano G Jr. Should we use the functional electrical stimulation-cycling exercise in clinical practice? Physiological and clinical effects systematic review with meta-analysis. Arch Phys Med Rehabil. 2024;22:S0003-9993(24)01057-8.
2. Sadamoto T, Bonde-Petersen F, Suzuki Y. Skeletal muscle tension, flow, pressure, and EMG during sustained isometric contractions in humans. Eur J Appl Physiol Occup Physiol. 1983;51(3):395–408.
3. Ferrante S, Pedrocchi A, Ferrigno G, Molteni F. Cycling induced by functional electrical stimulation improves the muscular strength and the motor control of individuals with post-acute stroke. Europa Medicophysica-SIMFER 2007 Award Winner. Eur J Phys Rehabil Med. 2008;44(2):159–67.
4. Johnston TE, Modlesky CM, Betz RR, Richard T, Lauer. Muscle changes following cycling and/or electrical stimulation in pediatric spinal cord injury. Arch Phys Med Rehabil. 2011;92(12):1937–43.
5. Backus D, Burdett B, Hawkins L, Manella C, McCully KK, Sweatman M. Outcomes after functional electrical stimulation cycle training in individuals with multiple sclerosis who are nonambulatory. Int J MS Care. 2017;19(3):113–21.
6. Sadowsky CL, Hammond ER, Strohl AB, Commean PK, Eby SA, Damiano DL, Wingert JR, Bae KT, McDonald JW III. Lower extremity functional electrical stimulation cycling promotes physical and functional recovery in chronic spinal cord injury. J Spinal Cord Med. 2013;36(6):623–31.
7. Ratchford JN, Shore W, Hammond ER, Gregory Rose J, Rifkin R, Nie P, Tan K, Quigg ME, de Lateur BJ, Kerr DA. A pilot study of functional electrical stimulation cycling in progressive multiple sclerosis. NeuroRehabilitation. 2010;27(2):121–8.
8. Brurok B, Helgerud J, Karlsen T, Leivseth G, Hoff J. Effect of aerobic high-intensity hybrid training on stroke volume and peak oxygen consumption in men with spinal cord injury. Am J Phys Med Rehabil. 2011;90(5):407–14.
9. Armstrong EL, Boyd RN, Horan SA, Kentish MJ, Ware RS, Carty CP. Functional electrical stimulation cycling, goal-directed training, and adapted cycling for children with cerebral palsy: a randomized controlled trial. Dev Med Child Neurol. 2020;62(12):1406–13.
10. Janssen TW, Beltman JM, Elich P, Koppe PA, Konijnenbelt H, de Haan A, Gerrits KH. Effects of electric stimulation-assisted cycling training in people with chronic stroke. Arch Phys Med Rehabil. 2008;89(3):463–9.
11. Bakkum AJ, de Groot S, Stolwijk-Swüste JM, van Kuppevelt DJ, ALLRISC, van der Woude LH, Janssen TW. Effects of hybrid cycling versus handcycling on wheelchair-specific fitness and physical activity in people with long-term spinal cord injury: a 16-week randomized controlled trial. Spinal Cord. 2015;53(3):395–401.
12. Kern H, Barberi L, Löfler S, Sbardella S, Burggraf S, Fruhmann H, Carraro U, Mosole S, Sarabon N, Vogelauer M, Mayr W, Krenn M, Cvecka J, Romanello V, Pietrangelo L, Protasi F, Sandri M, Zampieri S, Musaro A. Electrical stimulation counteracts muscle decline in seniors. Front Aging Neurosci. 2014;24:189.
13. Demchak TJ, Linderman JK, Mysiw WJ, Jackson R, Suun J, Devor ST. Effects of functional electric stimulation cycle ergometry training on lower limb musculature in acute sci individuals. J Sports Sci Med. 2005;4(3):263–71.
14. Baldi JC, Jackson RD, Moraille R, Mysiw WJ. Muscle atrophy is prevented in patients with acute spinal cord injury using functional electrical stimulation. Spinal Cord. 1998;36(7):463–9.
15. Dolbow DR, Credeur DP, Lemacks JL, Stokic DS, Pattanaik S, Corbin GN, Courtner AS. Electrically induced cycling and nutritional counseling for counteracting obesity after spinal cord injury: A pilot study. J Spinal Cord Med. 2021;44(4):533–40.
16. Yeh C-Y, Tsai K-H, Su F-C, Lo H-C. Effect of a bout of leg cycling with electrical stimulation on reduction of hypertonia in patients with stroke. Arch Phys Med Rehabil. 2010;91(11):1731–6.

17. Dhindsa MS, Merring CA, Brandt LE, Tanaka H, Griffin L. Muscle spasticity associated with reduced whole-leg perfusion in persons with spinal cord injury. J Spinal Cord Med. 2011;34(6):594–9.
18. Shang Y, Lin Y, Henry BA, Cheng R, Huang C, Chen L, Shelton BJ, Swartz KR, Salles SS, Yu G. Noninvasive evaluation of electrical stimulation impacts on muscle hemodynamics via integrating diffuse optical spectroscopies with muscle stimulator. J Biomed Opt. 2013;18:105002.
19. Zulbaran-Rojas A, Lee M, Bara RO, Flores-Camargo A, Spitz G, Finco MG, Bagheri AB, Modi D, Shaib F, Najafi B. Electrical stimulation to regain lower extremity muscle perfusion and endurance in patients with post-acute sequelae of SARS CoV-2: a randomized controlled trial. Physiol Rep. 2023;11(5):e15636.
20. Krause P, Szecsi J, Straube A. Changes in spastic muscle tone increase in patients with spinal cord injury using functional electrical stimulation and passive leg movements. Clin Rehabil. 2008;22(7):627–34.
21. Lo H-C, Tsai K-H, Su F-C, Chang G-L, Yeh C-Y. Effects of a functional electrical stimulation-assisted leg-cycling wheelchair on reducing spasticity of patients after stroke. J Rehabil Med. 2009;41(4):242–6.
22. Ralston KE, Harvey L, Batty J, Bonsan LB, Ben M, Cusmiani R, Bennett J. Functional electrical stimulation cycling has no clear effect on urine output, lower limb swelling, and spasticity in people with spinal cord injury: a randomised cross-over trial. J Physiother. 2013;59(4):237–43.
23. Nonoyama ML, Kin SM, Brooks D, Oh P. Comparison of cardiac rehabilitation outcomes in individuals with respiratory, cardiac or no comorbidities: a retrospective review. Can J Respir Ther. 2016;52(2):43–9.
24. Ward TJC, Plumptre CD, Dolmage TE, Jones AV, Trethewey R, Divall P, Singh SJ, Lindley MR, Steiner MC, Evans RA. Change in VO2peak in response to aerobic exercise training and the relationship with exercise prescription in people with COPD: a systematic review and meta-analysis. Chest. 2020;158(1):131–44.
25. Johnston TE, Smith BT, Mulcahey MJ, Betz RR, Lauer RT. A randomized controlled trial on the effects of cycling with and without electrical stimulation on cardiorespiratory and vascular health in children with spinal cord injury. Arch Phys Med Rehabil. 2009;90(8):1379–88.
26. Sansare A, Harrington AT, Wright H, Alesi J, Behboodi A, Verma K, Lee SCK. Aerobic responses to FES-assisted and volitional cycling in children with cerebral palsy. Sensors (Basel). 2021;21(22):7590.
27. Vanhorebeek I, Latronico N, Van den Berghe G. ICU-acquired weakness. Intensive Care Med. 2020;46(4):637–53.
28. Mulder E, Clément G, Linnarsson D, et al. Musculoskeletal effects of 5 days of bed rest with and without locomotion replacement training. Eur J Appl Physiol. 2015;115:727–38.
29. Waldauf P, Hrušková N, Blahutova B, Gojda J, Urban T, Krajčová A, Fric M, Jiroutková K, Řasová K, Duška F. Functional electrical stimulation-assisted cycle ergometry-based progressive mobility programme for mechanically ventilated patients: randomised controlled trial with 6 months follow-up. Thorax. 2021;76:664–71.
30. Berney S, Hopkins RO, Rose JW, Koopman R, Puthucheary Z, Pastva A, Gordon I, Colantuoni E, Parry SM, Needham DM, Denehy L. Functional electrical stimulation in-bed cycle ergometry in mechanically ventilated patients: a multicentre randomised controlled trial. Thorax. 2021;76:656–63.
31. Parry SM, Berney S, Warrillow S, El-Ansary D, Bryant AL, Hart N, Puthucheary Z, Koopman R, Denehy L. Functional electrical stimulation with cycling in the critically ill: a pilot case-matched control study. J Crit Care. 2014;29(4):695.e1–7.
32. Frazão M, de Lima Martins F, Cipriano G Jr. High-intensity low volume functional electrical stimulation-cycling exercise improves muscle performance and ambulation capacity in hospitalized patients: randomized controlled trial. Artif Organs. 2025;49:1756–64.
33. Maffiuletti NA, Gondin J, Place N, Stevens-Lapsley J, Vivodtzev I, Minetto MA. Clinical use of neuromuscular electrical stimulation for neuromuscular rehabilitation: what are we overlooking? Arch Phys Med Rehabil. 2018;99(4):806–12.

Technological Innovations and Future Perspectives in FES-Cycling

10

Murillo Frazão

Introduction

Functional Electrical Stimulation (FES) cycling has emerged as a transformative technology in the rehabilitation of individuals with mobility impairments. By using electrical impulses to stimulate muscle contractions, FES enables individuals to engage in cycling motions, even in the absence of voluntary muscle control. Over the years, advancements in FES technology have significantly improved its efficacy, accessibility, and adaptability, enhancing both rehabilitation outcomes and the overall user experience. As FES-cycling continues to evolve, it opens up new possibilities for improving physical health, promoting neuroplasticity, and offering greater independence for individuals with disabilities.

The next frontier of FES-cycling innovation lies in the integration of cutting-edge technologies such as artificial intelligence and wireless communication systems. These developments promise to enhance real-time adjustments to stimulation parameters, optimize cycling performance, and tailor rehabilitation programs to individual needs. Furthermore, the convergence of FES with other emerging fields like brain-computer interfaces and advanced robotics could potentially revolutionize the landscape of functional mobility, offering new hope for individuals with severe motor impairments. This chapter explores the current technological innovations driving the field of FES-cycling, as well as the future perspectives that hold the potential to redefine how we approach rehabilitation and mobility for people with disabilities.

M. Frazão (✉)
Lauro Wanderley University Hospital – EBSERH/UFPB, João Pessoa, PB, Brazil
e-mail: murillo.frazao@gmail.com

M. Frazão (ed.), *Functional Electrical Stimulation Cycling in Clinical Practice*,
https://doi.org/10.1007/978-3-032-23937-2_10

Advances in FES Hardware

Wireless FES Technology and Integration of Sensors for Real-Time Feedback and Control

Power delivery to implantable systems is a critical concern in wireless functional electrical stimulation devices. While implantable batteries offer a solution, they come with significant drawbacks, including high cost, larger size, and stringent safety requirements. Wireless power delivery via near-field inductive links has proven to be a more advantageous approach. The harvested power, operational range, and form factors can be optimized to suit specific neuronal applications and usage scenarios, enhancing both functionality and user convenience [1]. Additionally, a closed-loop system for real-time feedback and control plays a vital role in optimizing power utilization. It must be capable of recording evoked responses immediately after the stimulation pulses are terminated [2].

These two key features are essential for the successful application of wireless functional electrical stimulation in motor rehabilitation and health conditioning. First, it is critical to measure biomechanical variables to enable the implementation of closed-loop FES systems. Second, stimulation devices must be capable of delivering pulses to multiple channels, with amplitude and duration values that are dynamically adjusted based on the biomechanical variables.

Wireless systems that integrate these two features into a single device have been proposed, enabling the fully automated design and execution of stimulation protocols. The core principle of distributed architectures is to decentralize processing across a set of physically distributed units. These units' activities are coordinated at higher levels of the architecture, allowing for the delivery of complex functionalities and ensuring seamless operation. Below, we present two examples of wireless FES system architectures.

Cerone et al. proposed a system composed by two sets of wireless modules [3], combining the detection, conditioning and sampling of biomechanical signals (Sensor Unit) with the electric stimulation of skeletal muscles (Stimulation Unit) (Figs. 10.1 and 10.2). The detected signals are sent to a receiver through a Bluetooth link. The Stimulation Unit consists of a wireless (Wi-Fi link), programmable electrical stimulator. Both the Stimulation Unit and Sensor Unit modules communicate either with PC, mobile devices (Smartphone or Tablet) or a single board computer (e.g., Raspberry Pi) configured as a server. The server ensures the acquisition of signals, programming and customization of the stimulation pattern for each stimulation channel and the initiation and termination of the stimulation based on a user-defined program.

Abreu et al. [4] designed an external wireless FES architecture composed of Distributed Stimulation Units, Distributed Measurement Units, and a Control Unit. The Distributed Stimulation Units (Fig. 10.3) locally execute the stimulation profile, generating the stimulus. Meanwhile, the Distributed Measurement Units handle signal acquisition and data processing, which includes tasks such as digital filtering, envelope computation, and threshold detection. The Control Unit is

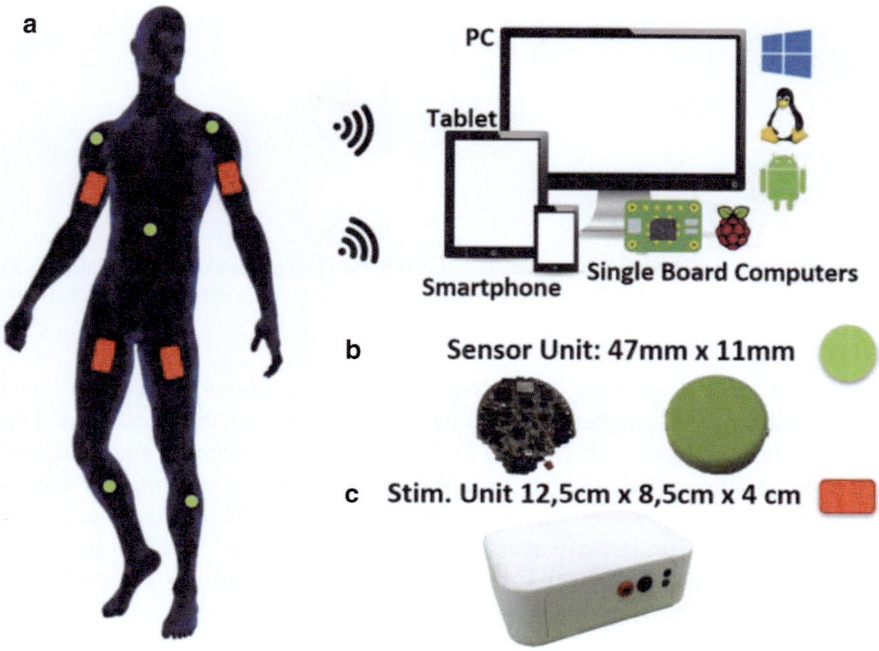

Fig. 10.1 (**a**) System Architecture composed by a set of wireless Sensor Unit (SEU, **b**) and a programmable Stimulation Unit (STU, **c**). (Cerone et al. [3])

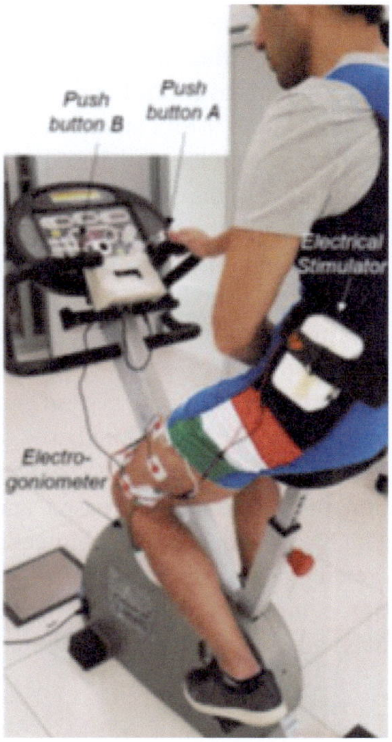

Fig. 10.2 Closed-loop FES-Cycling application of the system. Two STU modules have been programmed to stimulate bilaterally the quadriceps of a single healthy subject. Two SEU modules were used to acquire the stimulation trigger signals from two pushbuttons and the knee joint angles from two electrogoniometers. (Cerone et al. [3])

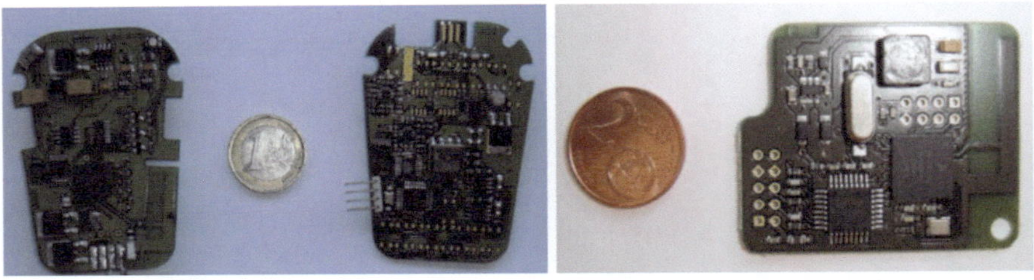

Fig. 10.3 (Left) A distributed stimulation unit is composed of a communication-dedicated board and a stimulation one. (Right) The controller board manages the wireless network and the real-time application. (Abreu et al. [4])

responsible for coordinating the activities of the Distributed Stimulation Units and Distributed Measurement Units to deliver high-level functionalities based on the running FES application (Fig. 10.4). It configures, coordinates, and schedules the tasks of all distributed units. Additionally, the Control Unit remotely modulates relevant parameters of the Distributed Stimulation Units and collects processed data from the Distributed Measurement Units for closed-loop control purposes. Finally, the Control Unit also supervises and ensures the quality of service across the network.

EMG-Driven System

Electromyography (EMG) is a technique used to evaluate and record the electrical activity generated by skeletal muscles, detecting the electrical potential produced by muscle cells when they are activated. An EMG-driven FES-cycling system utilizes EMG signals to control and modulate muscle stimulation during cycling exercises. In this system, EMG signals are collected and processed to detect the user's intent or muscle activity, and based on this information, the system delivers electrical stimulation to the corresponding muscles to assist or initiate movement (Fig. 10.5). The EMG-driven FES-cycling system offers a more natural and adaptive approach to rehabilitation, as it responds in real-time to the user's muscle activation patterns. By using the body's own muscle signals to guide stimulation, the system helps improve motor function, promotes neural plasticity, and enhances the effectiveness of rehabilitation.

During training, the system can adjust the intensity of electrical stimulation and cycling speed in real-time based on voluntary EMG signals [5]. Specifically, if the detected EMG signals are stronger than those from the previous cycle, the stimulation intensity can be increased, and the cycling speed be adjusted for the next cycle. The EMG signals provide biofeedback to the system, enabling real-time control and creating a dynamic, personalized interaction between the subject and the rehabilitation equipment. However, FES-generated artifacts can contaminate the EMG signals, making artifact removal a critical first step. To resolve this, the frequency of

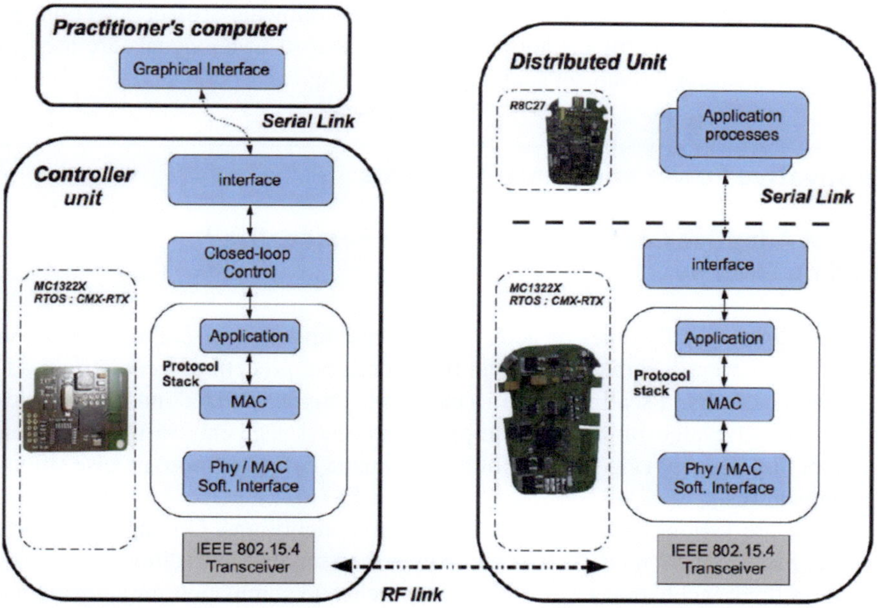

Fig. 10.4 Software modules deployment (Left) On the control unit board, embedded real-time software architecture manages both the wireless communication and the closed loop control. (Right) On the distributed unit board, the embedded micro-controller runs the real-time communication stack and controls the stimulation process. (Abreu et al. [4])

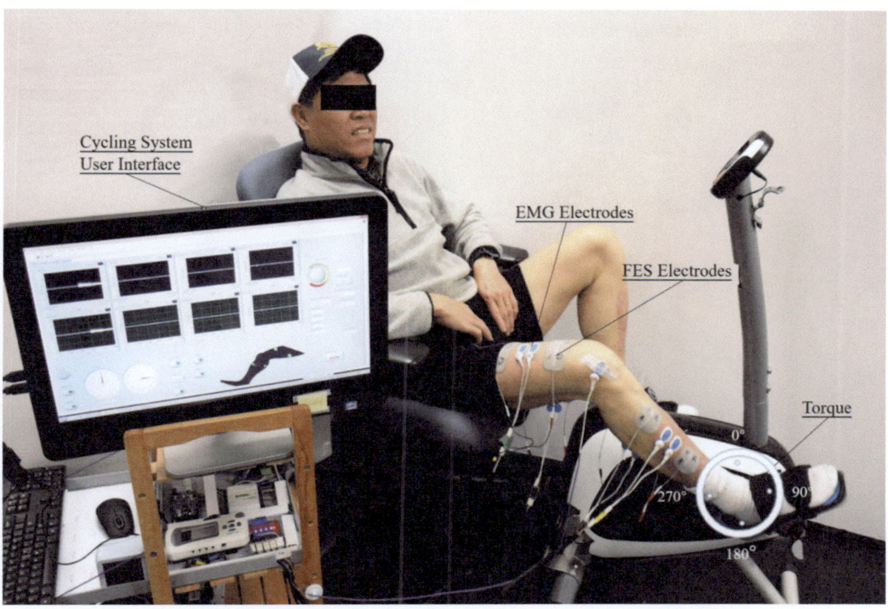

Fig. 10.5 A real-time EMG-driven FES cycling system. (Fang et al. [5])

the stimulus artifact is detected, and EMG signals following artifact detection are set to zero. Once the artifacts are removed, the cleaned EMG signals are used to accurately interpret the subject's intent during cycling.

Innovative Power and Control Systems

Use of Adaptive Control Algorithms for Personalized Cycling Therapy

FES-cycling typically relies on activation patterns linked to the crank angle of the pedals. However, dynamic changes in the underlying predefined geometric models (such as shifts in seating position) can cause desynchronized muscle contractions. Adaptive algorithms that interpret anatomical segments in real-time can prevent this issue, paving the way for the automatic design of more precise stimulation patterns.

There are various methodologies for adaptive algorithms. One approach uses inertial measurement units (IMUs) and, rather than relying on traditional methods, employs thigh inclination as the reference to generate stimulation timing patterns. The tilting angles of both thighs are estimated using an inertial sensor placed above each knee (Fig. 10.6). An IF–THEN rule algorithm then automatically detects the peak angles of the thighs in real time, triggering the start and stop of quadriceps muscle stimulation based on these events (Fig. 10.7) [6].

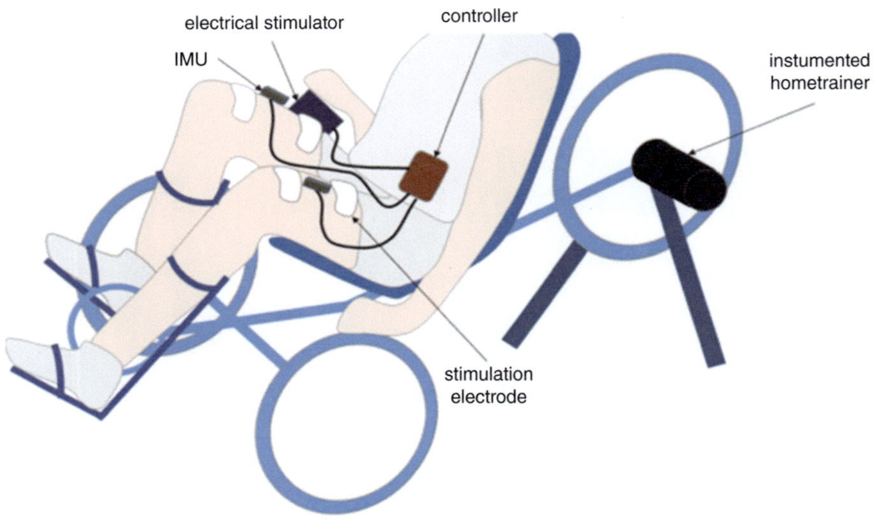

Fig. 10.6 Experimental setup designed to validate the proposed approach. The pilot was equipped with 2 IMUs located on each thigh. IMUs were wired to a Raspberry Pi3© (the controller) communicating with an electrical stimulator. An instrumented home trainer was set on the rear wheel to monitor power output during the experiment. *IMUs* inertial measurement units. (Sijobert et al. [6])

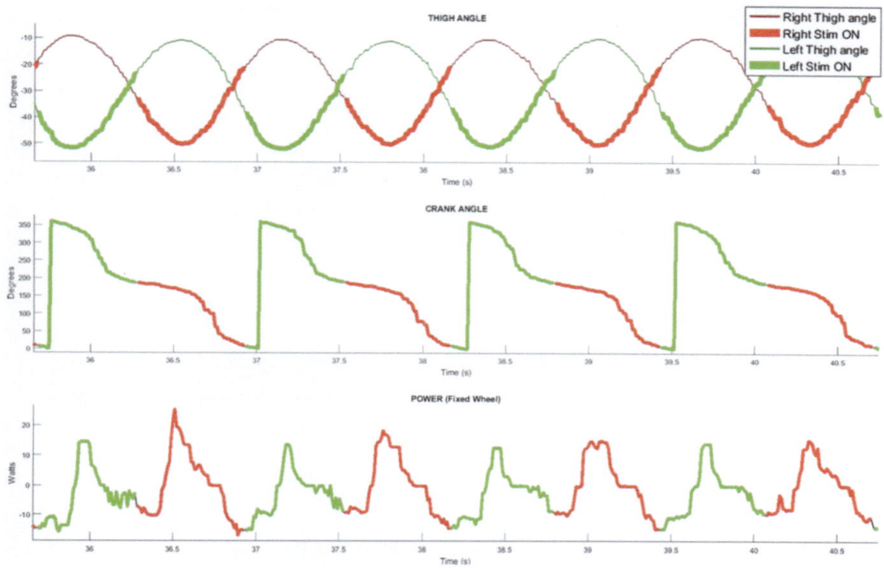

Fig. 10.7 Algorithm triggering process. (Top) Left (green) and right (red) thigh tilting angles; (middle) crank angle; (bottom) developed power. (Sijobert et al. [6])

Another approach is based on the instantaneous phase function [7], which estimates and interprets the instantaneous frequency of the signal using the Hilbert transform. This method generates a posteriori and interprets rhythmic signals as a cyclic phase. The Hilbert transform is a specific singular integral that takes a real-valued function and produces another real-valued function. In the frequency domain, the Hilbert transform has a simple representation: it imparts a phase shift of ±90° to every frequency component of a function, with the direction of the shift determined by the sign of the frequency. The Hilbert transform plays a crucial role in signal processing, as it is a key component of the analytic representation of a real-valued signal.

In this context of different methodologies for control algorithms, Le Guillou et al. [8] conducted an insightful study in which they analyzed three algorithms: Hilbert, BSgonio, and the Gait Cycle Index (GCI) Observer. The algorithms were evaluated on passive cycling inertial data of six participants with spinal cord injury. To ensure standardized comparison, a linear phase reference baseline was employed to define target events at 10%, 40%, 60%, and 90% of the cycling cycle's progress (Fig. 10.8). Limits of agreement of ±10% of the cycle's duration and Lin's concordance correlation coefficient (superior 0.99 indicates perfect agreement, 0.90–0.95 indicates a moderate strength of agreement) were used to assess the accuracy and precision of the event detection in the algorithms.

The delays in event detection were evaluated for each algorithm across 780 events. The analysis revealed that the Hilbert and BSgonio algorithms met the selected criteria, whereas the GCI Observer did not (Tables 10.1 and 10.2; Fig. 10.9).

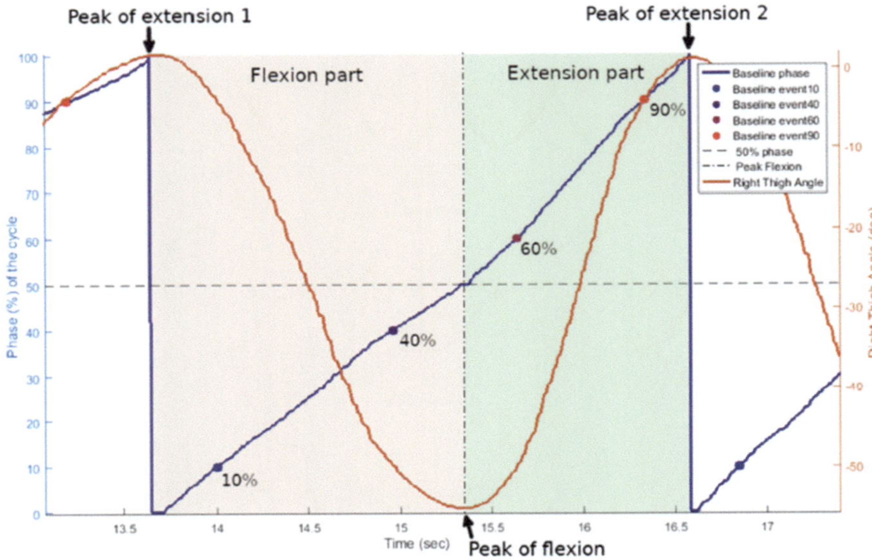

Fig. 10.8 Progression of the cycling movement as a linear phase increasing throughout a pedalling cycle and used as the baseline for reference in comparisons. Inclination angle of the right thigh in degrees during the cycling movement is shown in red (right axis). Phase in percentage of the cycle's progress is shown in blue (left axis). Events for threshold levels (10%, 40%, 60%, and 90%) from the baseline phase are shown in a gradient of colored dots. Flexion and extension phases of the pedalling cycle are highlighted, respectively, with light red and light green areas. (Le Guillou et al. [8])

Table 10.1 Algorithms respective results presented in percentage of cycle duration

	Hilbert ($n = 784$)	BSgonio ($n = 770$)	CGI ($n = 772$)
	Delay in % of cycle duration		
Median delay error	−0.20	0.05	−3.08
Mean delay error ± SD	−0.40 ± 3.16	−0.03 ± 2.22	−4.63 ± 8.70
99% upper LoA	5.17	2.25	8.59
99% lower LoA	−6.34	−2.51	−27.89
Absolute 95% LoA	5.59	2.44	21.57

Le Guillou et al. [8]
LoA limits of agreement

Table 10.2 Algorithms respective Lin's concordance correlation coefficients and confidence intervals

	Hilbert	BSgonio	GCI
Lin CCC	0.9941	0.9971	0.9440
Upper 95% of CI	0.9948	0.9975	0.9511
Lower 95% of CI	0.9932	0.9966	0.9360

Le Guillou et al. [8]
CCC concordance correlation coefficients; *CI* confidence interval

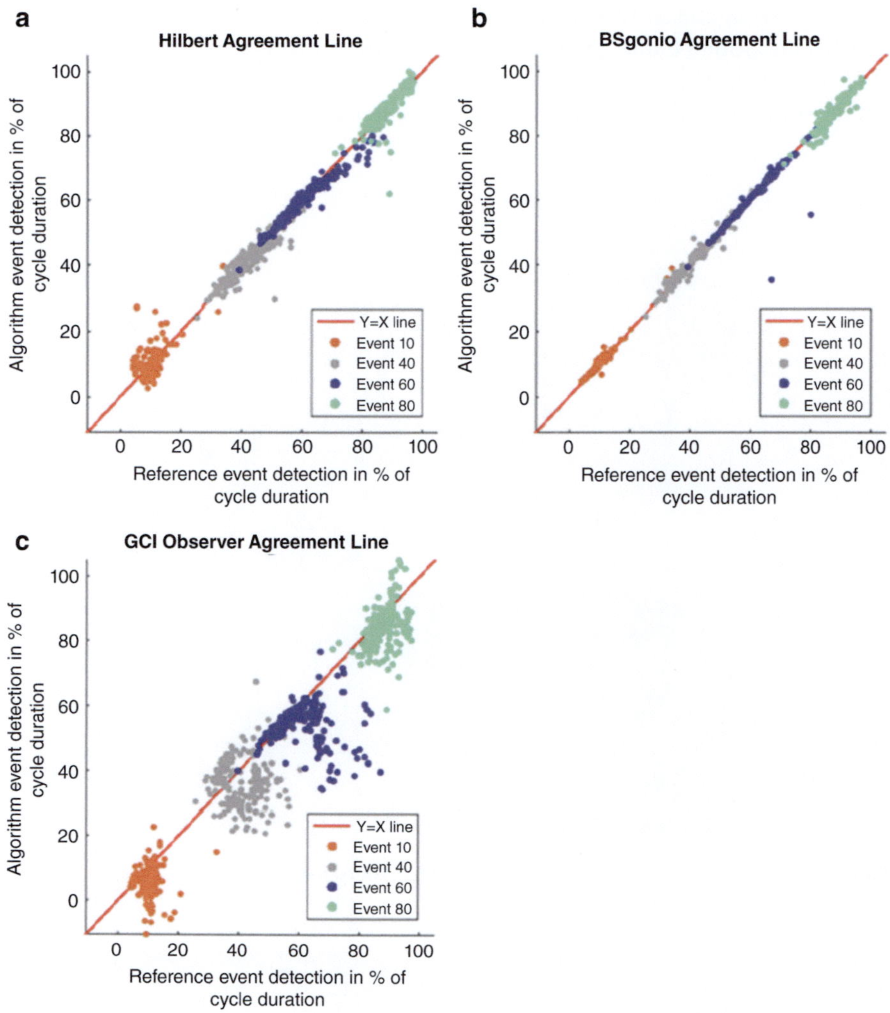

Fig. 10.9 Reference event detections against Algorithm event detections for the three algorithms. The red line is the 45° line through the origin where $Y = X$ corresponding to perfect agreement between the two methods. Presented from left to right: (**a**) Hilbert, (**b**) BSgonio, and (**c**) GCI Observer. Respective event types (10%, 40%, 60%, and 90%) are shown separately with dedicated colors. (Le Guillou et al. [8])

Integration with Other Assistive Technologies

Collaboration Between FES-Cycling and Exoskeletons or Robotic Devices

Functional electrical stimulation and robotic exoskeletons are two technologies that have become widely used to support rehabilitation. While each of these technologies has demonstrated positive outcomes on its own, their combination holds great potential to significantly enhance the rehabilitation process. Integrating robot-assisted lower limb training with FES (Figs. 10.10 and 10.11) appears to be a promising approach, offering more effective movement rehabilitation than either modality on its own [9]. FES activates the patient's muscles in a coordinated manner,

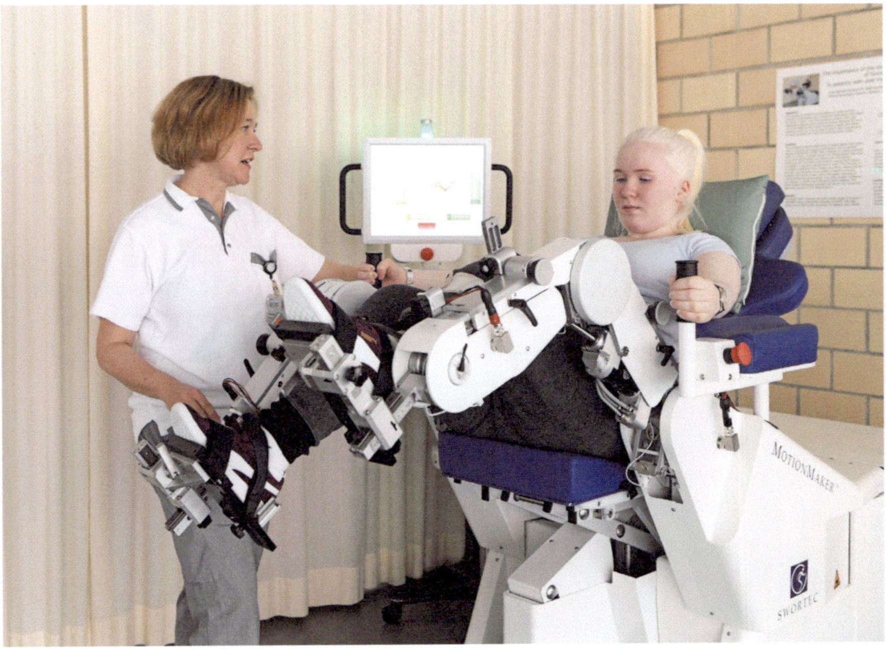

Fig. 10.10 MotionMaker™ stationary robotic device. (Bersch et al. [9])

Fig. 10.11 ROBERT® attached to the lower extremity of a volunteer. The lower leg was mounted into a brace, attached to the robot arm and then the electrodes to measure EMG (white and black nobs) and the electrodes to provide FES (grey pads) were placed on the thigh (knee exercise) or shank (ankle exercise). (Rikhof et al. [10])

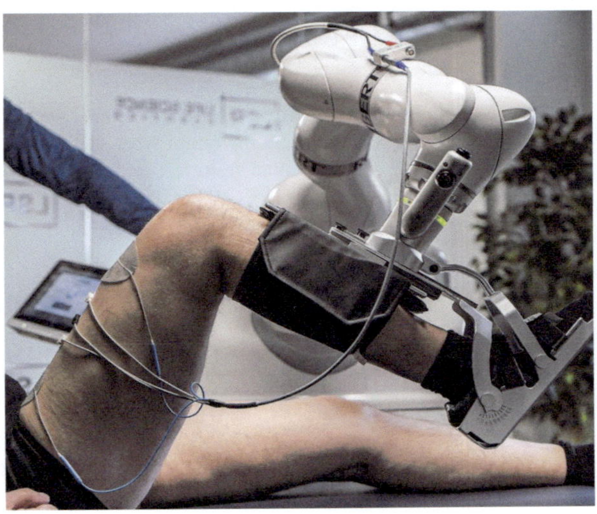

facilitating cortical reorganization, while mechatronic devices, such as robotic exoskeletons, assist in maintaining optimal lower limb movement and provide valuable quantitative assessments of the rehabilitation progress.

A growing area of interest is the development of hybrid exoskeletons that combine FES with active exoskeletons. These hybrid systems address some of the limitations of each individual technology, such as muscle fatigue and difficulties in joint trajectory control, which have previously hindered their widespread adoption in clinical practice. Fully active hybrid exoskeletons, which can dissipate and deliver power to the joints, have become a key focus. These systems compensate for insufficient muscle response in neurologically injured individuals and help mitigate muscle fatigue caused by FES. However, a significant drawback is their energy inefficiency and bulkiness. To improve these systems, future advancements should incorporate closed-loop FES control, which is based on indirect measures of muscle performance.

Assisting robotics enable patients to perform repetitive movements in a controlled manner, while FES-driven muscle activation aids the brain in relearning daily movements, a process known as neuroplasticity. This combination holds great promise in accelerating recovery and improving functional outcomes for individuals with neurological impairments [11].

Additionally, it has been shown that robotic rehabilitation can enhance the intensity of therapy by providing longer therapy durations with adjustable intensity, tailored to individual patients. When combined with FES, robotic rehabilitation can address the limitations of each approach when used separately. This integration can facilitate intensive and active therapy, particularly for patients with more severe impairments. These patients typically face challenges in designing effective, intensive rehabilitation programs. In this context, the combination of robotic therapy and FES presents a promising solution, as robotic exoskeletons provide precise force control and help delay muscle fatigue, while FES facilitates active engagement of the relevant muscles [10].

Use of Virtual Reality to Enhance Training and Rehabilitation Experiences

Virtual reality (VR) is a fully digital, computer-generated environment. There are three primary categories of VR simulations: non-immersive, semi-immersive, and fully-immersive experiences.

Non-immersive virtual experiences are often overlooked as a VR category due to their widespread use in everyday life. This type of VR creates a computer-generated environment but allows users to remain aware of and in control of their physical surroundings (Fig. 10.12). Non-immersive VR systems typically rely on a computer or video game console, a display, and input devices like keyboards, mice, or controllers. Video games serve as a classic example of non-immersive VR.

Semi-immersive virtual experiences provide users with a partially virtual environment. While users may feel as though they are in a different reality when

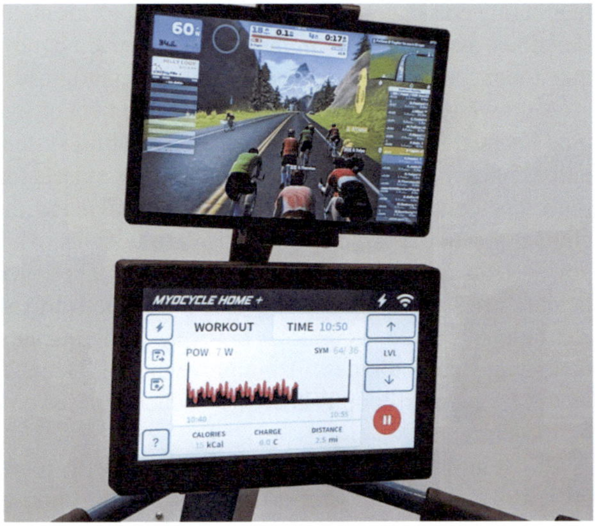

Fig. 10.12 Example of non-immersive virtual reality during FES-cycling exercise. (https://myolyn.com/virtual-reality-cycling-for-neurorecovery-myolyn/)

engaging with the digital imagery, they can still maintain awareness of their physical surroundings (Fig. 10.13). Semi-immersive technology enhances realism through 3D graphics, a concept referred to as "virtual reality depth." The more detailed the graphics, the more immersive the experience. This category of VR is often employed for educational or training purposes and relies on high-resolution displays, powerful computers, projectors, or specialized simulators that partially replicate real-world systems.

Fully immersive simulations offer the most realistic and engaging VR experience, combining both sight and sound (Fig. 10.14). To fully interact with these simulations, users need specialized equipment such as VR glasses or a head-mounted display. These VR headsets provide high-resolution content and a wide field of view. The display is typically split between the user's eyes to create a stereoscopic 3D effect, which, when combined with input tracking, results in a deeply immersive experience.

Rehabilitation activities that are more engaging, such as VR, can be more effective than conventional rehabilitation, as they have the potential to improve adherence and promote long-term use [12, 13]. This is particularly important for exercise therapies, where the benefits gained quickly diminish if the therapies are not performed regularly.

Linsey Duffel and colleagues were pioneers in the use of VR during FES-cycling exercises. They examined the effects of combining FES-cycling with a commercially available virtual reality cycle racing biofeedback system [14] (Fig. 10.15). Eleven participants with incomplete spinal cord injury (SCI) were recruited and completed a 12-session training program. Function was assessed using the bilateral International Standards for Neurological Classification of SCI (ISNC-SCI). Notably, two of the six participants with chronic injuries and four of the five participants with

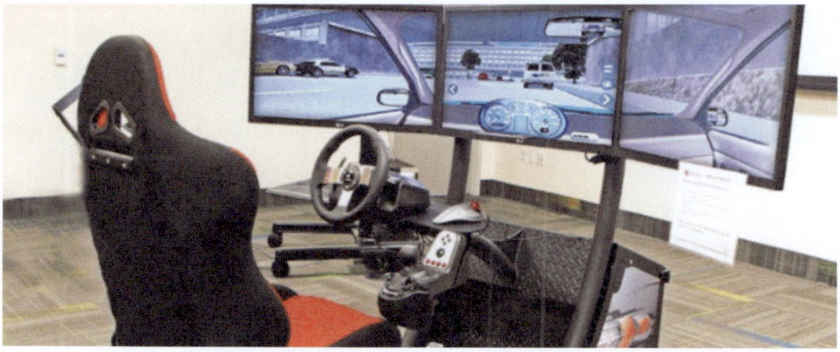

Fig. 10.13 Example of semi-immersive virtual reality. (https://www.google.com/imgres?imgurl=https%3A%2F%2Fmiro.medium.com%2Fmax%2F1388%2F1*YTmKF3spHW5EJMFuRMAdaA.png&tbnid=iRDR5IwtHifL_M&vet=12ahUKEwjj4OOJzpiMAxWWWLgEHfDzMEcQxiAoBXoECAAQJQ..i&imgrefurl=http%3A%2F%2Fwww.clarkeoutdoors.com%2F%3Fc%3Dcla5-111-13301152-3-19-82-semi%2Bimmersive%2Bvirtual%2Breality%2Bexample&docid=F0c3pFzRFZBooM&w=694&h=281&itg=1&q=Non-Immersive%20Virtual%20Reality&ved=2ahUKEwjj4OOJzpiMAxWWWLgEHfDzMEcQxiAoBXoECAAQJQ)

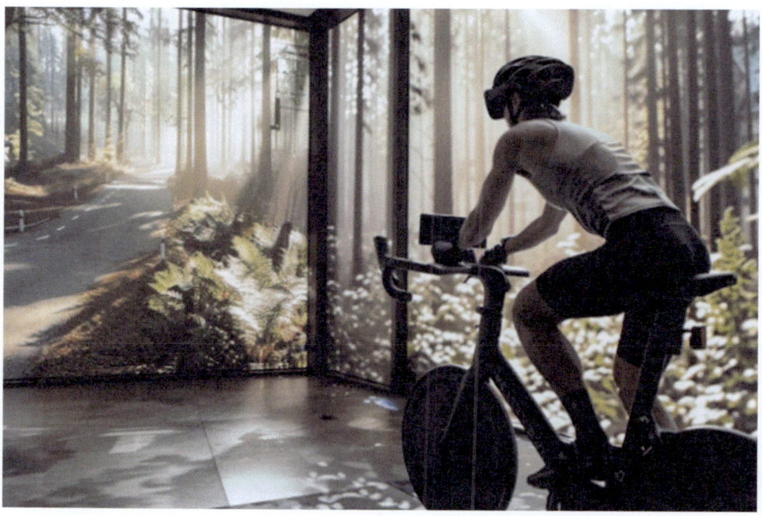

Fig. 10.14 Example of fully-immersive virtual reality. (https://www.nomtek.com/services/ar-vr-development/apple-vision-pro-development/use-cases/vr-indoor-cycling)

sub-acute injuries showed improvements in their ISNC-SCI motor scores, with increases of more than eight points.

Hasnan et al. investigated the exercise response during outdoor versus VR indoor hybrid FES-cycling in individuals with spinal cord injury (SCI) [15]. The mean 30-min VO2 was higher during indoor VR exercise (average VO2 for indoor VR exercise: 1316 ± 53 mL/min vs. outdoor cycling: 1255 ± 53 mL/min; highest VO2 for indoor VR exercise: 1615 ± 67 mL/min vs. outdoor cycling: 1725 ± 67 mL/min).

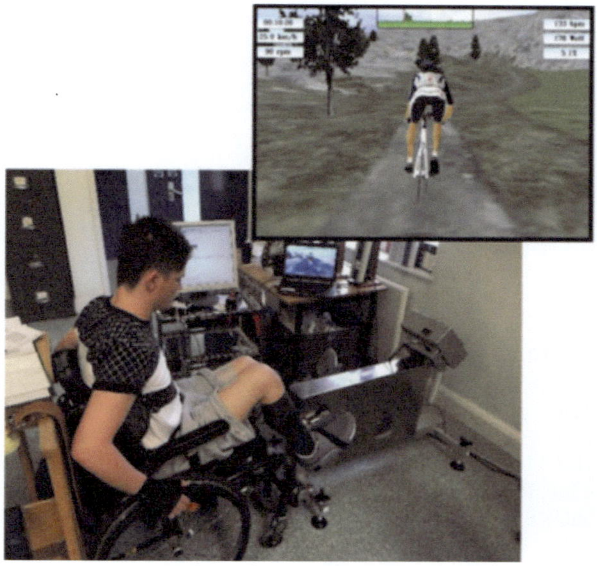

Fig. 10.15 FES-cycling exercise with participants sitting in their own wheelchairs in front of the VR screen. (Duffel et al. [14])

Arm and leg activity counts were significantly greater during indoor VR-assisted hybrid FES-cycling compared to outdoor cycling, with a 42% increase for the arms and a 23% increase for the legs, as well as improved mechanical efficiency. Similar responses were observed for exercise effort and perceptual-psychological outcomes in both modes. (Hasnan et al. [15])

FES and Brain-Computer Interface

Brain-computer interface (BCI) and functional electrical stimulation technologies can be integrated to enhance the rehabilitation process. In this approach, the user is first required to either imagine or perform specific movements. The resulting electroencephalogram (EEG) signals are captured by electrodes placed over the sensory-motor areas of the brain, then transmitted to an amplifier. After amplification and digitization, the signals are processed by a computer that analyzes the data and controls a 2D feedback display on the screen (Fig. 10.16). Similar to traditional therapy, users engage in motor imagery and receive real-time feedback. The key innovation in this system is the direct, real-time connection between brain activity and feedback. Visual and FES feedback is provided to the user only when they correctly imagine the movement, reinforcing accurate motor imagery [11].

Recent studies have demonstrated that combining a brain-computer interface system with functional electrical stimulation holds significant potential for creating an electronic neural bypass, capable of activating muscles affected by paralysis in individuals with stroke, spinal cord injuries, and potentially those with locked-in syndrome [16]. This integrated approach can enhance motor control by strengthening weakened muscles or restore motor function by reintroducing lost movements.

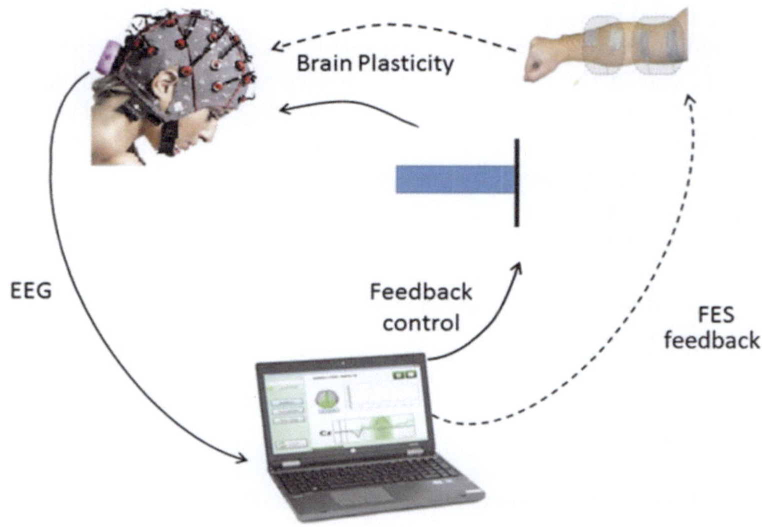

Fig. 10.16 The schematic view of the BCI and FES system. (Irimia et al. [11])

In a BCI-FES-cycling system, brain activity patterns associated with attempted movements are detected and used to trigger the delivery of FES to the corresponding muscles, facilitating coordinated movement and promoting rehabilitation.

Advancements in Artificial Intelligence

Predictive Analytics for Customizing FES-Cycling Protocols Based on Patient Data

Artificial Intelligence (AI) has shown significant promise in enhancing FES-cycling systems, offering a more personalized and adaptive approach to rehabilitation. By leveraging AI algorithms, such as reinforcement learning, these systems can continuously optimize and fine-tune the stimulation patterns based on real-time feedback, leading to improved cycling performance. AI can analyze complex data, including neural signals and muscle responses, to adapt the FES parameters to the individual needs of the user. This adaptability allows for more effective muscle activation, enhancing motor function and improving outcomes.

Moreover, AI in FES-cycling has the potential to reduce reliance on invasive sensors or additional hardware. AI-driven models can learn cycling patterns from limited data and then apply them to various cycling configurations. This can significantly reduce the time required for setup and calibration, making the technology more accessible and user-friendly for both patients and clinicians. By integrating AI into FES-cycling systems, rehabilitation can become more efficient and tailored to individual progress, enhancing recovery and overall quality of life for patients.

Wannawas and Faisal [17] proposed an AI-driven method for identifying patterns without the need for additional hardware or sensors. The approach begins by using reinforcement learning to identify model-based patterns in customized cycling models. The method then fine-tunes these patterns using real cycling data and offline reinforcement learning. The system was tested both in simulation and experimentally on a stationary tricycle, demonstrating its ability to robustly generate model-based patterns for various cycling configurations. In experimental trials, the model-based pattern resulted in higher cycling speeds compared to an EMG-based pattern. Furthermore, using just 100 seconds of cycling data, the method was able to fine-tune the pattern to achieve improved cycling performance.

Conclusions

The technological innovations in FES-cycling have already made significant strides in improving rehabilitation outcomes for individuals with mobility impairments. From advancements in stimulation protocols to the integration of real-time feedback mechanisms, these innovations have enhanced the precision, customization, and overall effectiveness of FES systems. As the field continues to evolve, the integration of cutting-edge technologies such as AI, machine learning, and brain-computer interfaces will open new pathways for personalized, adaptive therapies that are both more efficient and user-friendly. The future of FES-cycling holds the promise of not only improving physical function and health but also empowering individuals to regain independence and improve their quality of life.

However, the continued development of these technologies will require overcoming challenges related to cost, accessibility, and scalability, particularly in low-resource settings. As research and innovation progress, collaboration between engineers, clinicians, and patients will be crucial to ensure that FES-cycling systems are designed to meet the diverse needs of users. Looking ahead, the potential for FES-cycling to revolutionize rehabilitation and mobility for individuals with disabilities is immense, and with sustained effort, it may lead to breakthroughs that were once thought impossible, reshaping the future of functional mobility.

References

1. Nag S, Sharma D. Wirelessly powered stimulator and recorder for neuronal interfaces. In: Annual international conference of the IEEE Engineering in Medicine and Biology Society, Boston, MA, USA; 2011. p. 5612–6.
2. Lynch CL, Popovic MR. Functional electrical stimulation. IEEE Control Syst Mag. 2008;28(2):40–50.

3. Cerone GL, Vieira TMM, Botter A, Gazzoni M. Design of a Wireless, modular and programmable neuromuscular electrical stimulator. In: Annual international conference of the IEEE Engineering in Medicine and Biology Society; 2019. p. 3815–8.
4. Andreu D, Sijobert B, Toussaint M, Fattal C, Azevedo-Coste C, Guiraud D. Wireless electrical stimulators and sensors network for closed loop control in rehabilitation. Front Neurosci. 2020;14:117.
5. Fang Y, Chen S, Wang X, Leung KWC, Wang X, Tong K-Y. Real-time electromyography-driven functional electrical stimulation cycling system for chronic stroke rehabilitation. In: Annual international conference of the IEEE Engineering in Medicine and Biology Society; 2018. p. 2515–8.
6. Sijobert B, Le Guillou R, Fattal C, Coste CA. FES-induced cycling in complete SCI: a simpler control method based on inertial sensors. Sensors (Basel). 2019;19(19):4268.
7. Boashash B. Estimating and interpreting the instantaneous frequency of a signal. I. Fundamentals. Proc IEEE. 1992;80:520–38.
8. Le Guillou R, Schmoll M, Sijobert B, et al. A novel framework for quantifying accuracy and precision of event detection algorithms in FES-cycling. Sensors (Basel). 2021;21(13):4571.
9. Bersch I, Alberty M, Fridén J. Robot-assisted training with functional electrical stimulation enhances lower extremity function after spinal cord injury. Artif Organs. 2022;46(10):2009–14.
10. Rikhof CJH, Leerskov KS, Prange-Lasonder GB, et al. Combining robotics and functional electrical stimulation for assist-as-needed support of leg movements in stroke patients: a feasibility study. Med Eng Phys. 2024;130:104216.
11. Poboroniuc MS, Irimia DC. Intelligent functional electrical stimulation. In: Costin H, Schuller B, Florea AM, editors. Recent advances in intelligent assistive technologies: paradigms and applications, intelligent systems reference library. Cham: Springer Nature; 2020. p. 61–82.
12. Campo-Prieto P, Cancela-Carral JM, Rodríguez-Fuentes G. Wearable immersive virtual reality device for promoting physical activity in Parkinson's disease patients. Sensors (Basel). 2022;22(9):3302.
13. Doré B, Gaudreault A, Everard G, et al. Acceptability, feasibility, and effectiveness of immersive virtual technologies to promote exercise in older adults: a systematic review and meta-analysis. Sensors (Basel). 2023;23(5):2506.
14. Duffell LD, Paddison S, Alahmary AF, Donaldson N, Burridge J. The effects of FES cycling combined with virtual reality racing biofeedback on voluntary function after incomplete SCI: a pilot study. J Neuroeng Rehabil. 2019;16(1):149.
15. Hasnan N, Hamzaid NA, Magenthran V, Davis GM. Exercise responses during outdoor versus virtual reality indoor arm+FES-leg cycling in individuals with spinal cord. Injury. 2024;3:207–14.
16. Canny E, Vansteensel MJ, van der Salm SMA, Müller-Putz GR, Berezutskaya J. Boosting brain–computer interfaces with functional electrical stimulation: potential applications in people with locked-in syndrome. J Neuroeng Rehabil. 2023;20:157.
17. Wannawas N, Faisal AA. Towards AI-controlled movement restoration: learning FES-cycling stimulation with reinforcement learning. In: IEEE international conference on rehabilitation robotics; 2023. p. 1–6.

Index

A
Active-assisted cycling, 35
Advanced age
  effects of, 173, 174
  rationale for FES-cycling exercise, 174, 175
Aerobic enzyme activity, 160
Ageing, 174
Alternating current, 17
Aluminum electrodes, 18
Alveolar-capillary membrane, 159
Amperes (A), 13
Amplitude/intensity of current, 13, 14
Analgesic tolerance, 23
Apple™ game, 9
Artificial intelligence (AI), 229, 230
  predictive analytics, 229, 230
Ashworth scale, 89–91
Australian current, 17

B
BerkelBike, 192
Bicycle modifications, 8
Bicycles, 44
BioTone™ toolkit, 90
Biphasic currents, 15
Blood lactate, 79
  cardiorespiratory fitness, 79
Blood pressure, 56–57
  FES cycling, 56–57
Bone density, 170–171
  orthopedic conditions, 170–171
Bone health, 113–116
Brain-computer interface (BCI), 228, 229

C
Carbonic gas production (VCO_2), 52–53
Cardiac mechanics, 157
Cardiac output, 55–56
  cardiorespiratory fitness, 78, 79
Cardiopulmonary exercise test (CPET), 48, 71, 82–84
  ventilatory thresholds and determination of exercise intensity, 84, 86
Cardiorespiratory fitness (VO_2), 157
  FES-cycling technology, 71, 73, 75–77
    blood lactate, 79
    cardiac output, 78, 79
    heart rate, 77, 78
    peripheral oxygenation, 80
    stroke volume, 78
    ventilatory capacity, 80–82
Cardiorespiratory fitness improvement, 207, 208
  FES-cycling guidelines, 207, 208
Cardiovascular and metabolic function, 49–50, 110–112
  exercise on, 49–50
Cardiovascular and metabolic health
  stroke, 120
Cardiovascular disturbances, 110
Cardiovascular responses, FES cycling
  blood pressure, 56, 57
  cardiac output, 55, 56
  heart rate, 54, 55
  peripheral muscle oxygen extraction, 57
  stroke volume, 55

M. Frazão (ed.), *Functional Electrical Stimulation Cycling in Clinical Practice*,
https://doi.org/10.1007/978-3-032-23937-2

Caspase-3, 165
Cerebral palsy (CP)
  clinical application, challenges and future directions in, 125
  considerations with using FES-assisted cycling, 124, 125
  FES-assisted cycling, clinical benefits of, 124
  FES-assisted cycling with, 123
  impact of, 122
  issues with cycling as exercise, 123
  novel interventions, 122
Chronic kidney disease (CKD)
  impact of, 165
  rationale for FES-cycling exercise, 166
Chronic obstructive pulmonary disease (COPD)
  FES-cycling exercise, rationale for, 157, 158
  impact of, 156, 157
Circulation improvement, 24
Circulation/pressure injuries, 109, 110
Classical Russian Current, 16
Closed-loop control, 31, 32, 36, 40
Closed-loop FES-Cycling application, 217
Closed-loop system, 216
Competition, 183, 184
  competitive FES-cycling, equipment for
    controllers and stimulation units, 191
    electrodes, 190, 191
    stationary FES cycling ergometers for training, 191, 192
  international competitions
    Cybathlon, 192–194
    Lyon Cyber Days, 194, 195
  parameter sets/technology specificities
    parameter settings for, 188, 189
    technological specificities, 189
  and recreational FES-cycling, 190
    factors influencing performance, 190
  rules and regulations
    Cybathlon 2016, 195
    Cybathlon 2019, 195, 196
    Cybathlon 2024, 196
  training routine
    development of, 184, 185
    progress monitoring, 188
    training components, 187
    training frequency, 186
    training phases, 186, 187
Computer program, 8, 9
Continuous passive motion, 170
Continuous sensory input, 22
Control algorithms, 40
Controllers unit, 191
  competition, 191
Crank position sensors, 37
Cross-sectional area (CSA), 103
Cybathlon, 184, 192–194, 197
  Cybathlon 2016, 195
  Cybathlon 2019, 195, 196
  Cybathlon 2024, 196
Cycle ergometers
  with integrated feedback, 91
    feedback and progress monitoring, 92
    power measurement, 91
    resistance control, 92

D

Data analysis software, 92
Determination of exercise intensity, 84–86
Distributed stimulation units, 218

E

Eccentric contractions, 49
Electrical stimulation, 2, 22
  control algorithms, 40
  crank position sensors, 37
  electrode placement, 18–20
  inertial measurements units, 37–39
  modes, 40
  physiological basis of, 13
    amplitude/intensity of current, 13, 14
    frequency, 14, 15
    pulse width, 14, 15
    ramp time, 17, 18
    waveforms, 15–17
  physiological effects of, 20
    circulation improvement, 24
    muscle re-education, 22
    muscle spasticity, reduction of, 24, 25
    muscle strengthening, 20, 21
    pain management, 22–24
  principles of, 11, 12
  safety considerations and contraindications, 25, 26
  types of, 12, 13
Electrode inhomogeneities, 34
  skin and, 34
Electrode placement, 18–20
Electrodes, 32
  characteristics, 33-34
    material, 33
    requirements, 33, 34
    skin and electrode inhomogeneities, 34

Electromyography (EMG) sensors, 37–40, 218, 220
Electronic control systems, 35
Electrostimulator, 18
Electrotherapy, 11
Energy cost, 73
Energy expenditure, 53–54
Equipment types
  FES-cycling, 40
    non-static, 42–44
    static, 40–42
Ergometer devices interaction, 34–36
  control algorithms, 40
  crank position sensors, 37
  inertial measurements units, 37–39
  modes, 40
Exercise physiology
  metabolism, cardiovascular function and respiration, 49, 50
  muscular and neuromuscular responses, 49
  physical exercise and phases, 49
  principles of, 48, 49
Exoskeletons/robotic devices, 223, 225
External power, 51–52
  development of, 51–52

F

Fast-twitch type IIb fibers, 160
Feedback and progress monitoring, 92
FES-cycling, application of
  clinical benefits
    bone health, 113, 115, 116
    cardiovascular and metabolic function, 110–112
    pain, 116
    spasticity reduction and motor control, 112–114
  paralyzed muscles, stimulation of
    circulation/pressure injuries, 109, 110
    muscle health, 105, 106, 108, 109
  treatment protocols, 116, 117
FES-cycling, equipment
  competition
    controllers and stimulation units, 191
    electrodes, 190, 191
    stationary FES cycling ergometers for training, 191, 192
FES-cycling technology, 63, 64
  functional assessment
    cardiopulmonary exercise test, 82–84, 86
    mobility, 86–88
    spasticity, 89–91
  functional assessment, challenges in
    establishing consistent standards, 93
    physiological challenges, 94
  functional assessment, interpretation of, 93
  functional outcomes in
    cardiorespiratory fitness, 71, 73, 75–82
    muscle efficiency, 68, 71, 73
    muscle strength and power, 64–66, 68
    muscle synergy, 67–69
  technological tools for assessment
    cycle ergometers with integrated feedback, 91, 92
    data analysis software, 92
Frequency, 14, 15
Functional electrical stimulation (FES) cycling, 1, 3, 12, 31, 47, 101, 105, 195, 197, 215
  artificial intelligence, 229, 230
    predictive analytics, 229, 230
  application, 3
  cardiovascular responses, 48
    blood pressure, 56, 57
    cardiac output, 55, 56
    heart rate, 54, 55
    peripheral muscle oxygen extraction, 57
    stroke volume, 55
  characteristics, 32
    stimulation and control unit, 32
  dates, 1
  definition of, 2
  electrical stimulation and ergometer devices interaction, 36
    control algorithms, 40
    crank position sensors, 37
    electromyography sensors, 37, 39
    inertial measurements units, 37, 38
    modes, 40
  electrode characteristics, 32
    material, 33
    requirements, 33, 34
    skin and electrode inhomogeneities, 34
  equipment types
    non-static, 42–44
    static, 40–42
  ergometer devices, 34–36
  exercise physiology
    electrical stimulation and physical exercise, 50
    metabolism, cardiovascular function and respiration, 49, 50
    muscular and neuromuscular responses, 49

Functional electrical stimulation (FES)
cycling (*cont.*)
physical exercise and phases, 49
principles of, 48, 49
hardware
EMG-driven system, 218, 220
wireless FES technology and integration of sensors, 216–219
historical development of
bicycle modifications, 8
computer program, 8, 9
creation of, 5, 6
electrical stimulation and pathway, early beginnings of, 5
first device, 8
Glaser, Roger M., 7
Heaton, Harry H., 7
Petrofsky, Jerrold S., 6
Phillips, C.A., 7
innovation, 215
innovative power and control systems, 220–223
personalized cycling therapy, adaptive control algorithms for, 220–223
integration with assistive technologies
and brain-computer interface, 228, 229
and exoskeletons/robotic devices, 223, 225
virtual reality, 225, 226, 228
internal and external power development, 50–52
metabolic responses, 47
carbonic gas production, 52, 53
energy expenditure, 53, 54
lactate production, 53
oxygen uptake, 52
purpose, 3
in stimulating muscles, 2, 3
technology, 4
ventilatory responses, 48, 57, 59
Functional recovery, 120
stroke, 120

G
Gait, 120
speed, 86
stroke, 120
Gait Cycle Index (GCI) Observer, 221
Gate Control Theory of Pain, 22
Glaser, Roger M., 7
GLUT4, 164
Gross Motor Function Classification System (GMFCS), 88

H
Heart failure
FES-cycling exercise, rationale for, 160, 161
impact of, 159, 160
Heart rate, 54–55
cardiorespiratory fitness, 77–78
Heaton, Harry H., III, 7
Hemiplegia, 118
stroke, 118
High-intensity interval training (HIIT), 197
Hilbert, BSgonio, 221

I
Imbalance, 85
Implanted electrodes, 191
Implanted pulse generators (IPGs), 185
Inertial measurement units (IMUs), 37, 220
Intensive care unit (ICU), 168
Internal and external power development, 50–52
International competitions
Cybathlon, 192–194
Lyon Cyber Days, 194, 195
International Standards for Neurological Classification of SCI (ISNC-SCI), 226
Isokinetic dynamometry, 65
Isokinetic modes, 34, 35
Isopower exercise, 51

J
Joint mobility, 170
orthopedic conditions, 170

K
Knee extension, 87

L
Lactate production, 53
Lactic acid, 53
Left ventricular dysfunction, 159
Leisure, 183, 184
training routine
development of, 184, 185
progress monitoring, 188
training components, 187
training frequency, 186
training phases, 186, 187

Long COVID
  impact of, 167, 168
  rationale for FES-cycling exercise, 169
Lyon Cyber Days, 194, 195

M

Magnetic resistance units, 35
Maximal voluntary strength, 64
Mechanical activation of circulation, 24
Metabolic disease
  obesity and type 2 diabetes, 163
    rationale for FES-cycling exercise, 163–165
Metabolic gas analysis, 78
Metabolic responses, 47
  carbonic gas production, 52, 53
  energy expenditure, 53, 54
  lactate production, 53
  oxygen uptake, 52
Metabolism, 49–50
  exercise on, 49–50
Mobility
  gait speed, 86
  gross motor function, 87, 88
  motricity index, 86, 87
  physical function in intensive care test score, 87
  upright motor control test, 86, 87
Monophasic/direct current, 15
MOTOmed, 192
Motor control, 112–114
  stroke, 118
Motorized FES-cycling ergometers, 34
Motorized FES-cycling systems, 35
Motor neuron, 21
  afferent and efferent impulse of, 21
Motricity index, 86, 87
Multiple sclerosis (MS)
  application of functional electrical stimulation cycling, 126–132
  clinical benefits, 133, 134
  considerations for, 135
  future directions, 136
  impact of, 125, 126
  training effects, 133
  training protocols, 129, 133
Muscle damage, 167
Muscle efficiency, 68, 71, 73
  FES-cycling technology, 68, 71, 73
Muscle health, 105, 106, 108, 109
Muscle hypertrophy
  FES-cycling guideline, 203, 204
    recommendation, 204
Muscle mass
  FES-cycling effects on, 152, 153
  orthopedic conditions, 171–172
Muscle performance
  improvement, 209, 210
    FES-cycling guidelines, 209, 210
  orthopedic conditions, 172
Muscle re-education, 22
Muscle spasticity, reduction of, 24, 25
Muscle strength and power, 20, 21, 64–66, 68
  FES-cycling technology, 64–66, 68
Muscle synergy, 67–69
  FES-cycling technology, 67–69
Muscle trophism, 202
MyoCycle, 192

N

Nervous system, 117, 118
  pathophysiology and impact on, 117, 118
Neurological diseases, 101, 102
  cerebral palsy
    clinical application, challenges and future directions in, 125
    considerations with using FES-assisted cycling, 124, 125
    FES-assisted cycling, clinical benefits of, 124
    FES-assisted cycling with, 123
    impact of, 122
    issues with cycling as exercise, 123
    novel interventions, 122
  FES-cycling, application of
    clinical benefits, 110–116
    mobility with SCI, 105
    paralyzed muscles, stimulation of, 105, 106, 108–110
    treatment protocols, 116, 117
  multiple sclerosis
    application of functional electrical stimulation cycling, 126–132
    clinical benefits, 133, 134
    considerations for, 135
    future directions, 136
    impact of, 125, 126
    training effects, 133
    training protocols, 129, 133
  neuromuscular diseases, 136
    considerations and limitations, 139
    evidence and clinical applications, 137–139
    FES-cycling, rationale for, 136, 137

Neurological diseases (*cont.*)
spinal cord injury
complete and incomplete, 104, 105
impact of, 102
motor control, muscle strength, and mobility, 102, 103
stroke
cardiovascular and metabolic health, 120
gait and functional recovery, 120
motor control, hemiplegia, and functional limitations, 118
muscle strength and endurance, 119
nervous system, pathophysiology and impact on, 117, 118
quality of life and participation, 120
rehabilitation, application of, 119
spasticity, 120
treatment protocols and practical considerations, 120–122
Neuromuscular diseases (NMDs), 136
considerations and limitations, 139
evidence and clinical applications, 137–139
FES-cycling, rationale for, 136, 137
Neuromuscular electrical stimulation (NMES), 3, 12, 47
Neuroplasticity, 225
Neurorehabilitation, 139
Nitric oxide, 24
Non-invasive cardiac output monitors, 79
Non-motorized FES-cycling ergometers, 35
Non-neurological diseases, 151
advanced age
effects of, 173, 174
rationale for FES-cycling exercise, 174, 175
chronic kidney disease
impact of, 165
rationale for FES-cycling exercise, 166
chronic obstructive pulmonary disease
FES-cycling exercise, rationale for, 157, 158
impact of, 156, 157
heart failure
FES-cycling exercise, rationale for, 160, 161
impact of, 159, 160
hospitalized patients, 151, 152
muscle mass and performance, FES-cycling effects on, 152, 153
physical function and ambulation capacity, 153, 155
long COVID
impact of, 167, 168
rationale for FES-cycling exercise, 169
metabolic disease, 163–165
obesity and type 2 diabetes, 163–165
orthopedic conditions, 170
bone density, 170, 171
joint mobility, 170
muscle mass, 171, 172
muscle performance, 172
pain, 173
Non-static FES-cycling equipment, 42, 43
bicycles, 44
challenges, 44
resistance generation, 44
tricycles, 43
Non-stationary ergometers, 51

O

Obesity, 163
Opioids, 23
Orthopedic conditions, 170
bone density, 170, 171
joint mobility, 170
muscle mass, 171, 172
muscle performance, 172
pain, 173
Oxygen delivery, 159
Oxygen uptake (VO_2), 52

P

Pain, 116
management, 22–24
orthopedic conditions, 173
Paralysis, 1, 6
Paralyzed muscles
stimulation of
circulation/pressure injuries, 109, 110
muscle health, 105, 106, 108, 109
Pedulum test, 89
Peripheral muscle oxygen extraction, 57
Peripheral oxygenation, 80
Personalized cycling therapy, adaptive control algorithms for, 220–223
Petrofsky, Jerrold S., 6
Phillips, Chandler A., 7
Physical function, 153, 155
improvement
FES-cycling guidelines, 209, 210
non-neurological diseases, 153, 155
Physical Function in Intensive Care Test Score (PFIT-S), 87, 89
Power measurement, 91
Practical FES-cycling guideline, 201
cardiorespiratory fitness improvement, parameters sets and training routine for, 207, 208

muscle performance and physical function improvement, parameters sets and training routine for, 209, 210
parameters sets and training routine, 202, 205
muscle hypertrophy, 203, 204
power, 203
strength, 202, 203
spasticity reduction, parameters sets and training routine for, 206, 207
Pressure ulcers, 109
Pulse amplitude, 13
Pulsed current delivers, 17
Pulse width, 14, 15

Q
Quadratic monophasic current, 16
Quality of life, 120
stroke, 120

R
Ramp time, 17, 18
Recreational FES-cycling
competition and, 190
factors influencing performance, 190
Rectangular biphasic current, 16
Rehabilitation strategies, 151
Resistance control, 92
Respiration, 49–50
exercise on, 49–50
Restorative therapies, 192
ROBERT®, 224, 225

S
Safety, 25, 26
electrical stimulation, 25, 26
Sarcopenia, 158
Self-adhesive electrodes, 18
Self-adhesive hydrogel electrodes, 33
Silicone–carbon electrodes, 18
Sinusoidal biphasic current, 16
Skeletal muscle insulin resistance, 163
Skeletal muscle system, 156
Spasticity, 112
Ashworth scale, 89, 91
pendulum test, 89, 90
reduction, 112–114
FES-cycling guidelines, 206, 207
stroke, 120
Spinal cord injury (SCI), 183
complete and incomplete, 104, 105
impact of, 102
mobility with, 105
motor control, muscle strength and mobility, 102, 103
Sponges, 18
Static FES-cycling systems, 40–42
Stationary FES cycling ergometers, 191–192
Stimulation cost, 70
Stimulation unit, 191
competition, 191
Stroke
cardiovascular and metabolic health, 120
gait and functional recovery, 120
motor control, hemiplegia, and functional limitations, 118
muscle strength and endurance, 119
nervous system, pathophysiology and impact on, 117, 118
quality of life and participation, 120
rehabilitation, application of, 119
spasticity, 120
treatment protocols and practical considerations, 120–122
Stroke volume, 55
cardiorespiratory fitness, 78
Surface electrodes, 191
Symmetrical biphasic currents, 15
Systemic opioids, 24

T
Tachypneic breathing, 159
Torque sensors, 65
Training phases, 186–187
Transcutaneous electrical nerve stimulation (TENS), 3, 12
Transthoracic echocardiogram, 79
Tricycles, 43
Type 2 diabetes, 163
Type I fibers, 160

U
Ubiquitin–proteasome activation, 165
Upright motor control test, 86, 87

V
Ventilatory capacity, 80–82
Ventilatory responses, 48, 57, 59
FES cycling, 48, 57, 59
Ventilatory thresholds, 84–86
Virtual reality (VR), 225, 226, 228

W
Waveforms, 15–17
Wireless FES technology, 216–219

MIX
Papier aus verantwortungsvollen Quellen
Paper from responsible sources
FSC® C105338

If you have any concerns about our products,
you can contact us on
ProductSafety@springernature.com

In case Publisher is established outside the EU,
the EU authorized representative is:
Springer Nature Customer Service Center GmbH
Europaplatz 3, 69115 Heidelberg, Germany

Printed by Libri Plureos GmbH
in Hamburg, Germany